SILICON CARBIDE TECHNOLOGY FOR ADVANCED HUMAN HEALTHCARE APPLICATIONS

SILICON CARBIDE TECHNOLOGY FOR ADVANCED HUMAN HEALTHCARE APPLICATIONS

Edited by

STEPHEN E. SADDOW

College of Engineering, University of South Florida,
Tampa, FL, United States

ELSEVIER

Elsevier
Radarweg 29, PO Box 211, 1000 AE Amsterdam, Netherlands
The Boulevard, Langford Lane, Kidlington, Oxford OX5 1GB, United Kingdom
50 Hampshire Street, 5th Floor, Cambridge, MA 02139, United States

ISBN: 978-0-323-90609-8

For information on all Elsevier publications visit our website at https://www.elsevier.com/books-and-journals

Publisher: Matthew Deans
Acquisitions Editor: Sabrina Webber
Editorial Project Manager: Chiara Giglio
Production Project Manager: Anitha Sivaraj
Cover Designer: Matthew Limbert

Typeset by TNQ Technologies

Dedication

This book is dedicated to my love and life partner Vaine Angelo Saddow, whom I like "just a little bit," and who is always there for me as my consigliere. Watching you grow into a mamãe maravilhosa, being the best possible mother in the world for our children, has truly been inspiring to watch and learn from. I am eternally grateful that you are their mom and the heart of our family—thank you, love, you are the best partner I could ask for!

Contents

List of contributors

Evans Bernardin
Department of Medical Engineering, University of South Florida, Tampa, FL, United States

Mohammad Beygi
Institute of Electrical and Microengineering, École polytechnique fédérale de Lausanne, Lausanne, Switzerland

Jay Bieber
Nanotechnology Research & Education Center, University of South Florida, Tampa, FL, United States

Gabriele Bonaventura
Institute for Biomedical Research and Innovation, Italian National Research Council, Catania, Italy

William Chiappim
Departamento de Física, Laboratório de Plasmas e Processos, Instituto Tecnológico de Aeronáutica, São José dos Campos, Brazil

Stuart Cogan
University of Texas at Dallas, Richardson, TX, United States

Camilla Coletti
Center for Nanotechnology Innovation@NEST, Istituto Italiano di Tecnologia, Pisa, Italy

Domenica Convertino
Center for Nanotechnology Innovation@NEST, Istituto Italiano di Tecnologia, Pisa, Italy

William Dominguez-Viqueira
Moffitt Cancer Center, Tampa, FL, United States

Richard Everly
Nanotechnology Research & Education Center, University of South Florida, Tampa, FL, United States

Chenyin Feng
Department of Electrical Engineering, University of South Florida, Tampa, FL, United States; Department of Mechanical Engineering, University of South Florida, Tampa, FL, United States

Mariana Amorim Fraga
Escola de Engenharia, Universidade Presbiteriana Mackenzie, São Paulo, Brazil

Christopher L. Frewin
NeuroNexus LLC, Ann Arbor, MI, United States

Ludwig Galambos
Department of Electrical Engineering, Stanford University, Stanford, CA, United States

James Harris
Department of Electrical Engineering, Stanford University, Stanford, CA, United States

Alton Horsfall
Department of Engineering, University of Durham, Durham, United Kingdom

Philip Huie
Hansen Experimental Physics Laboratory, Stanford University, Stanford, CA, United States; Department of Ophthalmology, Stanford University, Stanford, CA, United States

Theodore Kamins
Department of Electrical Engineering, Stanford University, Stanford, CA, United States

Sheryl Kane
EIC Laboratories, Norwood, MA, United States

Ashok Kumar
Department of Mechanical Engineering, University of South Florida, Tampa, FL, United States

Francesco La Via
IMM-CNR, Catania, Sicily, Italy

Xin Lei
Department of Electrical Engineering, Stanford University, Stanford, CA, United States

Henri Lorach
Hansen Experimental Physics Laboratory, Stanford University, Stanford, CA, United States

Laura Marchetti
Center for Nanotechnology Innovation@NEST, Istituto Italiano di Tecnologia, Pisa, Italy; Department of Pharmacy, University of Pisa, Pisa, Italy

Keith Mathieson
Institute of Photonics, University of Strathclyde, Glasgow, Scotland, United Kingdom

Gokhan Mumcu
Electrical Engineering Department, University of South Florida, Tampa, FL, United States

Karthik Nagareddy
Department of Engineering, University of Durham, Durham, United Kingdom

Sukanya Pal
Department of Engineering, University of Durham, Durham, United Kingdom

Daniel Palanker
Hansen Experimental Physics Laboratory, Stanford University, Stanford, CA, United States; Department of Ophthalmology, Stanford University, Stanford, CA, United States

Rodrigo Sávio Pessoa
Departamento de Física, Laboratório de Plasmas e Processos, Instituto Tecnológico de Aeronáutica, São José dos Campos, Brazil

Amy Peters
Department of Engineering, University of Durham, Durham, United Kingdom

Kavyashree Puttananjegowda
Department of Electrical Engineering, University of South Florida, Tampa, FL, United States

Md Rubayat-E Tanjil
Department of Mechanical Engineering, University of South Florida, Tampa, FL, United States

Stephen E. Saddow
Departments of Electrical & Medical Engineering, University of South Florida, Tampa, FL, United States

Arash Takshi
Department of Electrical Engineering, University of South Florida, Tampa, FL, United States

Sylvia Thomas
Department of Electrical Engineering, University of South Florida, Tampa, FL, United States

Michael Cai Wang
Department of Mechanical Engineering, University of South Florida, Tampa, FL, United States

Massimo Zimbone
Institute for Microelectronics and Microsystems, Italian National Research Council, Catania, Italy

Foreword

When I was asked to introduce the third book edited by Prof. Stephen Saddow on the use of SiC in medicine, my first reaction was indecision about the type of preface I should write. Then I thought that, as a reader myself, I wished to know not only the scientific content of the book but also some more information about the man behind the scientist. So, I accepted the invitation to write a preface for Dr. Saddow's new book and hope that you, the reader, find it enlightening.

I first met Steve professionally several years ago. From the very beginning, looking at his research activity, I recognized the seminal work he was doing on the application of SiC thin films for biomedical devices and nanomedicine. I must say that his work was, for me, inspirational in starting my own research on SiC nanosystems for nanomedicine. Indeed, Steve spent a period of time as visiting professor in my group assisting me with my new activity on SiC nanowires.

It was during that period that I began to know the man behind the creative and deeply prepared scientist. He was serious and dedicated in the laboratory, but also cheerful, curious, and with a great sense of humor outside work. Nevertheless, regardless of whether we had had a beer together the night before, the following day he was again the creative and precise scientist we were used to meeting in the lab. Now, after many years, I am happy to be a part of his life and of his wonderful family.

Steve is a professor at the University of South Florida and does advanced research on SiC materials and devices, focusing on materials growth and innovative biomedical applications/devices.

The first book published by Steve was mostly documenting the bio- and hemocompatibility of SiC and some preliminary device concepts. The second book was more focused on the complete in vitro and in vivo assessment of SiC materials along with the disclosure of more advanced prototype devices. This third book now focuses on mature biomedical devices that will hopefully soon translate to clinical trial for eventual use in human healthcare. This is especially true for the neural probe work presented in several of the chapters.

The present volume is an up-to-date, accurate, well-referred, and flowing scientific compendium of a wide range of SiC applications in biomedical engineering and nanomedicine, that starts with a very nice, general introduction on healthcare applications of SiC. Going through the chapters, the reader finds a deep, comprehensive, and well-documented study of SiC applications in prosthetics, as well as the neural probe and biosensing fields.

In particular, Chapters 2–4 on prosthetic applications report on the biocompatibility of Si and SiC on neural stem cells, on graphene and SiC use for spinal cord repair, and on SiC protective coatings for implanted retinal prosthesis.

Following this impressive work, Chapters 5–7 describe how to design and engineer monolithic SiC neuronal interfaces, as well as how to develop a fully MRI-compatible SiC neuronal interface.

Finally, Chapters 8–10 present the latest detailed studies on a SiC nanoparticle-based electrochemical glucose nanosensors, on epitaxial graphene-based sensor technology, and on antibacterial and antifungal properties of SiC coatings.

I hope that this short preface has stimulated your curiosity to read through this excellent scientific book, and I hope that the work of Dr. Saddow will be inspirational for young scientists who wish to go deeper into the wonderful interdisciplinary research field of biomedical devices and nanomedicine, where materials scientists, physicists, engineers, chemists, biologists, and medical doctors meet not only to exchange ideas but also to develop new devices to improve future healthcare using advanced SiC biomedical technology.

Preface

The 21st century has long been hailed as the century of biology, as the extremely complex nature of the biological system is only now beginning to be more fully understood through the use of technology and the scientific tools which allow mankind to observe biological processes at the nano-scale. This has resulted in the ever pressing need to develop advanced 'smart materials and devices' for biomedical applications, and this important field of research has taken center stage worldwide as the new frontier of advanced scientific research. While biocompatible materials have been in use for decades, the quest to merge smart materials, such as those used in modern computer integrated circuits, with the biological system has proven to be much more difficult than originally imagined. If we take as one example the brain–machine interface, or BMI, which was first reported in the early 1970s and was based on silicon probes, we learn that mankind is not much closer to the prospect of long-term (multiple years or even decades) implantation of these devices. Why? Simply put most 'smart materials' such as semiconductors are typically toxic to the biological environment, and silicon is no exception. Therefore, what is needed to realize true nano-scale functionality is a material with the 'smart properties' of silicon and the 'biocompatible' properties of polymers. In prior books such a candidate material, silicon carbide (SiC), has been presented with the evidence that has been amassed, mostly over the last decade, indicating that this material system may prove to be the dream material for biomedical devices that must do more than simply provide structural support. Building on this important body of knowledge, this book now takes SiC biotechnology to the next level of prototype devices that are nearing clinical trial and, subsequently, commercial products for long-term human healthcare applications.

SiC has a long history as a robust and hard material, which was first used as an abrasive and cutting material in the 19th century and later as a high-temperature semiconductor for advanced applications in the 20th century. Indeed, the first solid-state blue light emission was observed from SiC in 1907, and this material has been under study ever since that time. One can consult the various available literature to fully understand all of the many aspects of SiC, from how it is formed, to its myriad crystal properties, and finally to the large number and types of applications it is being used in.

Fortunately, it is sufficient here to provide a brief overview of SiC so that the reader can understand why this material is so compelling for biomedical applications and may become one of the most used biomaterials in the future. Indeed, the purpose of this book is to build on the foundation of the first two books: ***Silicon Carbide Biotechnology: A biocompatible semiconductor for advanced biomedical devices***. The hope is that this will motivate biomedical engineers, medical professionals, and scientists, thus bringing together technologists from across many disciplines to help realize the ultimate use of SiC as one of the next generation of smart biomaterials for Human Healthcare applications.

The first edition of ***Silicon Carbide Biotechnology*** focused mainly on in vitro material studies in order to introduce the reader to the possibility that SiC can be an important player in the biomedical device community. Indeed, biocompatibility and hemocompatibility data were presented which either cleared up prior misconceptions of SiC in this arena or reinforced the known excellent performance of certain SiC material types, called polytypes, to the biological world. While prototype devices were introduced and discussed, the second edition focused mainly on the significant progress that has been made in development of SiC biomedical devices, ranging from neural implants to sensors to in vitro DNA assay systems. The organization ***Silicon Carbide Technology for Advanced Human Healthcare Applications*** starts with an updated introduction of SiC, with a particular emphasis on biomedical applications, and is then organized into four distinct sections. First, SiC as a platform for neural stem cells and spinal cord repair is presented. Next SiC for use in Neural Engineering applications is provided with chapters covering the use of SiC for retinal prostheses, neural implants for implantable neural interface (INI) applications, and the MRI compatibility of a cubic SiC monolithic which would allow for brain imaging before and after neuromodulation therapy. The book then moves to the use of SiC and graphene for biosensor applications. The final chapter, quite relevant in today's world, demonstrates the use of SiC as an antibacterial and antifungal coating to help reduce the spread of germs on man-made surfaces such as in hospitals and restaurants, etc.

Having completed the in vitro materials studies required by the FDA to allow for subsequent clinical trials in the second edition, we can now focus on the important topic of translating the latest research on SiC to clinical trial and then commercialization. Extremely comprehensive studies on the use of graphene on SiC, as well as surface functionalization of SiC, both for biosensor applications, were presented in the first two books, respectively.

We see that SiC, due to the fact that it is a compound semiconductor, provides more flexibility in terms of biosensor design simply by taking into account differences in how one can functionalize the Si and C surfaces of the material. This extra degree in design freedom is not possible with the mainstay smart biosensor material, silicon, which has proved to have issues with bio- and hemocompatibility.

The authors listed at the beginning of each chapter provided the content, including figures and text that comprise the majority of this book. The Editor both solicited these chapters and then edited the content in an effort to achieve a uniform and consistent text. This was done so that the reader could both focus on the very interesting subject matter contained within, and to also see the connection that many of the chapters have with each other. It is the Editor's hope that this endeavor was successful and that you, the reader of this book, will find this work both informative and enjoyable to read. Indeed, it was an extremely rewarding experience putting together ***Silicon Carbide Technology for Advanced Human Healthcare Applications***, which is the third book on this compelling subject, and the Editor hopes that you will find this as exciting as he did putting this all together.

At Academic Press/Elsevier Science, the project was coordinated by Louisa Hutchins and the Editor is grateful to her for all of her support and kind assistance throughout the project. In addition, Parvathy Bala very capably coordinated the production of the book and is gratefully acknowledged for all of her hard work in making sure galley proof corrections were made, copyright approvals completed, and for her overall help in pulling this book together. The Editor of ***Silicon Carbide Technology for Advanced Human Healthcare Applications*** hopes that users of this book, and especially the students who will become the next generation of biomedical practitioners and technologists, will find the subject matter of ***Silicon Carbide Technology for Advanced Human Healthcare Applications*** as interesting and exciting as the editor does.

Prof. Stephen E. Saddow, Editor
University of South Florida
Tampa, FL, USA

In memoriam

To my great friend and qualifying exam study partner, Dr. Kevin Boulais, who inspired me by earning his PhD while raising his three beautiful children mostly alone. And for his great advice to take lots of videos of my kids since I would miss hearing their sweet voices later in life. Thank you, Kevin, you left this world far too soon but we know you are cruising on your Harley in heaven smiling down at your legacy of 6 children and 13 grandchildren. R.I.P, my friend, you are forever missed.

Acknowledgments

This project was made possible by so many people that it is difficult to thank everyone sufficiently and completely, and if I forget to include anyone in this acknowledgment it is truly inadvertent. I am first grateful to my family who raised me to have real values—those of honest work and to always respect and appreciate others. Furthemore, I thank all of the chapter authors who contributed their great work to this book and helped to truly make it a comprehensive tome on the use of SiC for human healthcare applications. To them, I remain ever grateful. None of this would have been possible had it not been for all of the teachers and professors in my life, most notably my Ph.D. advisor, Prof. Chi Lee at the University of Maryland, who taught me that no matter how successful one is, or how famous one becomes, the true measure of a colleague is kindness and respect. Naturally, I am indebted to the dedicated students that I have had the good fortune to work with and advise over the past 25 years. It is upon the shoulders of many of these fine students that this work rests upon. A few deserve a special note of recognition as they were the SiC biomaterials pioneers who laid the foundation for this book. They are Dr. C. Coletti for her pioneering work on the in vitro biocompatibility of SiC and upon whose work Dr. N. Schettini (hemocompatibility) and Dr. C. Frewin (neuronal biocompatibility) directly followed. There is Dr. A. Oliveros, who continued this tradition and developed SiC biosensors along with exploring the biocompatibility of graphene and carbon-based conductors. Their work inspired the next generation of bio SiC researchers who took this to the device level: Dr. Evans Bernardin for the first proof-of-concept of the "all-SiC" INI, Dr. Mohammad Beygi for developing the first generation of 3C-SiC on SOI and demonstrating the MRI compatibility of this INI device, and Dr. Chenyin Feng, who developed a carbon-based flexible INI using sandwiching PPR-derived carbon in *a*-SiC insulators to enable a highly flexible and manufacturable INI. This core cadre of students made this work possible and I am eternally indebted to them. In addition, I wish to thank all of the present and former students of the USF SiC Group, as well as my close colleagues Dr. A. Hoff and Dr. S. Thomas of the Department of Electrical Engineering at USF. Dr. Hoff was my inspiration to enter the biomedical engineering field and introduced me to Dr. M. Jaroszeski of the Medical Engineering Department who opened his laboratory to my students thus making the work of the Bio-SiC group possible. A special thanks to Dr. S. Afroz in her pioneering on SiC in vivo glucose sensors, which Dr. Fabiola Araujo Cespedes continued toward the goal of continuous glucose monitoring (CGM). I wish to thank the USF NREC staff for their support and kind assistance to my students as well as my department chairman Dr. Christos Ferekides who has always been extremely supportive of my research activity and group. I especially want to thank Dr. William Dominguez Viqueira of the Moffitt Cancer Center for his invaluable time and expertise in evaluating 3C-SiC for MRI compatibility as well as Dr. Karl Muffly of the USF Morsani Medical School, for our very fruitful collaboration in the area of biomedical engineering and devices. I am especially indebted to my good friend and colleagues from IMEM in Parma, Dr. S. Iannotta, Dr. G. Salviati and Dr. F. Rossi, and Dr. Marco Nardi and Dr. Melanie Timpel in Trento for our continuing scientific collaboration in the area of SiC nanotechnology and its application to deep-tissue cancer therapy via NIR-PIT concept. I am particularly grateful to my colleagues at the National Cancer Institute, Dr. Peter Choyke, Dr. Stephen Adler, and Dr. Jurgen Seidel, for their incredible support and scientific knowledge as we explored the NIR-PIT concept in Bethesda at the NIH. I again thank Dr. C. Frewin for always being there to support and share my vision of SiC Biotechnology and for his ever-faithful friendship and dedication without which I doubt this book would be possible. A special thank you is in order for Editorial Project Manager Chiara Giglio. Not only did she provide essential assistance in the early stage of this book project but she helped to shape the scope and front cover art which are critical to the final book as you see here. Her never-ending willingness to assist me in the process and ensure maximum success of this book is truly appreciated. Finally, and most dear to my heart, is my partner in life and love, Vaine Angelo Saddow, with whom we have two amazing children, Luca Edward and Sophia Angelo, who provide all of the incentives that anyone needs to continue to strive for scientific and technological excellence—in some small way, I hope that all of this work will allow for their quality of life to be the best that man on earth can provide.

The Editor
Prof. Stephen E. Saddow
Tampa, FL, United States

CHAPTER 1

Recent advances in SiC biomedical devices: Healthcare applications

Stephen E. Saddow
Departments of Electrical & Medical Engineering, University of South Florida, Tampa, FL, United States

Contents

Silicon Carbide Technology for Advanced Human Healthcare Applications
ISBN 978-0-323-90609-8
https://doi.org/10.1016/B978-0-323-90609-8.00006-5

1. Introduction

Silicon carbide has a long history as a robust and hard material, first used as a cutting material in the 19th century and later as a high-temperature semiconductor for advanced applications in the 20th century. The history of silicon carbide (SiC) is quite interesting, and the reader is referred to the first chapter in a book dedicated to this subject [1]. It is best to consult the literature to fully understand all of the many aspects of SiC, from how it is formed, to its myriad of crystal properties, and finally to the large number and types of applications it has and is being used in. Fortunately, it is sufficient here to provide a brief overview of SiC so that the reader can understand why this material is so compelling for biomedical applications and may become one of the most used active biomaterials in the 21st century. Indeed, the purpose of this book is to lay the foundation for exactly this—to introduce silicon carbide to biomedical engineers, scientists, and medical professionals, thus bringing together technologists from across many disciplines to help develop the next generation of smart biodevices to realize advanced human healthcare solutions.

This book serves two important functions for those interested in modern human healthcare technology. First, it provides a brief review of silicon carbide technology from a material synthesis point of view. This is essentially an updated discussion from the first two books entitled *Silicon Carbide Biotechnology: A biocompatible Semiconductor for Advanced Biomedical Devices and Applications* (First Edition Elsevier ©2012 [2] and Second Edition Elsevier ©2016 [3]). These first books were actually distinct bodies of work despite the nomenclature used indicating that they were editions. Therefore, to provide the reader with both a fast review of these two works, as well as providing a road map as to where to look for information of specific interest, this chapter summarizes the key works reported in both books. In a general sense, the first book served the purpose to introduce SiC as a material that is extremely well suited for in vivo use in humans and was focused on research performed to describe the compatibility of SiC materials and rudimentary devices with animal and human tissue. The second book was focused on the next step in the process of developing next-generation biomedical devices from SiC for various applications. In this second book, further information on performing materials studies with strict coherence to ISO-10993 was provided, in addition to graphene and electrochemical biosensors, SiC Nanowire DNA detection and glucose sensing, advances in SiC neural implants, and finally SiC nanotechnology.

The present book is, again, completely distinct from the first two as the technology continues to advance at a very rapid pace. Here you will find chapters discussing advanced SiC-based devices, from neural implants to SiC used in antibacterial/antifungal applications. This book is organized as follows: First is this chapter a summary of SiC material technology and synthesis methods are discussed. This is followed by research highlights from the first two books that are very useful to understand the more advanced research presented here. Chapters 2 and 3 pertain to the use of SiC for neural stem cells and neuron regrowth—an extremely important area of neuroengineering with the ultimate goal to repair damaged/severed spinal cords and facilitate healing of damaged brain tissue. Chapter 4 provides an excellent overview of using amorphous SiC coatings for retinal implants to restore human vision. Chapters 5—7 involve the development of monolithic neural interfaces whereby only SiC, without any polymers or metals in contact with the brain, are used to fashion highly robust neural interfaces. Chapter 6 talks about the possibility that 3C—SiC is an MRI-compatible material whereby excellent performance in a 7 T MRI machine is reported. Chapter 7 involves the seamless integration of SiC and pyrolyzed photoresist film (PPF) as a carbon-based conducting medium in advanced, and highly flexible, neural interfaces. We then move on to sensor technology and discuss glucose sensing using SiC nanotechnology (Chapter 8) followed by epitaxial graphene on SiC (Chapter 9) sensor technology. The final chapter has ramifications for all SiC devices where research demonstrating the antibacterial and antifungal properties of SiC is presented. Let us begin our journey and I hope you enjoy reading this as much as we have putting this together for you.

2. Silicon carbide material synthesis and properties

2.1 Silicon carbide overview

SiC is first and foremost a material that consists of the covalent bonding of Si and C atoms, typically in biatomic layers as shown in Fig. 1.1. These form tetrahedrally oriented molecules of Si—C, with a very short bond length and, hence, a very high bond strength. This is the origin of the extremely high chemical and mechanical stability of SiC [4,5]. SiC can be formed in both amorphous, polycrystalline and monocrystalline solid forms and, due to the high bond strength and high-temperature operating potentiality of SiC, synthesis of SiC material normally requires high temperatures (greater than 1000°C), with the exception of amorphous SiC

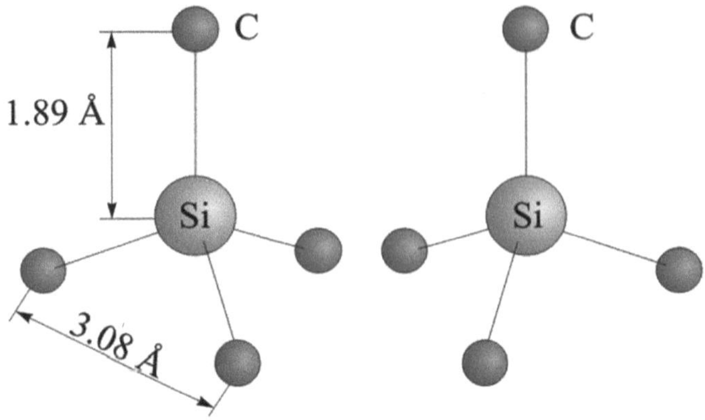

Figure 1.1 All SiC crystals are formed via bilayers of C and Si, covalently bonded to form a tetrahedron. Four carbon atoms are covalently bonded with a silicon atom in the center. Two types exist—one is rotated 180 degrees around the c-axis with respect to the other, as shown. This tetrahedrally bonded molecule then forms the basic building block of all SiC materials [1].

which can be deposited at temperatures between 200–300°C. The material can be grown in both bulk (boule) crystal form, currently with diameters up to 200 mm (8 inch) having been reported, and can be hetero-epitaxially grown on Si substrates (details of how this is accomplished are may be found in Ref. [5]).

One of the important characteristics of SiC is that the bilayers of Si and C (Fig. 1.1) can be stacked one upon the other in different crystal orientations: cubic, hexagonal, and rhombohedral. With more than 200 polytypes reported in the literature, the three technologically relevant forms are one purely cubic (β-SiC) and two hexagonal forms that actually have some cubic symmetry (α-SiC). These three polytypes are shown in Fig. 1.2. The cubic form has the designation 3C–SiC, where the 3 delineates that 3 bilayers of Si–C are needed to form the basic structure and C indicates that the crystal form is cubic. The hexagonal forms are 4H–SiC and 6H–SiC, where the 4 and 6 delineate that 4 and 6 bilayers are needed while the H indicates that the crystal form is hexagonal. While interesting in their own right, these various forms of SiC actually have varying applications, where the dominant power electronic device crystal of choice is 4H–SiC due to it having the highest band gap (3.2 eV). 6H–SiC is ideally suited for solid-state lighting (LEDs) as its lattice constant is close to the GaN family of alloys used in advanced LEDs that have enabled DVD and blue-ray technology, not to mention the solid-state lighting revolution that is currently

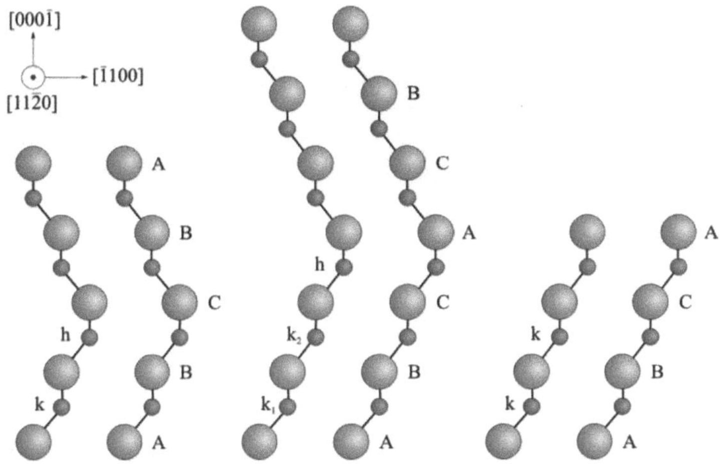

Figure 1.2 Atomic stacking sequence of the three technologically relevant SiC polytypes viewed in the [11−20] plane. From left to right, 4H−SiC, 6H−SiC, and 3C−SiC. *k* and *h* denote crystal symmetry points that are cubic and hexagonal, respectively [1].

leading to dramatic reductions in power consumption world-wide [6]. A comparison of the properties of SiC compared with Si is shown in Table 1.1 for reference.

2.2 Silicon carbide materials growth and processing

There is a long history of how to grow, process, and characterize SiC materials thus the reader is referred to several of the excellent references if further details are desired [7,8]. For this book, it is sufficient to provide an overview of the technology as it pertains to future biomedical devices, hence a simple discussion follows with sufficient references to fill in the details. We will first review how bulk hexagonal crystals of SiC are grown and, more importantly, what the state-of-the-art is and the key characteristics of these commercially available substrates. Next, the growth and synthesis of thin films, starting with homo-epitaxy on hexagonal substrates, followed by hetero-epitaxy on Si substrates, and finally polycrystalline growth on various surfaces will be presented. One of the great benefits of SiC is that it can be deposited in amorphous (*a*-SiC) form at lower temperatures using plasma-enhanced chemical vapor deposition (PECVD) than for film growth. This technology will be reviewed in this chapter, and the final section will be an introduction to how SiC can be micromachined and how this points to the potential of SiC as an excellent bioMEMS material.

Table 1.1 Basic properties of SiC compared with Si and Diamond [1].

Property	4H–SiC	6H–SiC	3C–SiC	Si	Diamond
Energy bandgap at 300 K (eV)	3.20	3.00	2.29	1.12	5.45
Intrinsic carrier concentration at 300 K (cm^{-3})	5×10^{-9}	1.6×10^{-6}	1.5×10^{-1}	1×10^{10}	$\sim 10^{-27}$
Critical breakdown electric field (MV/cm)	2.2	2.5	2.12	0.25	1–10
Saturated electron drift velocity ($\times 10^7$ cm/s)	2.0	2.0	2.5	1.0	1.5
Electron mobility (cm^2/V-s)	1000	600	800	1450	480
Hole mobility (cm^2/V-s)	115	100	40	470	1600
Thermal conductivity at 300 K (W/cm/K)	3.7	3.6	3.6	1.49	6–20
Coefficient of thermal expansion at 300 K (10^{-6}/K)	$4.3 \perp c$ $4.7 \parallel c$	$4.3 \perp c$ $4.7 \parallel c$	3.2	3.0	1.0
Lattice constant (a, c in Å)	$a = 3.0730$ $c = 10.053$	$a = 3.0806$ $c = 15.1173$	$a = 4.3596$	$a = 5.430$	$a = 3.5668$
Elastic coefficient* (GPa) *Calculated	$C_{44} = 600$	$C_{11} = 500$ $C_{12} = 92$ $C_{44} = 168$	$C_{11} = 352$ $C_{12} = 120$ $C_{44} = 233$	$C_{11} = 167$ $C_{12} = 65$ $C_{44} = 80$	$C_{11} = 1079$ $C_{12} = 124$ $C_{44} = 578$

2.2.1 Bulk growth

Single-crystal substrates of SiC have been in commercial production for over 3 decades, starting with Cree's first commercial 6H−SiC wafers, which were 25 mm in diameter in 1990 [9]. Much progress has been made worldwide since then, with both the quality and diameter of the wafers improving over the years; the current commercially available wafers are 200 mm (8 inches) and are available in both n-, p- and intrinsic (very high resistivity) form. Several manufacturers around the world sell SiC wafers and the crystal specifications are readily available [10]. In the research laboratory, 200 mm (8 inch) diameter wafers of quite high quality have been produced [11], which bodes well for the economic viability of SiC as an electronics technology (Fig. 1.3).

All SiC bulk wafers are grown in a high temperature (>2000°C) furnace that is either gas-fed (silicon and carbon-containing precursors transported in a carrier gas) or solid-fed with SiC powder that is sublimated (evaporated) and condenses on a single-crystal SiC seed [13,14]. Growth rates are typically 0.1−0.3 mm/h and a typical boule thickness is roughly 25−30 mm [15]. Typical resistivities range from 1×10^5 to 1×10^7 Ω-cm

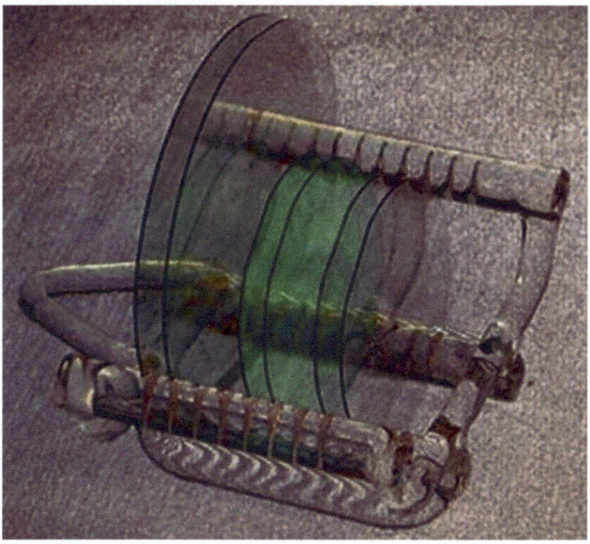

Figure 1.3 Commercially available SiC wafers can be found in off- and on-axis orientations, also with a Si or C terminated face. They can be either heavily doped or semiinsulating, depending on the application of use. Current wafers are 6 inches (150 mm) in diameter with 8 inch (200 mm) wafers demonstrated and ready for production in 2022. *(Photo courtesy of II-VI, Inc [12].)*

for semiinsulating crystals, and with high-temperature chemical vapor deposition (HTCVD) bulk growth intrinsic (high-purity, or HP) crystals with resistivities as high as 1×10^{11} Ω-cm have been reported [16]. The wafers are either cut parallel to the basal plane (i.e., perpendicular to the growth direction) or cut at a slight miscut angle, typically 3.5 and 4 degrees for 6H- and 4H−SiC, respectively. This is done to ensure that subsequent epitaxial growth replicates the proper polytype.

2.2.2 Thin films growth

Single crystalline SiC films can be grown epitaxially using a number of methods. The preferred method is chemical vapor deposition (CVD) [14], but liquid phase epitaxy [17] and molecular beam epitaxy [18] have been also used for some time. The application of HTCVD, which is used to also grow bulk crystals, has been used to achieve high growth rates [14]. The current state-of-the-art CVD reactors employ what is referred to as a hot-wall design whereas the growth substrate is surrounded by an actively heated graphite susceptor that allows for very high growth rates (typically as high as 100 μm/h with good crystal quality) [19]. The epitaxy of SiC is an active field of research, with numerous improvements in growth rate, crystal quality, doping control, etc. being made, which is critical for advanced device development. In addition, SiC crystals can be hydrogen polished via a hydrogen etching process that is somewhat dependent on both polytype and surface orientation (on-axis and off-axis) [20]. Hydrogen surface passivation using the same approach has been demonstrated which has an important role to play in the control of the SiC crystal surface chemical state, particularly when performing surface functionalization [21].

The growth of SiC thin films via homoepitaxy is a relatively straightforward process that involves the use of a silicon and a carbon-containing precursor transported to the growth surface via carrier gas, which is typically hydrogen. The silicon and carbon precursors have traditionally been silane and propane [22], and more recently chlorine-based silane precursors such as trichlorosilane have been used since the addition of Cl allows for higher growth rates with low Si-cluster defect levels [23]. When growing 3C−SiC, the only cubic polytype, on Si, this heteroepitaxy process typically involves three steps: first, hydrogen surface etching is performed to remove any native oxide that may be present, then a buffer layer is formed with the so-called carbonization step, which seeks to bond C to Si dangling bonds to create a first SiC layer, and finally the growth step which involves Si and C atoms delivered in the same process as described earlier for homoepitaxy [24]. Recently, this process was adapted by several groups to allow for use of the hot-wall CVD reactor and it was discovered that the removal of the hydrogen etching step and the inclusion of a small amount of silane between the carbonization and growth steps resulted in very high-quality films [25]. Use of this method has resulted in growth rates on the order of 10–30 μm/h, and the addition of chlorine has allowed for nearly double the growth rate in a large diameter reactor (Fig. 1.4) [26].

A new process that has been demonstrated uses a polycrystalline silicon film as a seed layer for poly-SiC growth [27]. While other groups have reported poly-SiC film growth this work involves the use of an oxide layer whereby the eventual release of poly-SiC MEMS structures can be easily facilitated [28], which will be discussed further in this Chapter. A study of the mechanical properties of both monocrystalline and polycrystalline 3C–SiC films grown on Si substrates was performed by Volinsky et al. [29]. The results demonstrated the mechanical durability of SiC, as expected, but also point out a very important property—3C–SiC films are more resistant to fracture and possess Young's modulus of nearly three times that of Si.

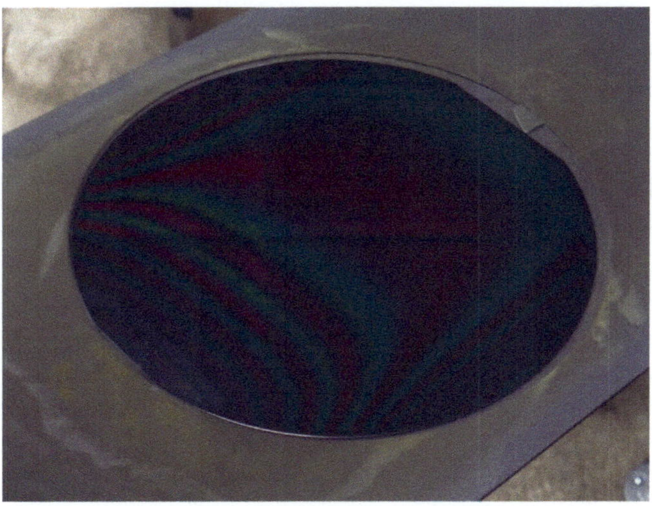

Figure 1.4 Monocrystalline and polycrystalline epi wafers of 3C–SiC are routinely grown using the CVD process. Typical epi-wafer diameters are 6 inches (150 mm) and make use of low cost and high quality of Si substrates, thus reducing the materials cost. 3C–SiC on Si allows for micromachining to be performed in a similar fashion to Si MEMS technology. Photo shows a 100 mm (4 inches) 3C–SiC epitaxial layer grown on (100)Si. Epi thickness ~3 μm. Note the reflection of ceiling tiles in the image due to highly specular morphology. *(Photo courtesy of USF SiC Group.)*

Using a Berkovich indenter the mechanical properties of thin (~1 μm thick) 3C−SiC films on (100)Si substrates were studied in our laboratory. Table 1.2 reports the average values of the measured hardness and modulus of elasticity of single crystal 3C−SiC, polycrystalline 3C−SiC, a 15R−SiC Lely platelet, and (100)Si substrate. At least five indents were performed at each maximum load. 15R−SiC was used as a comparison since this material is known to have a minimum number of dislocations. There is a relatively large absolute variation in measured elastic modulus (±50 GPa), not typically observed in the indentation of softer materials. One has to consider the relative variation, which is typically on the order of 10%. The reported mechanical properties are for a maximum indentation depth range between 60 and 250 nm, where quartz calibration is reasonable.

Wear tests on the single crystal 3C−SiC film were also performed in a 3 × 3 μm area using the low load transducer at 2 μN normal load and 1 Hz frequency. The objective of this procedure was to determine the wear resistance of the sample by repeated scanning of the poly-3C−SiC surface. After a certain number of wear cycles, the scans area was zoomed out to 5 × 5 μm to determine the material wear. The film topography of the mono- and poly-crystalline 3C−SiC film surface was measured before and after the tip-induced wear test, which was performed for 1045 scans. During this scanning, there was little to negligible wear, as only 1−2 nm of material depth was removed. This result confirms the high wear resistance of 3C−SiC films necessary for MEMS applications [30].

2.2.3 Amorphous SiC coatings

Amorphous SiC has long been studied and applied as a biomaterial. The amorphous form of SiC can be deposited using different techniques, most of which are familiar to the materials community such as PECVD, sputtering, pulsed laser deposition, evaporation, among others [2]. The advantage of amorphous SiC (*a*-SiC) is that it can be deposited at low temperatures which allows the coating of low-temperature materials such as

Table 1.2 Measured SiC mechanical properties versus Si [29].[a]

Material type	Hardness (GPa)	Elastic modulus (GPa)
(100)Si	12.46 + 0.78	172.13 + 7.76
Lely platelet 15R−SiC	42.76 + 1.19	442 + 16.34
3C−SiC on (100)Si	31.198 + 3.7	433 + 50
Poly-3C−SiC on (100)Si	33.54 + 3.3	457 + 50

[a]Measured via nanoindentation using a Hysitron Triboindenter with a Berkovich indenter tip.

polymers [30]. Another important advantage of *a*-SiC is that it can be electrically insulating, a property that many seek to exploit for numerous bio-electric devices [31]. One of the additional benefits, which is at the same time a challenge, is that line-of-sight coating of surfaces is usually the deposition mode, meaning that coating both sides of a material requires a rotation of the material during *a*-SiC coating. Issues that impact *a*-SiC functionality are the morphology of the film (smooth, rough, etc.) and the presence of any pinholes or cracks. In fact, one of the recent uses of *a*-SiC was in the coating of polyimide-based brain—machine interface (BMI) devices to overcome the problem of polymer swelling inside the brain [32]. Perhaps one of the best-known biomedical uses of *a*-SiC coatings was the very successful coating of coronary heart stents to reduce the serious problem of clotting in the cardiovascular system [32]. In this instance, Rzany and Schaldach at the University of Erlangen studied *a*-SiC:H (i.e., hydrogenated *a*-SiC [32]), as a candidate coating for stainless steel stents and reported that SiC appeared to be an ideal biomaterial due to its electronic properties in a physiological environment. They compared the performance of *a*-SiC:H coated and bare stainless steel in vitro and saw significantly improved performance for the SiC coated steel stent [33]. One of the top uses of *a*-SiC coatings is to improve the neurocompatibility of neural interfaces. Fig. 1.5 shows a commercially available nonfunctional single shank (NeuroNexus) probe that was coated with 0.5 μm of *a*-SiC using plasma-enhanced chemical vapor deposition. These implants have dimensions typical of implantable probes, that is, 5 mm in length, 15 μm thick, and 200 μm in width at the base and the widest part of the shank in contact with cortical tissue. Tissue response data is provided later in the chapter (Fig. 1.11) where the comparison with noncoated control probes demonstrated a significant reduction in immune system response.

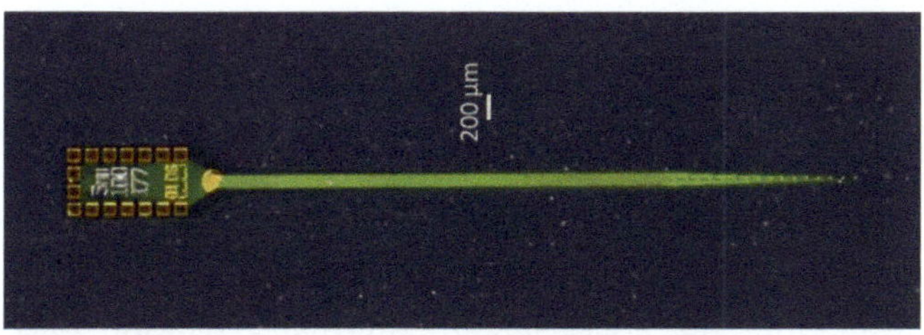

Figure 1.5 Photomicrograph showing nonfunctional Neuronexus probes used for testing the tissue response resulting from 4-week implantation in the rat motor cortex [3]. *(This figure was generously provided by Ms. Amy Davis of NeuroNexus Technologies (Ann Arbor, MI).)*

2.2.4 SiC micromachining

The realization of mechanical devices based on microelectronic circuit processing techniques is known as microelectro-mechanical systems or MEMS. While a full treatment of MEMS is not practical here, a brief summary of the salient features of this technology will allow the reader to have an adequate understanding of the technology. The thermal, mechanical, and chemical strength of the Si—C bond manifests itself in very high material hardness and Young's modulus. These values, as measured by Volinsky et al. [29], were ~31 and 433 GPa, respectively, for 1 μm thick monocrystalline 3C—SiC films grown on (100)Si substrates. Similar measurements made on polycrystalline 3C—SiC (i.e., poly-SiC) films of the same thickness and grown on the same substrate were comparable with ~33 and 457 GPa, respectively. For comparison purposes, the corresponding values for (100)Si in bulk-substrate (700 μm thick) form were only ~12 and ~172 GPa, respectively which is roughly 2/3 the value for the 3C—SiC films. As an example of a fairly routine micromachined device, 3C—SiC cantilevers, Fig. 1.6 shows a cross-section sketch of the process resulting in a free-standing cantilever [34]:

In Chapter 10 of [2], a more comprehensive discussion of BioMEMS technology based on SiC was presented. Basically, SiC MEMS are fabricated using the same micromachining technology of Si MEMS, so there is not the need to reinvent the processing required to make highly robust SiC MEMS. The basic process flow for SiC MEMS depends on whether one is using bulk SiC or 3C—SiC on Si as the MEMS material. One advantage to using the first option (all-SiC materials) is that there is no problem with differing thermal expansion coefficients during processing, but the cost and difficulty in forming mechanical structures in this highly robust material is an issue [35]. Moreover, 3C—SiC is grown heteroepitaxially on Si to form mono-crystalline 3C—SiC films. Mono-crystalline 3C—SiC on Si MEMS can be fabricated using standard Si MEMS techniques, as shown in Fig. 1.6, and allows for a much simpler MEMS process technology, in particular when poly-SiC on oxide release layers are utilized as described in the last section of this chapter. In this instance, the resulting MEMS structures were very straight and displayed a high durability during processing [36]. Subsequent 3C—SiC on Si MEMS devices did, however, display wafer bow issues resulting from the coefficient of thermal expansion mismatch between 3C—SiC and Si (about 8%) as well as the lattice mismatch (about 20%) between the two materials [37].

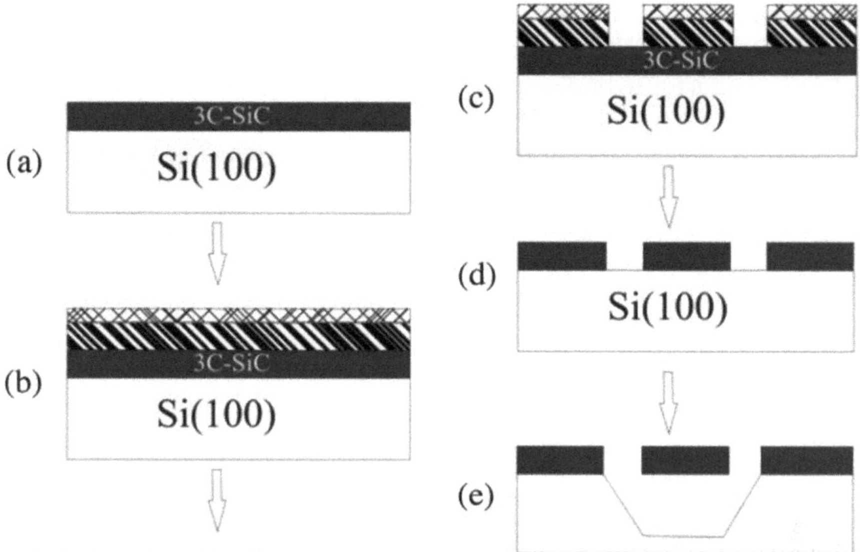

Figure 1.6 Free-standing cantilever formation. (A) CVD growth of the 3C—SiC film on the Si(100) substrate. (B). A 1-μm Al was deposited (second layer) through dc sputtering as a hard mask for SiC plasma etching, and about 1.8 μm of positive resist (first layer) was spun on the wafer. (C) Al layer etching with a wet solution of $HNO_3/H_3PO_4/CH_3COOH$. (D) ICP system with SF6/O2 chemistry was performed to transfer the Al pattern to the SiC layer. (E) A 20% KOH solution at 60°C for 60 min was used to selectively etch the Si substrate under the SiC structures [39].

2.3 SiC in vitro performance

Cell-semiconductor hybrid systems are a potential centerpiece in the scenery of biotechnological applications. The selection and study of promising crystalline semiconductor materials for biosensing applications are at the basis of the development of such hybrid systems. In this section, crystalline SiC is introduced as an extremely appealing material for bio-applications. For the first time, an in vitro biocompatibility study of the main three SiC polytypes was conducted (Chapter 4 of [2]). The obtained results document the biocompatibility of all principal SiC polytypes and their capability of directly interfacing cells without the need for surface functionalization. SiC polytypism and doping concentration had no influence on cell proliferation for the cell lines studied. Moreover, this study reported that SiC surfaces are a better substrate for mammalian cell cultures than Si in terms of both cell adhesion and proliferation. In the past, the fact that cells could be directly cultured on Si crystalline substrates led to a widespread use of this material in biotechnology [38–42]. The results reported in Ref. [2] define SiC as an even more promising substrate for future cell-semiconductor hybrid systems. A certain degree of bioactivity can even be observed for SiC when interacting with connective tissue cells. The main factors that have been shown to define SiC biocompatibility are its excellent tribological properties, hydrophilicity, and surface chemistry. SiC surface roughness variations within the nanometer scale have been shown to have minimal to no effect on cell adhesion and proliferation. On the other hand, surface micropatterning modifies the cellular adhesion pattern. Both HF treatment followed by a thorough deionized (DI) water rinse and hydrogen annealing is suitable to last steps in the SiC surface cleaning procedure before cell plating. However, a high presence of fluorine on the surfaces due to an insufficient water rinse negatively impacts cell proliferation. Piranha was found to be an excellent cleaning procedure in removing biomatter from SiC surfaces but the number of Piranha cleans on the same substrate should be limited to avoid surface chemistry modifications with a negative impact on cell proliferation. On the other hand, Radio Corporation of America (RCA) clean leaves cell adhesion sites and significant organic matter residue on the SiC surfaces further motivating piranha cleaning as the best method for SiC biological applications. The extremely promising results reported by Coletti in Ref. [43] are already sufficient to justify the choice of undertaking complete ISO 10993 testing, the necessary series of standards for evaluating the biocompatibility of a medical material before clinical trials. Indeed, amorphous SiC (*a*-SiC) and 3C–SiC were compared to other materials as part of a DARPA program to evaluate novel materials for neural probe applications, the details of which may be found in Chapter 3 of [2] and Chapter 2 of [3].

Numerous cell lines were studied to better understand literature reports that suggested that SiC was biopermissive or cytotoxic. Indeed, the work by Coletti was specifically aimed at trying to understand the apparent contradiction which, it turned out, was most likely due to nuances in how SiC should be prepared for cell culture. In the final analysis, SiC, and numerous polytypes and forms (amorphous, polycrystalline, monocrystalline, nano-structured, etc.), have all been shown to provide an excellent interface to the biological world (Fig. 1.7).

One of the important properties of implantable biodevices is hemocompatibility. This is particularly true for neural implants due to the dense nature of blood vasculature in the brain. Two studies were conducted to assess the interaction of platelet-rich plasma (PRP) with various SiC and

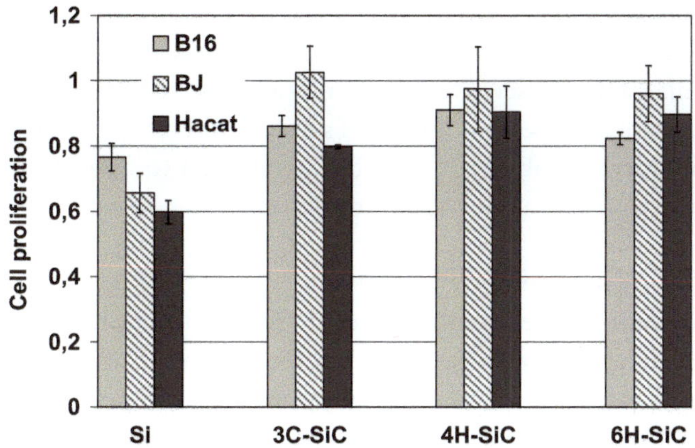

Figure 1.7 Cell proliferation of B16, BJ, and HaCaT cells expressed as $\overline{x} \pm \sigma_m$ measured via MTT assays at the third day. Cell proliferation is greater on SiC than on Si surfaces for all the cell lines studied [2].

control surfaces by both Schettini and Nezifati at the University of South Florida. In the first study by Schettini, it was observed that 3C–SiC was superior to Si when contacted with blood platelets, which was not surprising as Si is known to stimulate the clotting cascade (i.e., thrombosis). What was surprising was the observation that the hexagonal polytypes tested (4H- and 6H–SiC) were no better than Si when in contact with PRP (Fig. 1.8) [2].

These experiments were conducted under static conditions and *a*-SiC, an important material for subsequent SiC biomedical devices, was not

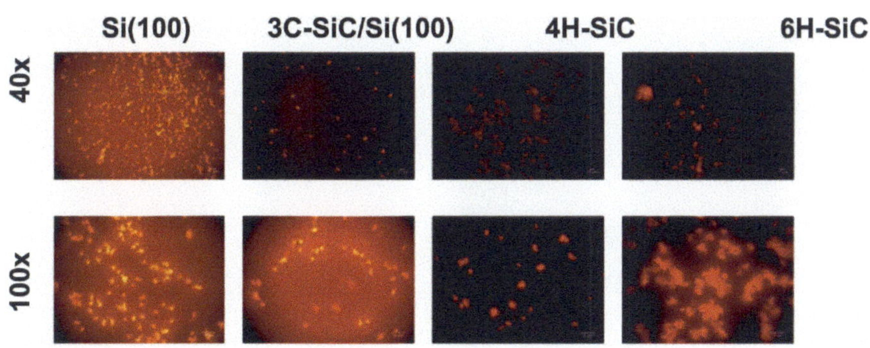

Figure 1.8 Fluorescent micrographs comparing adhered platelets on three different SiC polytypes and Si. 3C–SiC clearly shows lower adhesion and high circularity while Si presented the highest adhesion. 4H–SiC and 6H–SiC evidenced the presence of clumps and high degree of activation (Chapter 5 of [2]).

tested. Consequently, Nezifati conducted dynamic experiments using a flowing Chandler loop to mimic the actual blood flow condition in the cardiovascular system (see Chapter 3 of [3]). Fig. 1.9 shows a histogram comparing platelet adhesion to various surfaces and clearly demonstrates the superior hemocompatibility of 3C—SiC compared to Si and the excellent performance of *a*-SiC under these conditions:

2.4 SiC in vivo performance

Numerous studies have been conducted and reported in the literature. In this section, a brief review of in vivo studies performed at the University of South Florida is presented as further motivation for the development of SiC biomedical devices. Three (3) animal models were used (mouse, rat, and pig) and, in each case, a null immune system response to 3C—SiC was observed whereas a significant initiation of the immune system was observed for Si. The first involved nonfunctional 3C—SiC double-shank probes which were implanted into wild-type mice for 35 days. For the first time, a comprehensive analysis of 3C—SiC for neural device applications has been performed and reported in Chapter 7 of [3].

Perhaps the most important outcome of this pioneering work was the in vivo tissue comparison between identical form-fit Si and 3C—SiC passive double-shank devices. After harvesting tissue blocks from both the Si and 3C—SiC implant sites, which was performed on three (3) different mice, Fig. 1.10 shows the resulting tissue histology data:

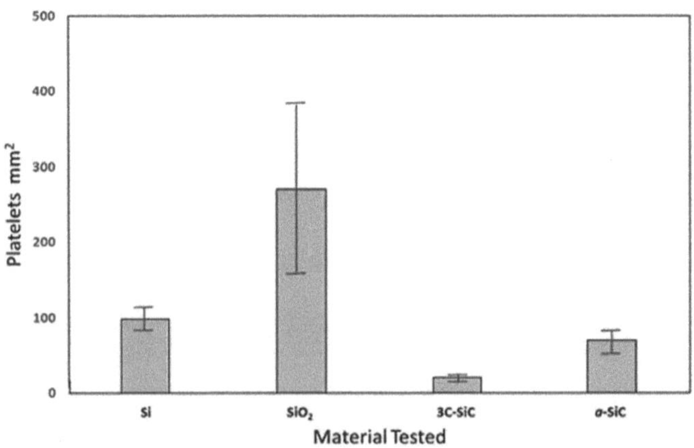

Figure 1.9 Dynamic hemocompatibility histogram of platelet activation of the Si, *a*-SiC on Si, SiO_2, and 3C—SiC using standard deviation as the error bar. Activated platelets per mm^2 were used to evaluate the hemocompatibility of the materials [3].

A number of important observations can be made from the images related to the implant location. A large area devoid of neural tissue (necrosis) is apparent around all of the Si implants, and the voids are often larger than 50 μm wide, a distance which is much larger than the implant thickness of ~20 μm. The left and right images are the same tissue slice for the Si and 3C−SiC implants, thus allowing for a meaningful direct comparison between the two materials within the same animal. The 3C−SiC material in animals one and two produced voids which are ~20 μm wide which is the same dimension as the device thickness indicating that no necrosis had occurred in the brain. Tissue from the third animal was an exception with a void width larger than 50 μm. This was the only animal that showed signs of increased glial fibrillary acidic protein (GFAP) + activity in relation to 3C−SiC.

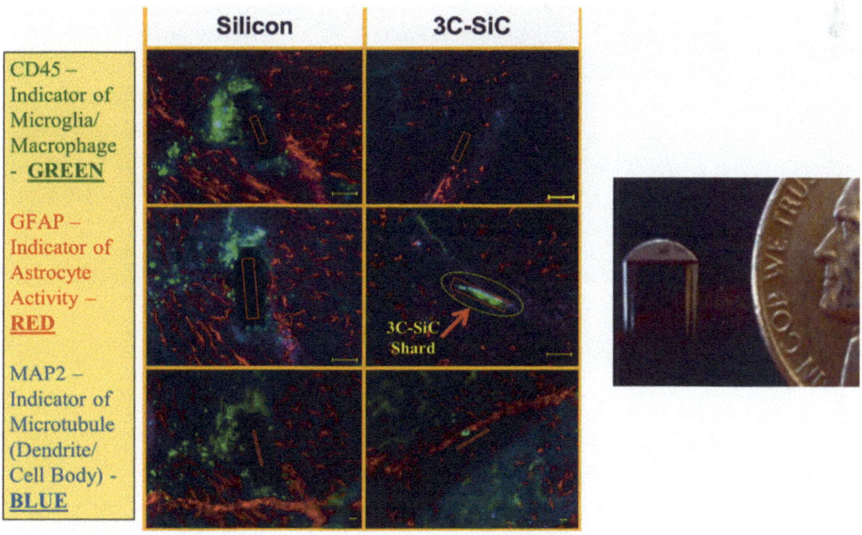

Figure 1.10 Selected digital photographs obtained from a Zeiss Axio Imager two microscope which was used for the immunofluorescence analysis of C57BL/6J mouse hippocampal tissue. Each row represents a selected tissue slice from a single animal ($N = 3$). The first column shows the tissue response within the left hemisphere of the hippocampus surrounding the Si implant and the second column presents the tissue associated with 3C−SiC within the right hemisphere. The legend on the left details the antibody stains used in the study. The orange boxes denote the approximate size of the implant at the tissue location. The scale bars are all 50 μm in length. Right photograph of implanted passive probes showing Si (left) and 3C−SiC (right) double-shanks glued together for simultaneous implantation into wild-type mice.\ *(Image from Ref. [3].)*

Based on this work functional SiC implants have been developed and will be presented later in this book (Chapter 5 All-SiC INI, Chapter 6 MRI compatibility of 3C–SiC INI, and Chapter 7 Carbon-electrode sandwiched with *a*-SiC INI).

While fully monolithic "All-SiC" neural interfaces, homogeneously integrated for long-term human use, has clear advantages over Si- or metal-based devices simply coated in SiC, for neuroscience applications (where long-term implantation is not a major issue) simply coating contemporary neural interfaces with *a*-SiC provides numerous benefits. The work done by Pancrazio et al. has shown a significant in vivo improvement of SiC-coated implants as shown in Fig. 1.11:

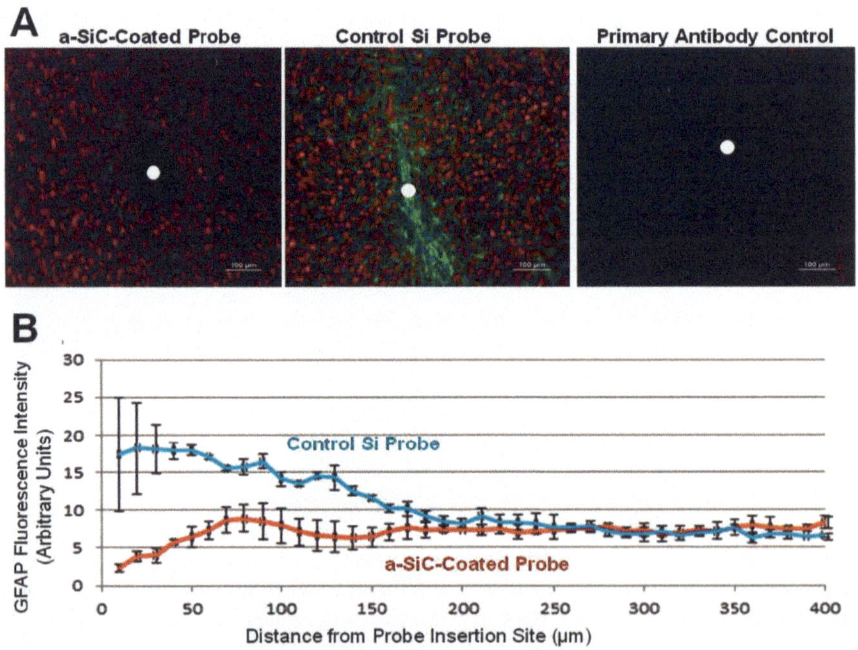

Figure 1.11 (A) Images from deep cortical tissue labeling NeuN in red (neurons), GFAP in green (astrocytes), and DAPI in blue (cell nuclei). White circles indicate center of probe locations. Left image is from tissue implanted with an *a*-SiC-coated probe, middle from a control Si probe, and the right image is the no primary control indicating little or no nonspecific antibody binding. (B) Immunohistochemistry summary data comparing results from an *a*-SiC-coated (red) and a control Si (blue) probes after implantation for 4 weeks. Data are mean ± SEM for $n = 2$ slices (Chapter 8 in Ref. [3]).

3. SiC biosensors

Numerous approaches to biosensing are available in the literature and is simply too exhaustive of a list to provide here. An overview of SiC biosensing that encompasses what is provided in this section may be found in [55]. Common to many biosensors is the need to functionalize the sensor surface to achieve adequate specificity (i.e., discrimination between target analyte and other components in the biosensor environment). Thus, we begin this section with a review of SiC surface functionalization followed by glucose and myoglobin sensing research. While this is not a complete review of all biosensor work in SiC, the objective is to provide some excellent examples of this important topic.

3.1 Surface functionalization

In recent years, striking advancements in SiC growth and processing have enabled the deployment of this wide bandgap semiconductor in high temperature, high power, and harsh environment applications. While important work toward improved solid-state devices continues, one of the most promising new frontiers for SiC lies at the inorganic/(bio) organic interface. To date, both silicon and diamond have taken on leading roles as materials for integrated biological applications. Although the technological maturity of silicon has made it an obvious choice for biosensors and implantable electrodes, it lacks the chemical stability required for long-term in vivo operation and its oxide is susceptible to in-diffusion of ions which can result in significant electronic drift current and high levels of electronic noise. Furthermore, it does not possess the mechanical strength required for implant coating materials. On the other hand, the chemical stability, mechanical hardness, and biocompatibility of SiC are practically unmatched by other materials studied to date.

A natural starting point for the development of functional silicon carbide for biomedical and biosensing applications is its surface termination, which defines the chemical reactivity, surface defect density, work function, and ambient stability of the material. Onto such surfaces a wide range of organic molecules can be covalently bound which possess specific head- and end-groups for defined chemical binding to the substrate, interactions with the surrounding environment, and grafting of biomolecules such as proteins and DNA. In Chapter 4 of [2], some examples of self-assembled monolayer (SAM) formation with organosilanes and short-chain alkenes, as well as direct surface photopolymerization using vinyl monomers, were reported. In fact, a case example of how SAM-modified surfaces can be used to control the spatial wettability of silicon carbide for future biomedical applications was provided, and the outcome of this work is shown in Figs. 1.12 and 1.13

3.1.1 SiC functionalization to enhance cell viability

In principle, a biocompatible substrate allows cells to perform required chemical processes on the surface, such as specific signal transduction responses that lead to cell attachment and proliferation [44,45]. These processes are mediated by the interactions between cell-surface integrin receptors and proteins from the extracellular matrix that are adsorbed on the substrate. Moreover, cytoskeletal filaments are fundamental to the spatial organization of the cell. For example, actin filaments assemble into dynamic cell structures, such as lamellipodia and filopodia, which provide the cells a means of locomotion [46]. Cells tend to spread and increase their attached area when a substrate promotes the adhesion of suitable proteins [47]. Likewise, if a substrate is attractive to a cell, the cell filopodia and lamellipodia extensions couple strongly with the surface [48,49]. Consequently, cell morphology provides an indication of substrate biocompatibility. The combination of surface wettability, roughness, and charge of the surface plays an important role in the appropriate assembly of the structures [44,50,51]. As described earlier, the use of SAMs to tune surface properties is particularly attractive for biotechnology and/or medical implant applications. SAMs can promote the immobilization of essential growth factors [52]

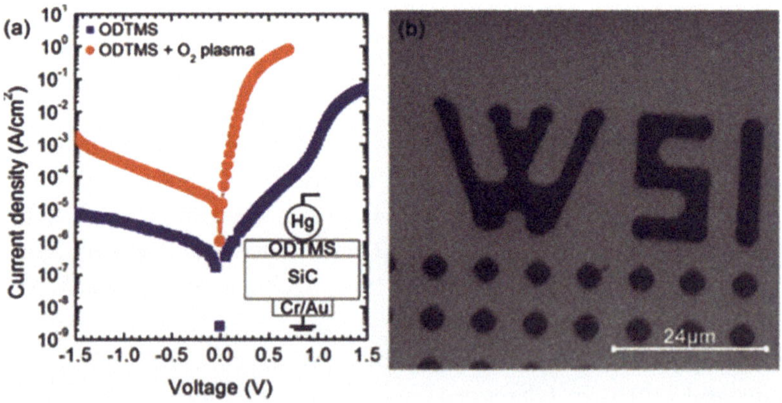

Figure 1.12 (a) IV curves of octadecyltrimethoxysilane (ODTMS)-functionalized 6H–SiC and (b) SEM micrograph of regions with different electrical conductivities. Dark areas indicate oxygen plasma-treated regions [2].

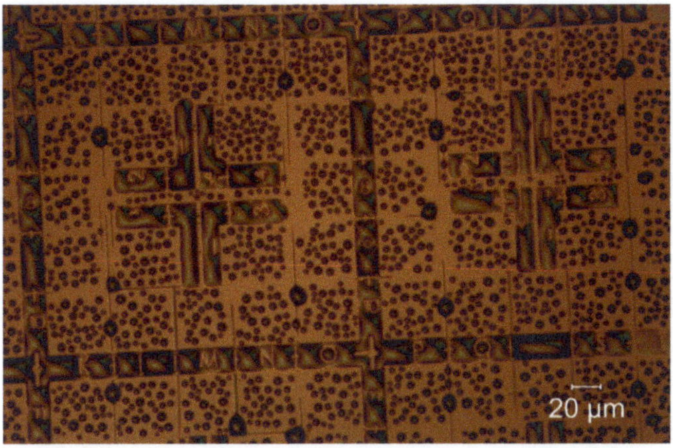

Figure 1.13 Wettability image of a micropatterned ODTMS-modified SiC surface. Water droplets condense preferentially in hydrophilic oxygen plasma-exposed regions [2].

and enhance cell proliferation [53], while maintaining close physical proximity and, therefore electrical coupling, between cells and the underlying substrate. SAM-based bio-functionalization of 6H–SiC was performed to assess its impact on cell morphology and substrate permissiveness. The SAMs were formed by reaction with aminopropyldiethoxymethylsilane and aminopropyltriethoxysilane (APTES) using the silanization techniques described in Chapter 8 of [2] to create moderately hydrophilic surfaces. Quantification of cell proliferation was achieved using 3-(4,5-dimethylthiazol-2-yl)-2,5-diphenyltetrazolium bromide (MTT) assays that were performed in accordance with the procedures outlined by Mossman [54] (Fig. 1.14).

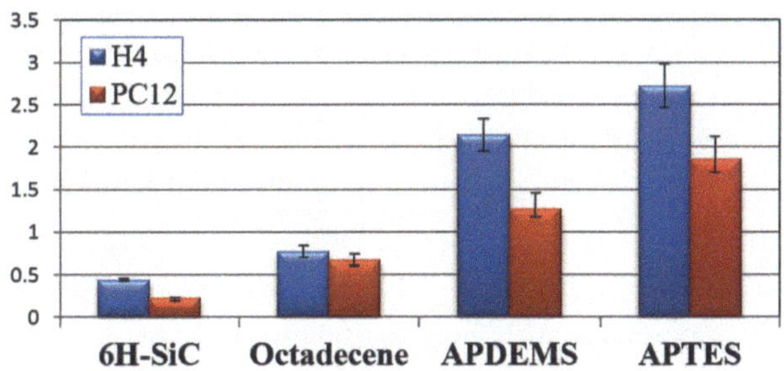

Figure 1.14 Proliferation of H4 and PC12 cell lines on (0001) 6H–SiC substrates versus surface termination, as determined by MTT assay analysis. The results are expressed as sample distribution of the mean ($\bar{\mathbf{x}}$) and standard error of the mean (σ_M) and normalized to the PSt readings, ($n = 3$) [2].

3.1.2 Myoglobin

Myoglobin is released into the blood when heart or skeletal muscle is injured. In principle the detection of Myoglobin can alert medical professionals to a pending heart attack. Thus, the development of a sensor to detect its presence in low concentrations is clearly needed for patients with a high risk of death by Myocardial infarction. Specificity of an immunosensor to the antigen of interest is one of the main properties that can be accomplished with immunosensors, as explained in Ref. [55]. For this reason, after performing characterization of antimyoglobin immobilized on APTE-modified 3C–SiC fluorescent microscopy was used to detect antimyoglobin/myoglobin binding.

To take the fluorescent images a Leica compound microscope with a CCD camera (SPOT5) and an exposure time of 5 s was used. Five (5) images for each of the surfaces tested were taken and the green intensity was quantified by calculating the integrated density of the images with ImageJ [56]. In order to process the data the background (SiC substrate without surface modification) was subtracted from surfaces A*–D*. In addition, the results were normalized with respect to the average integrated density obtained on the surface where the highest fluorescence was expected to be generated (Surface A*) and are reported in Fig. 1.15. The data are reported as the sample distribution of the mean $\overline{(x)}$ ($n = 9$) and the standard error of the mean (σ_M). A *t*-test was performed for each surface with respect to their controls.

3.2 Glucose

Silicon carbide has long been used in advanced radiofrequency systems due to its excellent carrier transport and high-power properties. Many of today's point-of-use healthcare systems are hybrid implantable systems that combine radio frequency (think WiFi) and biosensor technologies. Biosensors usually rely on relevant physiological parameters for continuous monitoring and an integrated antenna is employed to send the received data to an external receiver [58]. Therefore, implantable antennas have attracted considerable attention in recent years as a potential solution for communicating with these implantable biosensors. These hybrid systems combining radio frequency (RF) (antenna/wireless communication) and biosensor technologies are the key to developing the next generation of continuous monitoring systems including implantable pacemakers and defibrillators, glucose monitors, insulin pumps, hearing aids, health care facility communication, medical and emergency equipment tracking and remote patient monitoring just to name a few.

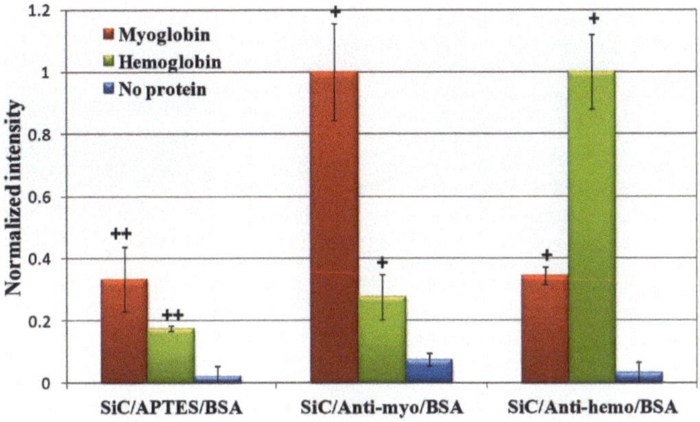

Figure 1.15 Normalized fluorescent intensity of Alexa-Fluor 488 labeled myoglobin and hemoglobin bound to APTES (left), antimyoglobin (center), and antihemoglobin immobilized on SiC (right) with their respective controls. The results are expressed as the sample distribution of the mean $\overline{(x)}$ and standard error of the mean (σ_M) and normalized to the positive control experiments in each test. $^{+}$ denotes *P*-values < .05 with respect to the antibody immobilized control and $^{++}$ denotes *P*-values < .05 with respect to the surface after APTES modification [57].

A continuous glucose monitoring sensor employing RF signals has been developed using the biocompatible material SiC [59]. The fabricated implantable RF antenna utilizes SiC as the material of choice due to its great potential benefit as a robust bio and hemocompatible material for long-term in vivo systems. Distinguished by its innovation to utilize SiC as the device material, this system removes the need to encase this biomedical device with biocompatible materials thus addressing the short lifetime issue of contemporary sensors.

Unlike biosensors that require direct contact with interstitial fluids to trigger chemical reactions to operate, this biocompatible SiC sensor does not require a direct interface to bodily fluids. The sensing mechanism is based upon a shift in the antenna resonant frequency as a function of change in glucose levels which electrically manifests itself as a change in blood permittivity and conductivity.

From these results, it was observed that the antenna response to blood mimicking liquid and pig blood had similar frequency shifting trends—the resonance frequency decreases with an increase of glucose levels. For a nondiabetic healthy person, the American Diabetes Association recommends a fasting plasma glucose level of 70–130 mg/dL, which is shown in Fig. 1.16 (*green shaded area*). Below 60–65 mg/dL is known as

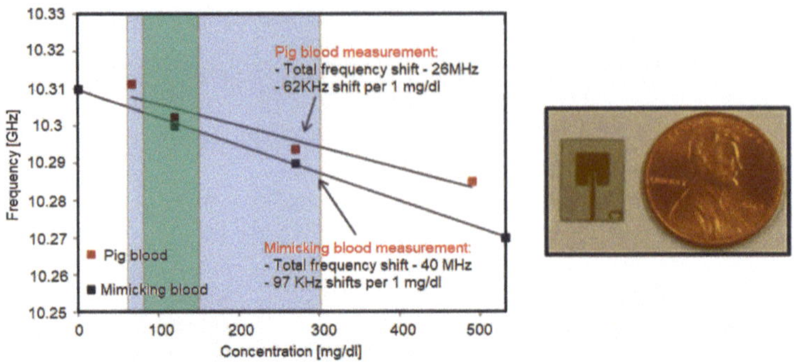

Figure 1.16 Measured relative resonance frequency shift dependence on glucose concentration. Photograph of the RF patch antenna on 4H–SiC. Note fairly linear response versus glucose concentration [3].

hypoglycemia and above 240 mg/dL is known as hyperglycemia (shown in *blue shaded areas*). Note that the SiC-based sensor covers the normal to critical care application regions with a reasonable slope in the frequency versus glucose response at 10 GHz. These results demonstrate the potential use of biocompatible SiC substrates for long-term, real-time continuous glucose monitoring of diabetic patients where the resonance frequency decreases with an increase of glucose levels with linear sensor performance. Due to limitations in the medical bands allocated for such a device, the sensor was redesigned to operate in the IMS band (2.45 GHz) and this work, while still ongoing, has been quite promising and is discussed next.

While these preliminary results are encouraging, they are not in the correct frequency band for biomedical devices. Following the work of Afroz et al. [59] another student in the University of South Florida (USF) SiC group continued the project with the specific objective of scaling the implantable sensor for the industrial, scientific, and medical radio (ISM) band [60]. In addition, a noninvasive solution would be much more convenient for the patient, would not require surgery, and lower power WiFi communication would be allowed due to no signal attenuation in human tissue. Fig. 1.17 depicts an antenna patch located above the upper arm. The antenna and the external circuitry are located outside the body.

The antenna and the electronic circuitry are located outside the body. The antenna is placed in a direct line of sight with a major (cephalic) vein. Measurements of the antenna patch were taken by placing the antenna 2 mm above the human phantom and in direct line of sight of the blood vessel and the blood glucose level varied. The sensor was simulated over the

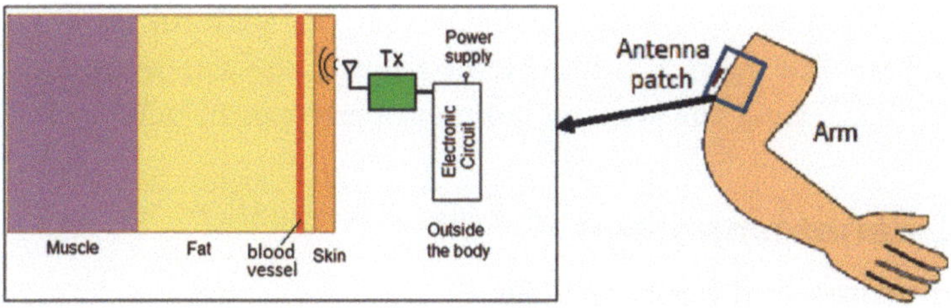

Figure 1.17 Noninvasive sensing antenna configuration on top of the arm to detect glucose changes in the cephalic vein showing HFSS simulation geometry [60].

0–2000 mg/dL glucose range using the equivalent relative permittivity calculated using the equation $\varepsilon_r\,(g_{5.8}) = 0.0596\,g_{5.8}^2 - 0.7416\,g_{5.8} + 52.642$ [59].

Fig. 1.18 summarizes the measured and experimental results from the noninvasive glucose sensor. The glucose variation from 0 to 2000 mg/dL resulted in a similar change in resonant frequency with a shift between simulated and experimental data observed. This shift can be due to tissue layers thickness variations used in the experimental setup, slight variations of the permittivity and conductivity thickness, as well as small variations during the antenna fabrication. Fortunately, the resonant frequency variation versus glucose level concentration has a similar trend.

Based on this data it seems feasible to use a single RF sensing antenna to extract glucose information from blood noninvasively. What is needed now

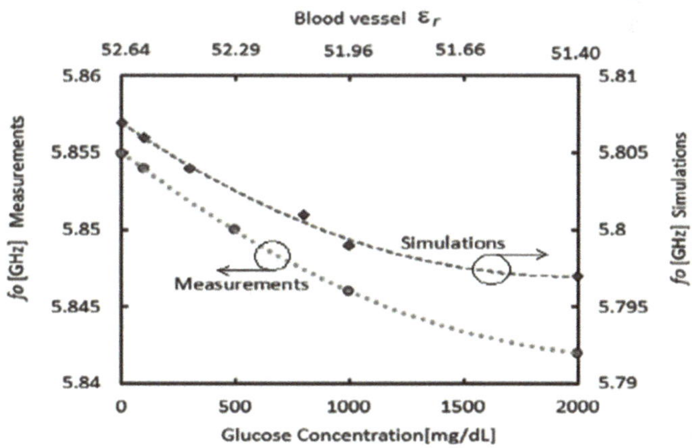

Figure 1.18 Measured and simulated resonant frequency versus glucose concentration [mg/dL] and blood ε_r. Note similar variation with an offset between experimental and simulated data [59].

is the development of a sensor platform that can perform these measurements in real-time with an automated output of the assessed glucose value provided that setting the sense antenna properly can be achieved.

4. SiC nanotechnology

4.1 Nanowires and nanoparticles

Nanotechnology is a very broad field of exploration and technical development which means different things to different people. In a broad sense systems/objects on the nanometer scale are considered and one definition may be found in Wikipedia which states "Nanotechnology, also shortened to nanotech, is the use of matter on an atomic, molecular, and supramolecular scale for industrial purposes." In the context of the present discussion, we present SiC nanotechnology using the classical definition with either three dimension (nanoparticle), two dimension (nanowire) or one dimension (nanowell) as the spatial feature(s) in the nanometer scale. Most of the reported works involving SiC nanotechnology use either nanoparticles or nanowires. Therefore, the following discussion relates to these types of nanostructures with their application to nanomedicine, in the present case, to treat cancer. For a more general discussion of SiC nanotechnology involving other applications an excellent review article is available [61].

Nanotechnology promotes the research and development of innovative systems with unique properties and applications in several fields, from sensors to nanomedicine [62]. For health care applications, the ability to tailor the material properties allows for the design of new nanosystems with enhanced performance for diagnostics, imaging, and oncotherapy [63,64]. Nanowires (NWs) based on cubic silicon carbide (3C−SiC) have a strong potential to pave the way for the development of a novel generation of implantable nano-devices since they are chemically inert and compatible in the biological environment. Indeed, 3C−SiC is a proved bio- and hemocompatible material, and some biomedical device prototypes have been successfully realized by micromachining of thin films, as reviewed by Zorman et al. in Ref. [2]. The combination of 3C−SiC with silicon dioxide in core/shell NW structures (i.e., core/shell 3C−SiC/SiO_2 NWs) opens more ways to engineer the surface via functionalization and decoration with macro-molecules and nanoparticles [65,66]. The potential use of core/shell NWs in nanomedicine is driven by the presence of the amorphous shell, as it can modify the material behavior in the biological environment. For instance, for blood-contacting applications, silicon oxide could induce a stronger aggregation and activation of platelets, promoting clot formation and acute inflammatory processes [67,68]. Further, a peculiar feature of the core/shell NWs is their optical emission: the oxide shell enhances the core luminescence [69–71] when the nanosystem is excited by highly energetic sources, such as electron beams or X-rays. This property opens the possibility to exploit 3C–SiC/SiO_x NWs as radiation-resistant scintillation nanostructures, which can be properly functionalized to play an active role for new oncotherapies, for example, X-ray excited photodynamic therapy [72], in nanomedicine.

4.1.1 Photodynamic therapy to treat deep-tissue cancer using nanowires

In the field of clinical oncotherapy, the standard protocols to control cancer growth and spread are still based on chemo- and radio-therapy combined with surgical resection. New strategies, such as the genetic approach, are expected to deeply change cancer treatments in the near future. Alternative approaches aimed at killing tumors while minimizing side effects could be allowed by new classes of multifunctional nanomaterials and are presently under study. For instance, scintillation nanoparticles (NPs) were recently proposed in pilot studies [73,74] to activate self-lighted photodynamic therapy (SLPDT) to treat deep cancer. SLPDT is a variation of the well assessed photodynamic therapy (PDT) usually used to "treat tumors on or just under the skin or on the lining of internal organs or cavities through the generation of an active form of oxygen (singlet oxygen, $^1O_2$) that destroys nearby cancer cells" (definition from the US-National Cancer Institute [75]). In the previously mentioned pilot studies on SLPDT, photosensitizers are attached to the scintillation NPs and allow light generation under X-ray irradiation. The photosensitizer (e.g., organic dyes, aromatic hydrocarbons, porphyrins, phthalocyanines, and related tetrapyrroles) [76] promotes, through singlet oxygen generation, oxidative stress to kill cancer cells [77]. Since X-rays can penetrate through body tissue, deep tumors can be reached and treated with this method (Fig. 1.19).

The work by Salviati et al. [2]. provides an overview of the growth and optical properties and some in vitro applications of core/shell 3C–SiC/SiO_2 NWs and bare SiC NWs. It was shown, by the analysis of cell proliferation, cell cycle progression, and oxidative stress, that the core/shell NWs are cytocompatible over a time of up to 10 days. They are effectively internalized by cells through the macropinocytosis mechanism

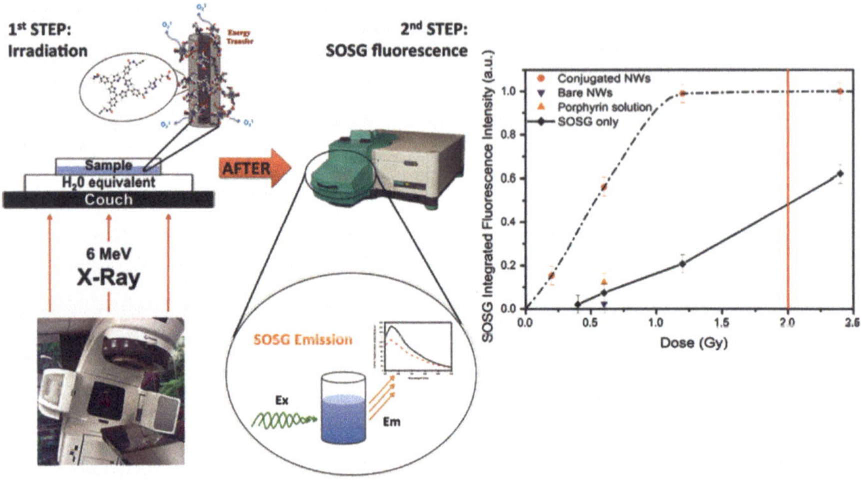

Figure 1.19 $^1O_2$ production excited by X-rays in a radiation therapy setup. Sketch of the experimental steps: a dish containing the sample solution is put on the couch and irradiated from the bottom, then it is transferred to a spectrophotometer to acquire the fluorescence spectrum of the SOSG marker. The plot reports the measured integrated fluorescence intensity, proportional to $^1O_2$ generated, as a function of the radiation dose. The experimental points are obtained from a SOSG kit in water, with H_2TPACPP-functionalised NWs (*red circles*) or without NWs (*black diamonds*). The orange up-triangle at 0.6 Gy is the experimental point obtained from SOSG kit in a water solution of mere porphyrin, while the blue down-triangle is obtained from SOSG kit in a water suspension of NWs as grown. The usual dose for clinical treatment (2 Gy) is indicated by the *red vertical line. (From Ref. [71].)*

(phagocytosis only in the THP-1 model) and sporadically by direct penetration. In all the cell lines studied, the intracellular presence of NWs induces the same molecular events: peroxidation of membrane lipids and oxidation of proteins. These effects are late stage and may be limited by the activation of protection systems, for instance, the effect of ROS is not acute and effectively countered by the intracellular scavenger. These results highlight that the core/shell 3C–SiC/SiO_2 NWs do not elicit either midterm (72 h) or long-term (10 days) cytotoxic activity leading to irreversible cellular damages or death.

4.1.2 *Near-infrared photo-immune therapy using SiC nanostructures*

While singlet oxygen generation does kill cancer cells, it also kills healthy cells within close proximity. An alternate approach, proposed by a research team led by Saddow and colleagues from Italy, Hungary, and the NCI

(Bethesda, MD), is seeking to use SiC nanostructures to facilitate cancer treatment via photo-immune therapy (PIT). This research is ongoing, and details may be found on the National Institutes of Health Grantome website (https://grantome.com/grant/NIH/R21-CA223969-01A1). The research grant abstract is provided in quotes below which states the promise of PIT using near IR (NIR) illumination for the treatment of recurring and untreatable surface cancer. The concept in the work by Saddow et al. is to enable "deep-tissue" cancer treatment by using X-ray irradiation to simulate 690 nm NIR from SiC nanostructures to activate the PIT process for such pernicious cancers as liver, pancreas, etc. So far, a very promising nanostructure system has been developed and reported by Beke et al. from this project [78].

Current methods of cancer treatment such as surgery, radiation, and chemo-immuno-therapy strive to balance cancer treatment against adverse effects. Several treatments that aim to kill cancer cells while sparing normal cells are in development. However, no such therapies have been developed for locally advanced, deep visceral cancers. Photo-immune therapy (PIT) is a targeted therapy for cancer with highly selective cell killing based on the use of an antibody-photoabsorber (IR700DX) conjugate (APC) and targeted low energy light therapy. Developed by the National Cancer Institute, this therapy is termed near-infrared PIT (NIR-PIT). The antibody can be chosen for optimal binding to a particular cancer based on its cell surface expression. IR700DX is only toxic to cells when the APC is bound to the cell membrane. When exposed to near-infrared light ($\sim$690 nm) rapid cell necrosis occurs in tumor cells due to changes in cell membrane permeability, but no damage is observed in normal cells that have no or minimal expression of the target antigen. NIR-PIT is in clinical trials in inoperable recurrent head/neck cancers using the conjugate Cetuximab-IR700. A Phase I study has demonstrated minimal adverse events with substantial effects on the tumor including several complete responses. Our strategy relies on silicon carbide (SiC) nanostructures to enable deep-tissue treatment of cancer via NIR-PIT. While a single exposure of APC followed by a single dose of NIR light is effective in knocking down cancer cells, it is not adequate to completely kill the tumor likely due to incomplete penetration of the APC within the tumor. However, multiple exposures of light separated by hours to days are effective and have often resulted in cures in models. The APC demonstrates a relatively long circulation time thus, after first light exposure, additional circulating APCs enter the tumor and bind to remaining tumor cells. Since NIR-PIT kills tumor cells but not vascular endothelium, the vessels are left intact with a 24-fold increase in the permeability of tumor vessels to macromolecules as large as 200 nm, an effect termed Super Enhanced Permeability and Retention (SUPR). This project takes advantage of SUPR after an initial NIR-PIT treatment for delivering X-ray activatable nanoparticles to the tumor.

4.1.3 Room-temperature DNA assays using a-SiC coated Si nanowires

Semiconducting nanowires are of a growing interest in nanoelectronic devices, in particular for sensing applications [79]. While silicon is the most widely used material in this field, it lacks long-term stability in an aqueous solution [80—82] and, therefore, is not suited for most liquid environments. Indeed, chemical resistance to the medium is essential for device reliability and signal stability. Silicon carbide appears as a promising material for these applications [5,6], thanks to its semiconducting properties as well as its very high chemical stability and biocompatibility [83]. However, SiC is much more difficult to etch due to its high physical and chemical stability, compared to Si material. Thus, core—shell Si/SiC nanowires could be an advantageous compromise between these two approaches [84]. The applications include ion-sensitive field effect transistors (FETs) (ISFETs), chemical FETs (ChemFETs), and other related sensing devices. These devices would benefit from the strong chemical and physical stability of the SiC shell and from the superior electron transport within the Si core.

In this work [85], transmission electron microscopy (TEM) analysis was conducted to investigate the structural and crystallographic differences between the two methods. Fig. 1.20 depicts the full stack obtained after Si NW etching and *a*-SiC coating using PECVD. Si NWs exhibit a rectangular shape after dry etching of the patterned topmost Si film and are coated with a thin layer of *a*-SiC. Despite the low contrast between *a*-SiC, SiO_2, and the glue matrix, TEM images show that the *a*-SiC coating is conformal and covers the entire exposed Si and SiO_2 surfaces with a thickness of about 12.5 nm, decreasing to 10 nm on the NW sidewalls. As amorphous SiC behaves like an insulator, devices remain electrically isolated from one another despite the SiC layer covering the SiO_2 surface. The high-resolution image (Fig. 1.20B) shows no voids or defects at the Si/*a*-SiC interface and a low constraint on the first five atomic layers of the Si crystal.

Devices were characterized electrically using current-voltage measurements after defining the metal contacts. Typical I_D-V_G transfer characteristics resulting from the PECVD process are shown in Fig. 1.21 and plotted versus

(a) 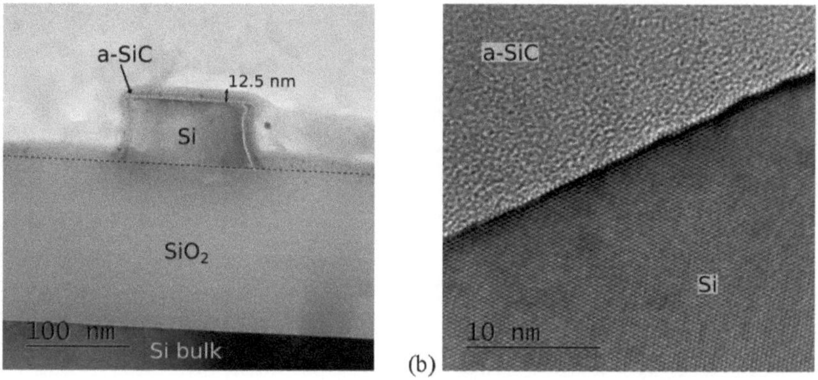

(b)

Figure 1.20 SiC-coated Si nanowire DNA sensor data. (A) TEM cross-section image of a Si NW etched from SOI substrate and covered with amorphous SiC deposited by PECVD, and (B) zoomed-in HR-TEM image at the Si/*a*-SiC interface [85].

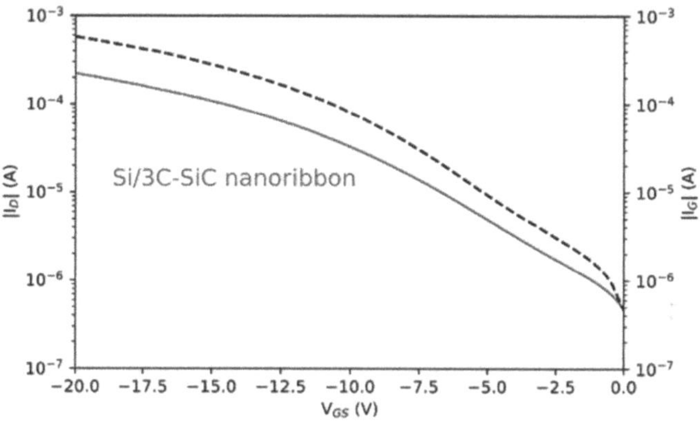

Figure 1.21 Transfer characteristics of back-gated core–shell Si/*a*-SiC nanoribbon devices: *a*-SiC SOI device resulting in thin SiC shell. Drain current plotted with *solid line* and gate current with *dashed line* [85].

gate current I_G. Electrical characterization was conducted on nanoribbons (NRs) only because they provided higher reproducibility than NWs. The devices were back-gated from the Si substrate and biased with a drain voltage $V_D = -4$ V.

In this study, PECVD of a passivating *a*-SiC layer allowed for the development of potentially high durability core–shell Si/*a*-SiC devices designed to be operated in liquid environments. Based on these results, further research will focus on core–shell Si/*a*-SiC FETs using PECVD of *a*-SiC, hence benefitting from the reproducible electrical performances exhibited throughout the process.

4.2 Epitaxial graphene and pyrolyzed photoresist film on SiC surfaces

Single-layer and few-layer graphene are obtained on SiC substrates via a thermal decomposition process. To this end, the SiC crystal was heated at temperatures above 1000°C. As a result, Si desorbs from the surface in gaseous form and carbon atoms that are left behind rearrange in the hexagonal lattice that is the hallmark of graphene. Epitaxial graphene on SiC has been seen as a leading contender for post-complimentary metal oxide semiconductor (CMOS) electronics because the substrate can, if properly doped, be semi-insulating. This is clearly a practical and scalable approach for 2D electronics [86]. Hexagonal SiC crystals, namely 4H- and 6H−SiC, provide an ideal template for graphene growth and thus have evolved as the substrates of choice. In contrast, limited attention was initially given to the possibility of growing graphene on the cubic SiC polytype (3C−SiC), although the (111) orientation of this crystal would also naturally accommodate the sixfold symmetry of graphene. Notably, when using 4H- and 6H−SiC substrates, graphene grows differently on the Si-face (i.e., SiC(0001)), and C-face (i.e., SiC $(000\,\overline{1})$), of SiC. For instance, vacuum annealing of SiC crystals leads to small graphene domains typically 30−100 nm in diameter on Si terminated (0001) SiC, whereas on the C-terminated $(000\,\overline{1})$ face larger domains (~200 nm) of multilayered rotationally disordered graphene (i.e., turbostratic growth) have been produced [87,88]. The epitaxial graphene produced under ultra-high vacuum conditions was the initial approach to grow graphene on SiC, but it lacked continuity on the films. Such inhomogeneous films do not meet the demands of large-scale device production, which requires larger domains and tighter thickness control. In 2009, Emtsev and colleagues demonstrated that by growing under Ar atmosphere the quality and homogeneity of graphene grown on the SiC(0001) could be drastically improved [89].

The first carbon layer that grows on top of SiC(0001) is what is known as zero-layer (or buffer layer) graphene [86]. It is in part covalently bonded to the SiC substrate and, hence, electronically inactive. The second carbon layer grows on top of the zero-layer without interlayer bonds and acts like monolayer graphene (Fig. 1.22).

Graphene films were epitaxially grown on 6H−SiC(0001) substrates. Initially, the 6H−SiC samples were H_2 etched to remove any polishing damage and to obtain a well-ordered surface [90]. Subsequently, graphene growth was performed in an Ar atmosphere at temperatures of ~1650°C

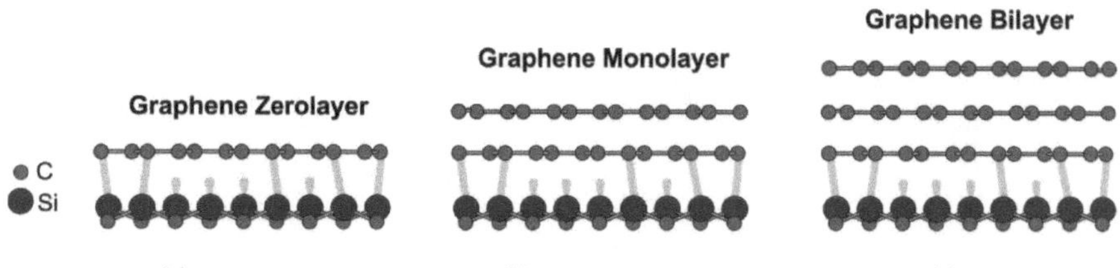

Figure 1.22 Side view model of epitaxial graphene on SiC. (A) Zero-layer graphene, Bb) monolayer graphene, and (C) bilayer graphene configurations [2].

with a pressure of ~900 mbar as described in Ref. [89]. The quality and thickness of the graphene films were evaluated by angle-resolved photoemission spectroscopy and X-ray photoelectron spectroscopy. All of the samples presented monolayer thickness and homogeneity similar to that reported in Ref. [90].

Carbon films may be synthesized by pyrolyzation of photoresist and are referred to as pyrolyzed photoresist film, or PPF. This was produced after spinning S1813 photoresist at 3000 rpm on a Si wafer (~1.7 μm thick) and annealing in Ar at 750°C in a CVD reactor for 30 min at 900 mbar pressure. Atomic force microscopy (AFM) and surface water contact angle (SWCA) analysis were used to assess the surface morphology and wettability of SiC, PPF, and graphene. The surface topography analysis was done using an XE-100 Advanced Scanning Microscope from Park Systems. The SWCA measurements were obtained from the average of 10 μL droplets deposited on three different areas of the sample. A KSV CAM101 system from KSV Instruments was used for this task, and the contact angle (θ) was estimated by measuring the angles between the baseline of the droplet and the tangent at the droplet boundary.

In vitro (MTT) assays were conducted using human keratinocyte (HaCaT) cells on both carbon surfaces as described in Ref. [2]. After 72 h, the morphology of the HaCaT cells on graphene, PPF, and 6H—SiC was similar to that on the PSt control (data not shown) with signs of cell—cell interaction and cell—substrate interaction. The cells were found to be flattened (indication of good adhesion with the substrate) and with a cuboidal shape typical of this cell type. An assessment of the cell viability was obtained via MTT after 72 h of incubation and with respect to the PSt control. The viability values were 0.35 ± 0.18 (standard deviation of the mean) for graphene and 0.41 ± 0.08 for 6H—SiC. On the other hand, cell viability on the PPF substrates was found to be 0.91 ± 0.13, hence

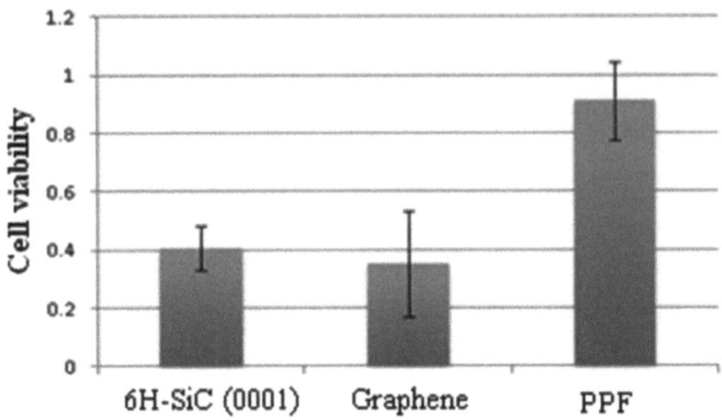

Figure 1.23 MTT assay results of HaCaT cells on graphene. Average cell viability on each substrate normalized to PSt readings (P-value $< .05$). Results expressed as sample distribution of the mean ($\overline{\mathbf{x}}$) and standard error of the mean (σ_M) and normalized to the PSt readings [2].

significantly higher than that obtained for the other two substrates (see Fig. 1.23).

4.3 Luminescent cell markers

When performing in vitro studies it is critical to have luminescent cell markers to study cellular processes and function. Normally fluorescent markers are biochemical in nature and, thus, have a limited lifetime (often minutes to hours maximum). Having a longer-lasting optically active marker is very attractive, especially for the long-time frame in vitro studies. The application of SiC Quantum Dots (QDs) for fluorescent cell labeling was reported in Ref. [2] by Bluet et al. Two different top-down processes were investigated to produce SiC QDs from bulk or polycrystalline SiC substrates: electrochemical etching and laser ablation.

Stable dispersion of the SiC QDs was obtained in water (as in other polar solvents) due to their negative charges, thus cell incubation with these solutions was realized. To obtain a visible fluorescence, the cubic SiC polytype has been chosen for these experiments. A strong fluorescence from the SiC QDs, which undoubtedly penetrated inside the cell, was observed. The expected cytocompatibility of SiC QDs has been checked by MTT assays for reasonably low QD concentrations, that is, below 0.25 mg/mL. This demonstrates the efficiency of noncytotoxic cell labeling with SiC QDs. Furthermore, a preferential location of the QDs in the cell nuclei has been evidenced. A possible explanation is the electrostatic attraction of negatively charged SiC QDs by the chromatin. Maybe due to this specific localization, high SiC QD concentration hinders cell proliferation. Consequently, a cytotoxicity comparison has been performed between epithelial healthy and cancer cells that reveal a selective cytotoxicity with the preferential killing of tumoral cells in a large proportion (up to three cancer cells for one healthy).

The magnified fluorescence photo in Fig. 1.24 shows two single cells marked by the 3C–SiC QDs and confirms that the QDs are indeed strongly localized in the intracellular environment with a brighter nucleus indicating that the QDs crossed the nuclear membrane. This detailed picture also highlights a heterogeneous distribution of the QDs in the cytoplasm. In particular, we can notice that the QDs are more localized inside and near the cell nucleus rather than at the cell peripheries.

Efficient cell labeling by 3C–SiC QDs is demonstrated without cell toxicity for concentrations up to 250 μg/mL. At higher concentrations, the very efficient uptake of the QDs in the cell nucleus induces a decreasing cell proliferation. When speaking about cell proliferation reduction, one

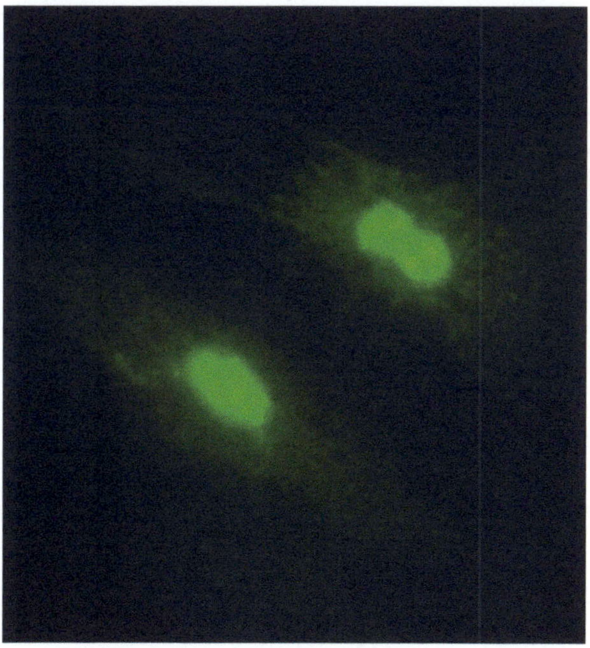

Figure 1.24 High magnification fluorescence microscopy image of 2 cells showing heterogeneous marking using 3C–SiC quantum dots with preferential targeting of the nuclei [2].

immediately thinks about cancer therapy provided that cancer cells are more affected than healthy ones.

5. SiC implants

Implants refer to the general class of devices/materials that are surgically inserted into the human body. They typically involve dental prostheses such as artificial teeth, cardiovascular stents to prevent vascular collapse after angioplasty, or biosensors such as those used in modern glucose monitoring systems. There are also skeletal (bone) implants traditionally made with metals for such common applications as artificial knees and the like and have a limited lifetime [96]. In the case of bone implants, they are often treated to display a ceramic surface to tissue to reduce and/or eliminate irritation and thus reduce body rejection. Perhaps the most interesting application of SiC implants involves the human nervous system, namely either the central (brain) or peripheral (limbs) system. In this section, we will review some excellent examples of the use of SiC both in bone and to provide a bi-directional signal pathway to the nervous system.

5.1 Bone growth

Polycrystalline SiC has been extensively used in the ceramics industry and is mainly known for its mechanical strength and refractory characteristics. Hence it is used extensively as a grinding agent as well as for refractory high-strength machining tool coatings. As we have seen SiC is highly biocompatible and, when implanted, is known to cause minimal inflammation or tissue response [91–94]. However, while some earlier reports indicated that SiC does not support the growth of cells in vitro the misconception was mainly due to a lack of understanding of the complex crystal structure of SiC, where the polytype chosen for study and the cell line evaluated do impact the resulting cell adhesion to SiC surfaces [2]. To explore the potential of SiC as a substrate for bone growth, the nanoporous SiC (np-SiC) surface was mineralized with sol-gel coatings of hydroxyapatite (HA), under various deposition conditions, as described in Ref. [2].

Hydroxyapatite is among the most ubiquitous phases of calcium phosphate-based materials and has been widely used as a bone substitute material for orthopedic and dental applications due to the biological and chemical similarity between HA and the mineralized bone matrix of the human tissue [95–98]. The ability of HA to form a chemical bond with the host bone tissue renders HA very advantageous as a synthetic bone substitute for clinical applications. The osteoconductive characteristics of HA also make it more popular compared to other ceramic or metal-based bone substitutes. Furthermore, HA is biocompatible which makes it a preferred synthetic material compared to other existing bone-implant systems such as allografts and xenografts [5–8]. Synthetic HA has been synthesized in bulk form from powders and sintered ceramics, as well as thin-film coatings on metal and ceramic substrates using a variety of solid-state, chemical, and vapor phase techniques.

HA films of different thicknesses (0.7–4 μm) were synthesized on commercial, as well as in-house synthesized, nanoporous SiC comprising nanometer-sized pores (~10, ~16 and ~50 nm) using a sol–gel method employing phosphorus pentoxide (P_2O_5) and calcium nitrate ($Ca(NO_3)_2$, $4H_2O$) as precursors. The formation of nanostructured HA with grain sizes close to the dimension of the pores on the underlying substrate has been identified up to the calcination temperature of ~500°C in air. A smooth, dense, and crack-free HA film with low porosity has been obtained after sintering the nanostructured HA film at ~900°C in air. The HA film of ~1.4 μm thickness showed good cohesive strength between the particles. The cohesive strength, however, decreases with an increase in film thickness above ~2 μm. Cell attachment studies revealed that for an HA film of ~1.4 μm thickness good adhesion with the custom made ~16 and

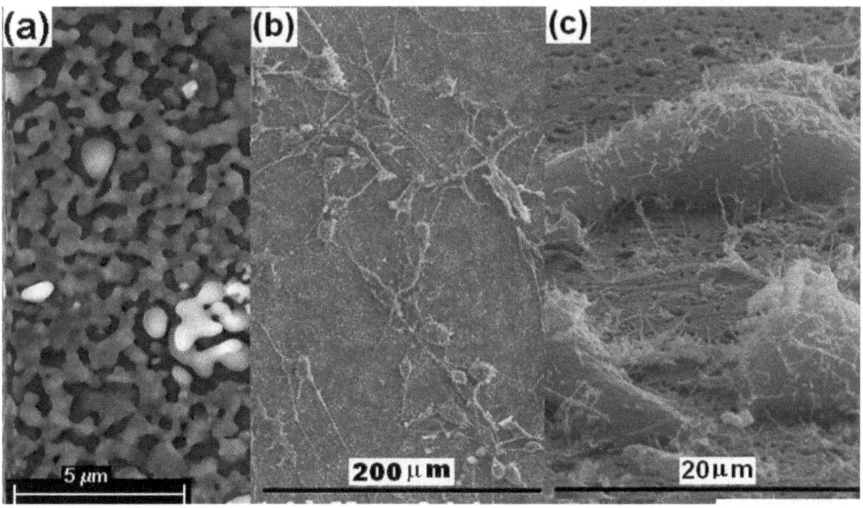

Figure 1.25 SEM micrograph (A) of ~1.4 μm of HA film on custom-made ~16 nm np-SiC obtained after thermal treatment at ~900°C for 1 2 h. The MG-63 cell attachment to 1.4 μm thick HA on ~16 nm np-SiC at lower magnification (B) and higher magnification (C) [2].

~50 nm np-SiC was exhibited throughout the cell culture due to the improvement in the adhesive strength of the HA film with the substrate with the increasing pore size (Fig. 1.25).

5.2 Dental and orthopedic implants

Dental implants are perhaps one of the most common devices implanted in the human body for long-term use. There are several issues, mostly relating to the osseointegration and biocompatibility of the implant to tissue (soft and bone). Some examples of superior implants using SiC are shown below (Fig. 1.26).

One of the important observations of using SiC for dental implants is the natural bio-fouling resistance of this material, which will be discussed in detail by Franca et al. in Chapter 10. Not only are biofilms inhibited when SiC surfaces are presented to biological material [99], cell viability of HA mixed with SiC before the coating of surfaces is enhanced [100]. Both of these properties, along with the structural properties of SiC, make this an ideal material for dental implant applications (Fig. 1.27).

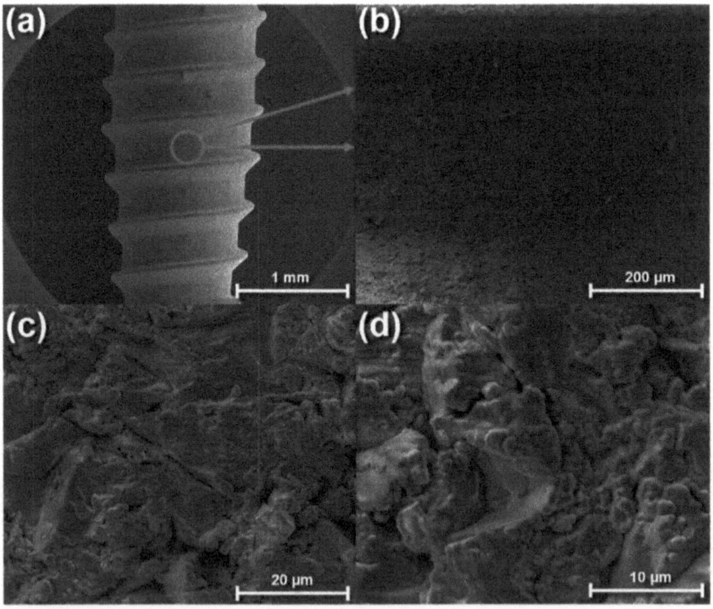

Figure 1.26 Scanning electron microscope images of a SiC-coated titanium implant at various magnifications. Image (A) shows the overall surface of the implant, whereas images (B—D) show detailed images of the implant surface morphology at increasing magnifications [99].

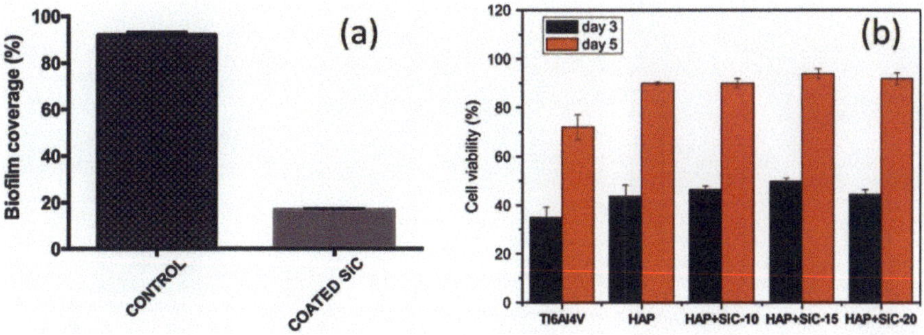

Figure 1.27 (A) Live coverage of *Streptococcus mutans* and *Streptococcus sanguinis* after 24 h of culture on the noncoated (control) and coated surfaces [100]. (B) The cell viability of the investigated samples as shown. Here, SiC was added to the hydroxyapatite and the impact on cell viability was observed [99].

5.3 SiC neural implants

The potential impact of neurocompatible implantable devices to assist millions who suffer from brain and spinal cord injury or limb loss is tremendous, both in restoring patient health, as well as the quality of life. Until now, no known reliable solution to this challenge has been found, with most of the current technology relying on nonneurocompatible materials such as silicon, tungsten, or platinum, along with polymer-based insulators. SiC and, in particular 3C—SiC, appears to be an ideal material to meet this challenging application: the evidence of bio- and hemocompatibility is increasing; it is a semiconductor that allows for tailored doping profiles and the seamless integration of electronics with the implants; it is highly durable, even within harsh, corrosive environments; SiC is also an excellent thermal conductor [1].

The only neural implant approved for humans to date is based on the University of Utah intracortical array [101]. Unfortunately, due to numerous challenges, long-term reliable performance has yet to be achieved with the silicon shank and parylene-C/platinum materials used to create the recording/stimulating tip (Fig. 1.28):

Fortunately, numerous instances of SiC being used as a robust material for INI applications have been reported [102—105]. In the USF SiC group, we have been working on this challenge for nearly 2 decades and have developed several possible solutions to address long-term in vivo INI issues such as an all-SiC monolithic micro-electrode array (MEA) constructed using 4H—SiC [103], an alternate device based on 3C—SiC on either bulk Si or silicon on insulator (SOI) substrates [104], and most recently an ultra-

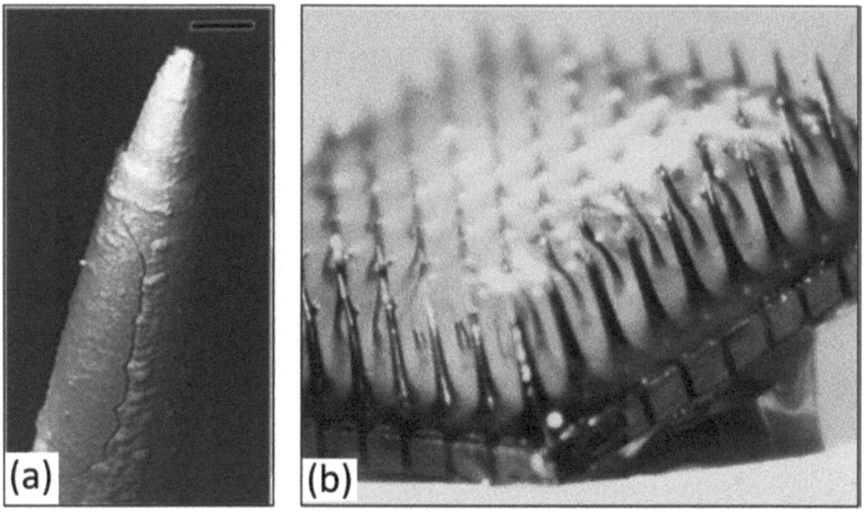

Figure 1.28 In vivo failures common in today's heterogeneously integrated silicon-based neural probes. The Utah Intracortical Array (Blackrock), (a) Side view of an electrode with a large longitudinal crack in the parylene-C insulation adjacent to surface irregularities (20 um scale). (b) Explanted UIEA array at 10 months. The array was completely encapsulated. SiC Intracortical Neural Interface (INI) devices may be a great solution to this challenge thus allowing for long-term human use in BMI systems.

thin interface using *a*-SiC as the base and capping insulation which sandwiches a carbon electrode created using PPF [106]. Not only has excellent electrical performance been demonstrated in phosphate-buffered sailine (PBS), but in the case of the 3C−SiC all-SiC interface on SOI excellent MRI compatibility has been observed in a 7T animal bore MRI system at the Moffitt Cancer Center located on the USF campus [105]. Details of this research are included in Chapter 5 (all-SiC INI) and Chapter 6 (MRI compatibility of an all-SiC INI comprised of 3C−SiC). A preview of these results is shown below (Fig. 1.29):

In Chapter 7, Table 7.4, the electrochemical performance of commonly used electrode materials for mINP is compared to the SiC devices reported in this book (Chapter's 5, 6 and 7). Of the various forms of SiC mINI developed, the PPF electrode demonstrated a low impedance at 1 kHz and the largest CSC among the other materials, which further indicate that PPF is a promising candidate for next-generation mINP devices. One remaining issue is to assess the long-term stability of this material system which is work that will be reported in the near future.

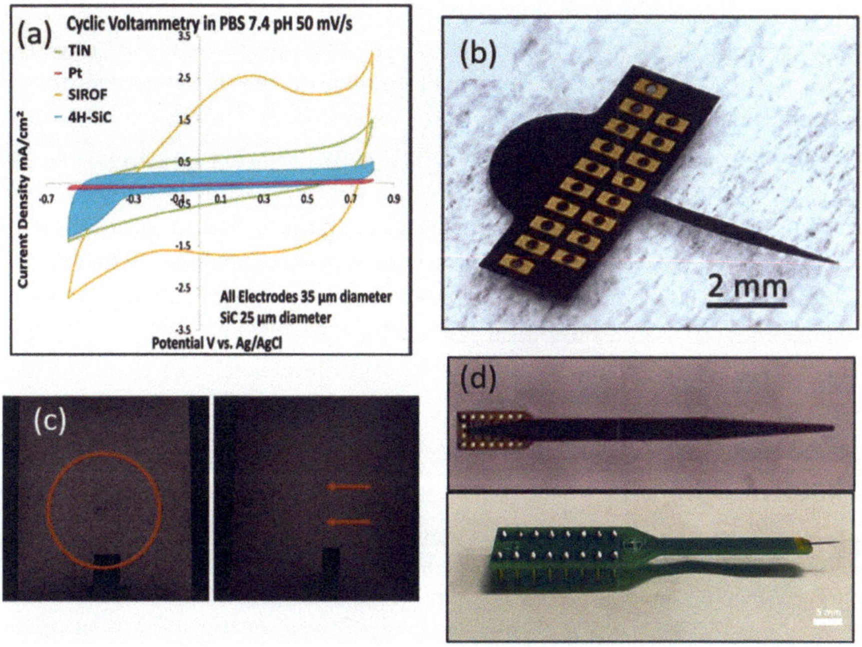

Figure 1.29 Examples of SiC INI devices developed in the USF SiC Group. (A) CV performance comparison of an all-SiC (4H–SiC polytype) MEA showing superior performance to Pt electrodes of the same form-fit [103]. (B) Free-standing all-SiC (3C–SiC on SOI) 16 channel functional INI used to assess the MRI compatibility [104]. (C) sagittal (left) and coronal (right) MRI images @7T showing no image artifacts and ~transparent performance in a brain-tissue phantom [105]. (D) Photographs of C-based a-SiC INI showing released device ~1 μm thick (top) and packaged device with Si backing for structural support mounted on a NeuroNexus 16 channel package header for future in vivo testing [106].

6. Summary

In this introductory chapter of *Silicon Carbide Technology for Advanced Human Healthcare Applications*, we have introduced SiC as a robust and highly useful material for biomedical devices and applications. A review of the basic material structure was made followed by a discussion of the various forms of SiC that are in use today including a snapshot of the many ways that SiC materials are grown/synthesized/formed. Following the SiC materials discussion, the second half of the chapter focused on biomedical devices which primarly consisted of highlights from two previous books on this compelling subject [2,3]. Based on this introduction, the reader should be able to continue reading the next chapters in this book with an impression of the overall SiC biotechnology landscape. The hope is that this will allow one to gain in-depth and comprehensive information on why SiC is ideally poised to lead the way to the development of the next generation of biomedical devices, especially for long-term chronic human implant applications. We hope you enjoy the following discussion as much as we enjoyed putting it together. In fact, once completed this book has motivated us even further to accelerate the development and incorporation of SiC in advanced "next-generation" biomedical devices. The future of biomedical devices continues to look bright. By working at the nexus of advanced materials and biological systems/devices it is our sincere hope that this will lead to better lives for many around the planet once these devices reach the marketplace.

Acknowledgments

None of this would have been possible without the dedication and hard work of many of my doctoral students. Their contribution to the SiC biomedical device story is impressive, and I sincerely acknowledge all of these pioneering researchers here: Camilla Coletti (connective tissue compatibility), Christopher Frewin (neural compatibility and interfaces), Norelli Schettini and Maysam Nezifati (hemocompatibility), Alexandra Oliveros, Shamima Afroz and Fabiola Araujo (biosensors), Evans Bernardin and Chenyin Feng (neural interfaces), and Mohammad Beygi (neural interfaces and MRI compatibility). I gratefully acknowledge all of the contributors to the first two books on this subject who I have referenced throughout this chapter to highlight the tremendous depth and breadth of R&D in this growing field of biomedical devices for healthcare applications. Their contribution is greatly appreciated and acknowledged. It is on the shoulders of all of these fine contributors that this book stands on and I am truly grateful to them all. Finally, for this chapter, I would like to thank the NIR-PIT research team for such a tremendous project interaction as we seek to find a selective cancer treatment for deep-tissue cancer: In Parma G. Salviati, F. Begi and F. Rossi; in Trento M. Nardi and Melanie Timpel; in Budapest David Beke and Adam Gali; in Bethesda MD P. Choyke, S. Adler and J. Seidel.

References

[1] S. E. Saddow and A. Agrawal, Editors, Advances in Silicon Carbide Processing and Applications, © 2004 Artech House ISBN 1-58053-740-5.
[2] S.E. Saddow, Silicon Carbide Biotechnology: A Biocompatible Semiconductor for Advanced Biomedical Devices and Applications, Elsevier Science, Netherlands, 2012.
[3] S.E. Saddow, Silicon Carbide Biotechnology: A Biocompatible Semiconductor for Advanced Biomedical Devices and Applications, second ed., Elsevier Science, Netherlands, 2016.
[4] H. Guo, Y Wang, S Chen, G Zhang, H Zhang, Z Li, "PECVD SiC as a chemical resistant material in MEMS," Proceedings of the 1st IEEE International Conference

on Nano/Micro Engineered and Molecular Systems, January 18-21, 2006, Zhuhai, China.
[5] I. Yonenaga, Thermo-mechanical stability of wide-bandgap semiconductors: high temperature hardness of SiC, AlN, GaN, ZnO and ZnSe, Physica B: Condensed Matter 308–310 (2001) 1150–1152.
[6] http://www.forbes.com/2008/02/27/incandescent-led-cfl-pf-guru_in_mm_0227energy_inl.html. Accessed 8 May 2011.
[7] S.Y. Karpova, A.V. Kulika, I.A. Zhmakina, Y.N. Makarovb, E.N. Mokhovc, M.G. Rammc, M.S. Ramm, A.D. Roenkovc, Y.A. Vodakov, Analysis of sublimation growth of bulk SiC crystals in tantalum container, Journal of Crystal Growth 211 (1–4) (2000) 347–351.
[8] S. Saddow, F.La Via (Eds.), Advanced Silicon Carbide Devices and Processing, BoD—Books on Demand, 2015.
[9] http://www.cree.com/about/milestones.asp accessed 24 May 2010.
[10] S.G. Müller, R.C. Glass, H.M. Hobgood, V.F. Tsvetkov, M. Brady, D. Henshall, J. R Jenny, D. Malta, C.H. Carter Jr., The status of SiC bulk growth from an industrial point of view, Journal of Crystal Growth 211 (1–4) (2000) 325–332.
[11] http://compoundsemiconductor.net/csc/news-details.php?cat=news&id=19732335. Accessed 8 May 2011.
[12] http://www.iiviwbg.com/.
[13] S.A. Sakwe, M. Stockmeier, P. Hens, R. Müller, D. Queren, U. Kunecke, K. Konias, R. Hock, A. Magerl, M. Pons, A. Winnacker, P. Wellmann, Bulk growth of SiC – review on advances of SiC vapor growth for improved doping and systematic study on dislocation evolution, in: P. Friedrichs, T. Kimoto, L. Ley, G. Pensl (Eds.), Silicon Carbide, Vol. 1: Growth, Defects, and Novel Applications, Copyright © 2010 WILEY-VCH, 2009.
[14] A. Ellison, B. Magnusson, N.T. Son, L. Storasta, E. Janzén, High temperature CVD growth of SiC, Materials Science and Engineering B 61–62 (1999) 113–120.
[15] T. Kimoto, Bulk and epitaxial growth of silicon carbide, Progress in Crystal Growth and Characterization of Materials 62.2 (2016) 329–351.
[16] A. Ellison, B. Magnusson, N.T. Son, L. Storasta, E. Janzén, HTCVD grown semi-insulating SiC substrates, Materials Science Forum 433–436 (2003) 33–38.
[17] M. Syvajarvi, R. Yakimova, H.H. Radamson, N.T. Son, Q. Wahab, I.G. Ivanov, E. Janzen, Liquid phase epitaxial growth of SiC, Journal of Crystal Growth 197 (1999) 147–154.
[18] J. Chen, A.J. Steckl, M.J. Loboda, Molecular beam epitaxy growth of SiC on Si(111) from silacyclobutane, Journal of Vacuum Science & Technology B: Microelectronics and Nanometer Structures 16 (3) (1998) 1305–1308.
[19] O. Kordina, C. Hallin, A. Henry, J.P. Bergman, I. Ivanov, A. Ellison, N.T. Son, E. Janzén, Growth of SiC by "hot-wall" CVD and HTCVD, physica Status Solidi (B) 202 (1) (1997) 321–334.
[20] C.L. Frewin, C. Coletti, C. Riedl, U. Starke, S.E. Saddow, A comprehensive study of hydrogen etching on the major SiC polytypes and crystal orientations, Materials Science Forum 615–617 (2009) 589–592.
[21] C. Coletti, C.L. Frewin, A.M. Hoff, S.E. Saddow, Electronic passivation of 3C-SiC(001) via hydrogen treatment, Electrochemical and Solid-State Letters 11 (10) (2008) H285–H287.
[22] D.J. Larkin, P.G. Neudeck, J.A. Powell, L.G. Matus, Site-competition epitaxy for superior silicon carbide electronics, Applied Physics Letters 65 (13) (1994) 1659–1661.

[23] F. La Via, G. Izzo, M. Mauceri, G. Pistoneb, G. Condorelli, L. Perdicaro, G. Abbondanza, L. Calcagno, G. Foti, D. Crippa, 4H-SiC epitaxial layer growth by trichlorosilane (TCS), Journal of Crystal Growth 311 (1) (2008) 107–113.
[24] S. Nishino, J.A. Powell, H.A. Will, Production of large-area single-crystal wafers of cubic SiC for semiconductor, Applied Physics Letters 42 (1983) 460–462.
[25] M. Reyes, Y. Shishkin, S. Harvey, S.E. Saddow, Development of a high-growth rate 3C-SiC on Si CVD process, Materials Research Society Meeting Proceedings 911 (2006) 79.
[26] M. Reyes, Y. Shishkin, S. Harvey, S.E. Saddow, Increased growth rates of 3C-SiC on Si(100) substrates via HCl growth additive, Materials Science Forum 556–557 (2007) 191–194.
[27] C.L. Frewin, C. Locke, J. Wang, P. Spagnol, S.E. Saddow, Growth of cubic silicon carbide on oxide using polysilicon as a seed layer for micro-electro-mechanical machine applications, Journal of Crystal Growth 311 (17) (2009) 4179–4182.
[28] C. Locke, C. Frewin, L. Abbati, S.E. Saddow, Demonstration of 3C-SiC MEMS structures on poly-Si on-oxide substrates, Materials Research Society Proceedings 1246 (2010), 1246–B08-05.
[29] J. Deva Reddy, A.A. Volinsky, C. Frewin, C. Locke, S.E. Saddow, Mechanical properties of single and polycrystalline SiC thin films, Materials Research Society Symposium Proceedings 1049 (2008).
[30] R. Yakimova, R.M. Petoral Jr., G. R Yazdi, C. Vahlberg, A. Lloyd Spetz, K. Uvdal, Surface functionalization and biomedical applications based on SiC, Journal of Physics. D: Applied Physics 40 (2007) 6435.
[31] S.F. Cogan, D.J. Edell, A.A. Guzelian, Y. Ping Liu, R. Edell, Plasma-enhanced chemical vapor deposited silicon carbide as an implantable dielectric coating, Journal of Biomedical Materials Research Part A 67A (2003) 856–867.
[32] K. Hattori, T. Mori, H. Okamoto, Y. Hamakawa, Photothermal modulation spectroscopy of multilayered structures of amorphous silicon and amorphous silicon carbide, Physical Review Letters 60 (1988) 825–827.
[33] A. Rzany, M. Schaldach, Smart material silicon carbide: reduced activation of cells and proteins on a SiC: H coated stainless steel, Progress in Biomedical Research 4 (2001) 182–194.
[34] R. Anzalone, G. D'Arrigo, M. Camarda, C. Locke, S.E. Saddow, F. La Via, Advanced residual stress analysis and FEM simulation on heteroepitaxial 3C–SiC for MEMS application, Journal of Microelectromechanical Systems 20 (3) (June 2011) 745–752, https://doi.org/10.1109/JMEMS.2011.2127451.
[35] M. Mehregany, C.A. Zorman, N. Rajan, W. Chien Hung, Silicon carbide MEMS for harsh environments, Proceedings of the IEEE 86 (8) (1998) 1594–1609.
[36] R. Anzalone, A. Severino, C. Locke, S.E. Saddow, F. La Via, G. D'Arrigo, 3C-SiC hetero-epitaxial films for sensor fabrication, Advances in Science and Technology 54 (2008) 411–415. Trans Tech Publications, Switzerland.
[37] R. Anzalone, M. Camarda, G. D'Arrigo, C. Locke, A. Canino, N. Piulso, A. Severino, A. La Magna, S.E. Saddow, F. La Via, Advanced stress analysis by microstructures realization on high-quality hetero-epitaxial 3C-SiC for MEMS application, Materials Science Forum 679-680 (2011) 133–136.
[38] S.C. Bayliss, L.D. Buckberry, P.J. Harris, M. Tobin, Journal of Porous Materials 7 (2000) 191–195.
[39] A.H. Mayne, S.C. Bayliss, P. Barr, M. Tobin, L.D. Buckberry, Physics Status Solidi. (A) 182 (2000) 505.
[40] R. Thewes, C. Paulus, et al., in: ESSDERC Proceedings 2004, 2004, pp. 19–28.
[41] J.F. Rizzo III, J. Wyatt, S. Kelly, D. Shire, Investigative Ophtalmology & Visual Science 44 (2003) 5362–5369.

[42] M.S. Humayun, et al., Vision Research 43 (2003) 2537–2581.
[43] S.E. Saddow, C.L. Frewin, C. Coletti, N. Schettini, E. Weeber, A. Oliveros, M. Jarosezski, Single-crystal silicon carbide: a biocompatible and hemocompatible semiconductor for advanced biomedical applications, Materials Science Forum 679 (2011) 824–830 (Trans Tech Publications Ltd).
[44] S. Miyamoto, S. Akiyama, K. Yamada, Synergistic roles for receptor occupancy and aggregation in integrin transmembrane function, Science 267 (1995) 883.
[45] R. Juliano, S. Haskill, N. Carolina, Mini-review signal transduction from the extracellular matrix. Cell 120 (1993) 577.
[46] B. Alberts, et al., Molecular Biology of the Cell (2002) 1463.
[47] R.G. Richards, The effect of surface roughness on fibroblast adhesion in vitro, Injury 27 (1996) SC38–43.
[48] I. Levitan, L. Kaczmarek, Adhesion molecules and axon pathfinding, The Neuron Cell and Molecular Biology (2002) 435.
[49] C. Goodman, Mechanisms and molecules that control growth cone guidance, Annual Review in Neuroscience 19 (1996) 341.
[50] P. Underwood, J.G. Steele, B. Dalton, Effects of polystyrene surface chemistry on the biological activity of solid phase fibronectin and vitronectin, analysed with monoclonal antibodies, Journal of Cell Science 104 (1993) 793.
[51] K.B. McClary, T. Ugarova, D.W. Grainger, Modulating fibroblast adhesion, spreading, and proliferation using self-assembled monolayer films of alkylthiolates on gold, Journal of Biomedical Materials Research 50 (2000) 428.
[52] M. Mrksich, G.M. Whitesides, Using self-assembled monolayers to understand the interactions of manmade surfaces with proteins and cells, Annual Review of Biophysics and Biomolecular Structure 25 (1996) 55.
[53] D. Stenger, C.J. Pike, J.J. Hickman, C.W. Cotman, Surface determinants of neuronal survival and growth on self-assembled monolayers in culture, Brain Research 630 (1993) 136.
[54] T. Mossman, Rapid colorimetric assay for cellular growth and survival: application to proliferation and cytotoxicity assays, Journal of Immunological Methods 65 (1983) 55.
[55] A. Oliveros, A. Guiseppi-Elie, S.E. Saddow, Silicon carbide: a versatile material for biosensor applications, Biomedical Microdevices 15 (2013) 353–368.
[56] https://en.wikipedia.org/wiki/ImageJ.
[57] Alexandra Oliveros Villalba, Myoglobin Detection on SiC: Immunosensor Development for Myocardial Infarction, PhD Dissertation, University of South Florida, ©2013.
[58] R.D. Beach, R.W. Conlan, M.C. Godwin, F. Moussy, Towards a miniature implantable in vivo telemetry monitoring system dynamically configurable as a potentiostat or galvanostat for two- and three-electrode biosensors, IEEE Transactions on Instrumentation and Measurement 54 (1) (2005).
[59] S. Afroz, S.W. Thomas, G. Mumcu, S.E. Saddow, Implantable SiC based RF antenna biosensor for continuous glucose monitoring, in: Sensors, IEEE, 2013.
[60] Fabiola Araujo Cespedes, RF Sensing System for Continuous Blood Glucose Monitoring, Dissertation, PhD Dissertation, University of South Florida, ©2017.
[61] T. Sahu, B. Ghosh, S.K. Pradhan, T. Ganguly, Diverse role of silicon carbide in the domain of nanomaterials, Int. J. Electrochem 2012 (2012) 271285.
[62] I. Linkov, M.E. Bates, L.J. Canis, T.P. Seager, J.M. Keisler, A decision directed approach for prioritizing research into the impact of nanomaterials on the environment and human health, Nature Nanotech 6 (2011) 784–787.
[63] M. Ferrari, Cancer Nanotechnology: opportunities and challenges, Nature reviews/ Cancer 5 (2005) 161–171.

[64] T.L. Doane, C. Burda, The unique role of nanoparticles in nanomedicine: imaging, drug delivery and therapy, Chemical Society Reviews 41 (2012) 2885–2911.
[65] F. Fabbri, F. Rossi, M. Melucci, I. Manet, G. Attolini, L. Favaretto, M. Zambianchi, G. Salviati, Nanoscale Research Letters 7 (1) (2012) 1–8.
[66] F. Rossi, F. Fabbri, M. Tallarida, D. Schmeisser, M. Modreanu, G. Attolini, G. Salviati, Structural and luminescence properties of HfO_2 nanocrystals grown by atomic layer deposition on SiC/SiO_2 core/shell nanowires, Scripta Materialia 69 (2013) 744.
[67] J.J. Corbalan, C. Medina, A. Jacoby, T. Malinski, M.W. Radomski, International Journal of Nanomedicine 7 (2012) 631.
[68] H. Steuer, R. Krastev, N. Lembert, Journal of Biomedical Materials Research Part B: Applied Biomaterials 102 (5) (2014) 897–902.
[69] F. Fabbri, F. Rossi, G. Attolini, G. Salviati, S. Iannotta, L. Aversa, R. Verucchi, M.V. Nardi, N. Fukata, B. Dierre, T. Sekiguchi, Enhancement of the core near-band-edge emission induced by an amorphous shell in coaxial one-dimensional nanostructure: the case of SiC/SiO_2 core/shell self-organized nanowires, Nanotechnology 21 (2010) 345702.
[70] F. Fabbri, F. Rossi, G. Attolini, G. Salviati, B. Dierre, T. Sekiguchi, N. Fukata, Luminescence properties of SiC/SiO_2 core–shell nanowires with different radial structure, Materials Letters 71 (2012) 137.
[71] F. Fabbri, F. Rossi, P. Lagonegro, M. Negri, J.S. Ponraj, M. Bosi, G. Attolini, G. Salviati, 3C-SiC Nanowires luminescence enhancement by coating with a conformal oxides layer, Journal of Physics D: Applied Physics 47 (2014) 394006.
[72] F. Rossi, E. Bedogni, F. Bigi, T. Rimoldi, L. Cristofolini, S. Pinelli, R. Alinovi, M. Negri, S. Dhanabalan, G. Attolini, Scientific Reports 5 (2015) 7606.
[73] W. Chen, J. Zhang, Using nanoparticles to enable simultaneous radiation and photodynamic therapies for cancer treatment, Journal of Nanoscience and Nanotechnology 6 (2006) 1159–1166.
[74] Y. Liu, W. Chen, S. Wang, A.L. Joly, Investigation of water-soluble x-ray luminescence nanoparticles for photodynamic activation, Applied Physics Letters 92 (2008) 043901.
[75] https://en.wikipedia.org/wiki/Photodynamic_therapy.
[76] M.C. DeRosa, R.J. Crutchley, Photosensitized singlet oxygen and its applications, Coordination Chemistry Reviews 233–234 (2002) 351–371.
[77] R. Bonnet, Photosensitizers of the porphyrin and phthalocyanine series for photodynamic therapy, Coordination Chemistry Reviews 24 (1995) 19–33.
[78] D. Beke, et al., Enhancement of X-ray-excited red luminescence of chromium-doped zinc gallate via ultrasmall silicon carbide nanocrystals. Chemistry of Materials 33.7 (2021) 2457–2465.
[79] R. Ahmad, T. Mahmoudi, M.S. Ahn, Y.B. Hahn, Biosensors Bioelectronics 100 (2018) 312–325.
[80] W. Zhou, X. Dai, T.M. Fu, C. Xie, J. Liu, C.M. Lieber, Nano Letters 14 (2014) 1614–1619.
[81] R. Bange, E. Bano, L. Rapenne, S. Labau, B. Pelissier, M. Legallais, B. Salem, V. Stambouli, Materials Science Forum 897 (2017) 638–641.
[82] R. Bange, E. Bano, L. Rapenne, V. Stambouli Bange, Romain, et al., Superior long term stability of SiC nanowires over Si nanowires under physiological conditions. Materials Research Express 6.1 (2018) 015013.
[83] S.E. Saddow, C.L. Frewin, M. Reyes, J. Register, M. Nezafati, S. Thomas, ECS Transactions 61 (2014) 101–111.

[84] M. Ollivier, L. Latu-Romain, B. Salem, L. Fradetal, V. Brouzet, J.H. Choi, E. Bano, Integration of SiC-1D nanostructures into nano-field effect transistors, Materials Science in Semiconductor Processing 29 (2014) 218–222.
[85] R. Bange, E. Bano, L. Rapenne, A. Mantoux, S.E. Saddow, V. Stambouli, Development of SOI FETs based on core-shell Si/SiC nanowires for sensing in liquid environments, ECSCRM, Materials Science Forum 963 (2019).
[86] J. Hass, W.A.D. Heer, E.H. Conrad, The growth and morphology of epitaxial multilayer graphene, Journal of Physics: Condensed Matter 20 (2008) 1–27.
[87] C. Riedl, C. Coletti, U. Starke, Structural and electronic properties of epitaxial graphene on SiC (0 0 0 1): a review of growth, characterization, transfer doping and hydrogen intercalation, Journal of Physics D: Applied Physics 43 (37) (2010) 374009.
[88] H. Kageshima, H. Hibino, M. Nagase, H. Yamaguchi, Theoretical study of epitaxial graphene growth on SiC(0001) surfaces, Applied Physics Express 2 (May. 2009) 065502.
[89] K.V. Emtsev, A. Bostwick, K. Horn, J. Jobst, G.L. Kellogg, L. Ley, J.L. McChesney, T. Ohta, S. a Reshanov, J. Röhrl, E. Rotenberg, A.K. Schmid, D. Waldmann, H.B. Weber, T. Seyller, Towards wafer-size graphene layers by atmospheric pressure graphitization of silicon carbide, Nature Materials 8 (Mar. 2009) 203–207.
[90] C.L. Frewin, The Neuron-Silicon Carbide Interface: Biocompatibility Study and BMI Device Development, PhD Dissertation, University of South Florida ©2009.
[91] X. Li, W. Cai, J. An, S. Kim, J. Nah, D. Yang, R. Piner, A. Velamakanni, I. Jung, E. Tutuc, S.K. Banerjee, L. Colombo, R.S. Ruoff, Large-area synthesis of high-quality and uniform graphene films on copper foils, Science (New York, N.Y.) 324 (Jun. 2009) 1312–1314.
[92] N. Nurdin, P. Francois, Y. Mugnier, J. Krumeich, M. Moret, B.O. Aronsson, P. Descouts, Haemocompatibility evaluation of DLC and SIC coated surfaces, European Cells & Materials 5 (2003) 17–28.
[93] A. de Carlos, J.P. Borrajo, J. Serra, P. Gonzalez, Behaviour of MG-63 osteoblast-like cells on wood-based biomorphic SiC ceramics coated with bioactive glass, Journal of Materials Science: Materials Medicine 17 (2006) 523–529.
[94] P. Gonzalez, J. Serra, S. Liste, S. Chiussi, B. Bion, M. Perez-Amor, J. Martinexz-Fernadez, A.R. de Arellano-Lopez, F.M. Varela-Feria, New biomprphic SC ceramics coated with bioactive glass for biomedical applications, Biomaterials 24 (2003) 4827–4832.
[95] S. Monnink, A. van Boven, H. Peels, I. Tigchelaar, P. de Kam, H. Crijns, W. van Oeveren, Silicon carbide coated coronary stents have low platelet and leukocyte adhesion during platelet activation, Journal of Investigative Medicine 47 (1999) 304–310.
[96] L.L. Hench, Biomaterials: a forecast for the future, Biomaterials 19 (1998) 1419–1423.
[97] S. Itoh, S. Nakamura, M. Nakamura, K. Shinomiya, K. Yamashita, Enhanced bone ingrowth into hydroxyapatite with interconnected pores by electrical polarization, Biomaterials 27 (2006) 5572–5579.
[98] C.E. Wen, W. Xu, W.Y. Hu, P.D. Hodgson, Hydroxyapatite/titania sol–gel coatings on titanium–zirconium alloy for biomedical applications, Acta Biomaterialia 3 (2007) 403–410.
[99] C. Fares, S.-M. Hsu, M. Xian, X. Xia, F. Ren, J.J. Mecholsky Jr., L. Gonzaga, J. Esquivel-Upshaw, Demonstration of a SiC protective coating for titanium implants, Materials 13 (2020) 3321, https://doi.org/10.3390/ma13153321.
[100] S.E. Afonso Camargo, A.S. Mohiuddeen, C. Fares, J.L. Partain, P.H. Carey IV, F. Ren, S.-M. Hsu, A.E. Clark, J.F. Esquivel-Upshaw, Anti-bacterial properties and

biocompatibility of novel SiC coating for dental ceramic, Journal of Functional Biomaterials 11 (2020) 33, https://doi.org/10.3390/jfb11020033.
[101] E.M. Maynard, T. Craig, Nordhausen, R.A. Normann, The Utah intracortical electrode array: a recording structure for potential brain-computer interfaces, Electroencephalography and Clinical Neurophysiology 102.3 (1997) 228–239.
[102] J.C. Barrese, J. Aceros, J.P. Donoghue, Scanning electron microscopy of chronically implanted intracortical microelectrode arrays in non-human primates, Journal of Neural Engineering 13 (January 29, 2016) 026003.
[103] E.K. Bernardin, C.L. Frewin, R. Everly, J. Ul Hassan, S.E. Saddow, Demonstration of a robust all-silicon-carbide intracortical neural interface, Micromachines 9 (2018) 412, https://doi.org/10.3390/mi9080412.
[104] M. Beygi, J.T. Bentley, C.L. Frewin, C.A. Kuliasha, A. Takshi, E.K. Bernardin, F. La Via, S.E. Saddow, Fabrication of a monolithic implantable neural interface from cubic silicon carbide, Micromachines 10 (2019) 430, https://doi.org/10.3390/mi10070430.
[105] M. Beygi, W. Dominguez-Viqueira, C. Feng, G. Mumcu, C.L. Frewin, F. La Via, S.E. Saddow, Silicon carbide and MRI: towards developing a MRI safe neural interface, Micromachines 12 (2021) 126, https://doi.org/10.3390/mi12020126.
[106] C. Feng, C.L. Frewin, M.R.-E. Tanjil, R. Everly, J. Bieber, A. Kumar, M.C. Wang, S.E. Saddow, A flexible a-SiC-based neural interface utilizing pyrolyzed-photoresist film (C) active sites, Micromachines 12 (2021) 821, https://doi.org/10.3390/mi12070821.

CHAPTER 2

Silicon carbide as a highly permissive surface for neural stem cells

Gabriele Bonaventura[1] and Massimo Zimbone[2]
[1]Institute for Biomedical Research and Innovation, Italian National Research Council, Catania, Italy;
[2]Institute for Microelectronics and Microsystems, Italian National Research Council, Catania, Italy

Contents

1. Introduction

1.1 A focus on regenerative medicine

The scientific interest in regenerative medicine based on stem cells therapies has paved the way to regenerate, modify, and restore human organ functions altered by trauma and diseases, especially for which current clinical therapeutic outcomes are not effective. Stem cells represent the common denominator for all types of regeneration in every living organism [1]. These particular cells exhibit the specific properties to proliferate indefinitely through an asymmetrical cell division, by self-renewal properties, and by the ability to drive their differentiation toward specific cell phenotypes of all tissues [1,2]. Stem cells can be cataloged in accordance with both their developmental competence as totipotent, pluripotent, and

Silicon Carbide Technology for Advanced Human Healthcare Applications
ISBN 978-0-323-90609-8
https://doi.org/10.1016/B978-0-323-90609-8.00014-4

multipotent and their tissue origin as adult, fetal, or embryonal stem cells [2].

In particular, totipotency indicates the capability to produce all cell types of the entire fetus, including placenta. Pluripotency refers to the capacity to form cell types of all three germ layers (endoderm, mesoderm, and ectoderm), but not the whole organism [3]. Multipotency is the property to differentiate into a specific cell phenotype related to tissues in which stem cells reside [3].

Especially in the context of neurodegenerative disorders, stem cells have attracted researchers' interest as a tool for the repair and regeneration of the damaged nervous system that is considered to be extremely limited in the self-repairing capacity of adult neural tissue [4]. Neurodegenerative diseases are usually described by loss of function leading to apoptosis of neuronal and glial cells. These neurological conditions can be classified according to primary clinical features (e.g., dementia, parkinsonism, or motor neuron disease), anatomic distribution of neurodegeneration (e.g., frontotemporal degenerations, extrapyramidal disorders, or spinocerebellar degenerations), or principal molecular abnormality.

The lack of self-restoring capability of adult neural tissue justifies the search for alternative sources of cells to introduce new intervention protocols in neurodegenerative diseases [4]. To this end, different stem cell tissue sources have been examined to determine the most efficacious and productive method for cell replacement therapy in neurodegenerative disorders [5]. Among the different types of currently available stem cells, neural stem cells (NSCs) have been widely applied as suitable cells for neuro-regeneration. NSCs can be differentiated from different sources, including dental pulp stem cells (DPSCs) [6]. Previous research showed the innate neurogenic potential of DPSCs, which are derived from the neural crest [6–8]. Another interesting cell type, due to their ability to promote axonal regeneration and functional restoration in lesioned neural areas, is olfactory ensheathing cells (OECs). OECs are a type of glial cell that shows phenotypic properties with both Schwann cells (SCs) and astrocytes and possess peculiar characteristics such as plasticity and the ability to secrete several growth factors, such as neurotrophins and neuregulins [9].

Recently, OECs and DP-NSCs have been recognized as an interesting alternative source of stem cells for cellular transplantations strategies [8,9] and the management of neurodegenerative diseases and spinal cord injury, which is one of the most devastating forms of injury leading to disability and death [10,11]. Moreover, the combination of stem cells and nanotechnologies seems to be a promising approach for the development of clinically translatable cell-based therapies enhancing neural repair.

1.1.1 Biomaterials in transplantation approach

Semiconductor-based biomaterials have opened new scenarios for important biomedical applications [12], including heart stent coatings, brain implants, tissue implant scaffolds, and in vivo biosensors [12–16]. The main concern is to find a suitable material that produces low or no adverse effects when grafted into the body. Such a material could be implanted for the long term and be capable of interfacing with electronic devices. In the brain, semiconductor-based biomaterials are used for neural prosthetics, with stimulating and recording electrodes, or as a scaffold to enhance neuronal repair [17]. Stimulation-based electrodes are used to restore vision, hearing or alleviate the symptoms of Parkinson's disease [18,19]. Recording-based prosthetics hold great promise for movement restoration [20,21], such as in patients affected by traumatic brain injury, stroke, or amyotrophic lateral sclerosis [22–24]. Semiconductor-based biomaterials are also used in neural tissue engineering as a scaffold to control axonal growth through the lesion site, improve cell survival rate and maintenance of grafted cells, or drive host cell migration (e.g., Schwann cells and astrocytes) [25–28]. Recent investigations reported that transplantation of NSCs, SCs, and OECs showed encouraging effects on neural regeneration and functional recovery in some neurodegenerative diseases.

Thus, the study of neural cell behavior, such as adhesion, viability, and biocompatibility, to different semiconductor-based surfaces is fundamental to develop new novel biomedical devices, as different studies reported that biomaterial supports can serve multiple functions in transplantation approaches. Recently, silicon carbide has attracted the attention of researchers due to its higher biocompatibility compared to Si, as assessed through in vitro and in vivo studies as reviewed in Chapter 1 and [29]. In this context, many candidate semiconducting materials for biotechnological applications have been investigated for their tissue compatibility and sensing potentiality. The main concern is to find a suitable material that produces low or no adverse effects when grafted in the body that can be implanted for long term and is capable of interfacing with electronic devices. In the field of semiconductors, Silicon (Si) has been the preferred substrate material for microdevices due to its low cost and ready availability. However, it presents several drawbacks that limit its use in biomedical applications, specifically a cytotoxic interaction with the body and a resulting short period of stability when used in vivo. Especially, for permanently implanted devices (such as glucose sensors, brain−machine-interface devices, smart bone, and organ implants), a more compatible material is required that is not rejected by the body and not recognized as a foreign material [10]. Silicon carbide (SiC) and, in particular, cubic silicon carbide (3C−SiC) has been proven to be a good substrate for this purpose, being both bio- and hemocompatible, and useable for the manufacture of implantable devices [29,30].

3C−SiC is a wide bandgap semiconductor ($Eg = 3.2$ eV) with extraordinary chemophysical properties. It is both extremely stable and inert, and it is able to work at high frequency, high-temperature, and in harsh environments, with better performance than silicon-based devices. It is a polymorphic material with more than 200 different known polytypes, among which the most used are the cubic 3C−SiC and the hexagonal 4H- and 6H−SiC [31−33]. 4H−SiC is used for high power electronic devices, 6H−SiC for optoelectronic devices as a substrate for GaN, while 3C−SiC has a surface with chemical-physical properties that makes it highly suitable for biotechnological applications. Previously, the main drawbacks of 3C−SiC were the high cost and the low quality of the substrate (compared with Si). Nevertheless, the cost has considerably decreased in recent years, and material quality has achieved very high standards, therefore implantable radiofrequency devices for real-time and in vivo measurements of the glucose and neuronal interface devices have already been manufactured [14,34]. 3C−SiC is thus considered a suitable bridge between internal neural networks and external electronic devices [34].

The aim of the work presented in this chapter was to test the biocompatibility of Si and 3C−SiC in an in vitro model of human neurons derived from dental pulp mesenchymal stem cells, and in OECs derived from mouse olfactory bulbs.

2. In vitro biocompatibility of DP-NSC with 3C−SiC

2.1 Material characterization

3C-silicon carbide epitaxial wafers were synthesized through an epitaxial chemical vapor deposition process on silicon as substrates as described in Chapter 1. 3C−SiC is the only polytype that is stable at temperatures lower than the silicon melting point making it unique in that it can be grown on silicon substrates. The lattice mismatch between silicon and SiC is of the order of 20%, and so a high number of defects are present at the heterointerface. These defects propagate into the epilayer, and they may induce a nonflat morphology on the SiC surface. This is observed via optical microscopy in Fig. 2.1. In Fig. 2.1A and B, the Si and 3C–SiC surface are shown, respectively. A perfectly flat surface is observed for the Si substrate, while undulations are apparent for 3C–SiC grown on Si. Nevertheless, excellent crystal quality can be achieved by controlling the surface orientation, epitaxial growth conditions, and growth chemistry to reduce defect generation. In Fig. 2.1C, the 3C–SiC photoluminescence band at 540 nm (2.3 eV) is shown. The presence of this band is related to the high quality of the crystal and is associated with both the band-to-band transition and the nitrogen doping (n-type dopant) level. The Si substrate has a negligible luminescence intensity and is not shown. Another crystal quality benchmark is related to the Raman spectra.

The Raman spectra of the 3C–SiC (black) and the Si (red) samples are shown in Fig. 2.1D. 3C–SiC Raman spectra are composed of Transversal

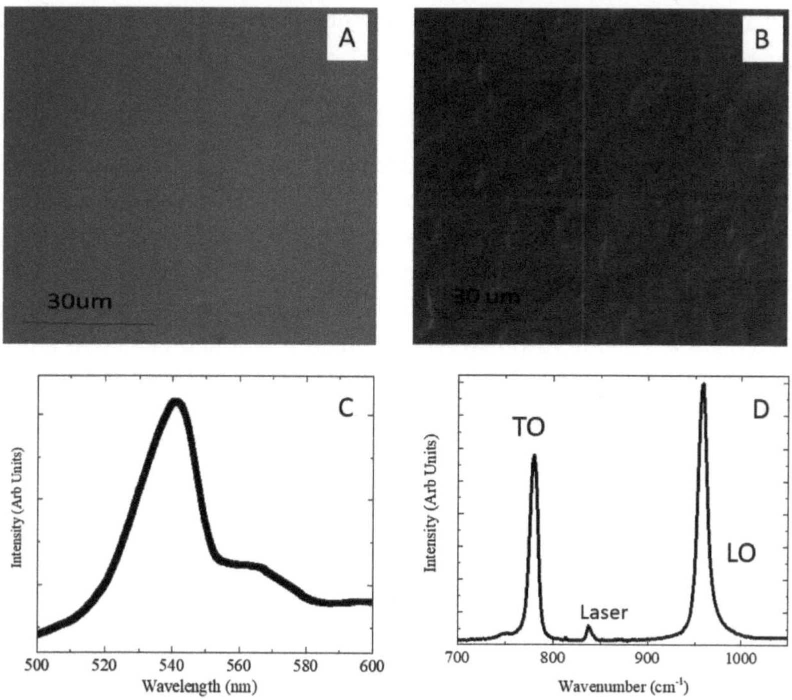

Figure 2.1 Characterization of Si and 3C–SiC wafers. Optical images of silicon (A) and 3C-silicon carbide (B) surfaces. Si (red) and 3C–SiC (black) Raman spectra (C). In the same figure, TO and LOPC peaks are labeled. Photoluminescence spectra of 3C–SiC (D).

Optical (TO) and Longitudinal Optical Plasmon Coupled (LOPC) vibrations at 769 and 972 cm^{-1}, respectively. The information on the crystal quality, orientation, stress, and donor density of the synthesized material can be deduced by the shape and position of these peaks. In particular, the position intensity and width of the TO peak are related to the presence of stress and to the quality of the sample. Indeed, in our experimental configuration (in backscattering configuration), TO vibration is not allowed (for 001 crystal direction) because of the selection rules, and the presence of small amount defects gives the peak observed in Fig. 2.1D. Unfortunately, it is not possible to have a quantitative measure of the amount of defects that presumably are stacking faults. The TO spectral position gives information on the wafer residual stress induced by the Si substrate. Indeed, a spectral shift of the TO line is linearly related to the lattice compression. By using the formula $W_{TO} = 796.5 - 3734\ (Da)/a$, a negligible tensile stress was observed due to the high quality of the sample. Moreover, the donor density was measured by accurately fitting the LOPC peak with a suitable model as reported elsewhere. The fitting procedure allows us to estimate a donor concentration of less than $1 \times 10^{17}\ cm^{-3}$.

2.2 Dental pulp stem cells isolation and neuronal differentiation

DPSCs were obtained from five extracted teeth from five patients. Briefly, to isolate the pulp tissue, the freshly extracted teeth were splayed to remove the pulp tissue, then cut into small fragments of 1 mm, and treated for enzymatic digestion with 3 mg/mL collagenase type I (Gibco Invitrogen, Carlsbad, CA) for 1 hour at 37°C. The tissue pellet was then suspended in Dulbecco's Modified Eagle's Medium (DMEM) to which was added penicillin (100 U/mL), streptomycin (100 mg/mL), and 15% fetal bovine serum (FBS). The DPSCs were then cultured at 37°C in a humidified atmosphere of 5% CO_2, and the medium was replaced every 3 days. The cells were cultured for 6 days in vitro (DIV) in basic cell medium (DMEM), and subsequently to the medium was added the following neural induction cocktail: 0.5 mM isobutyl methyl xanthine, 20 ng/mL human epidermal growth factor, 1 mM dibutyrylcAMP (dbcAMP), 10 ng/mL nerve growth factor, 10 ng/mL brain-derived neurotrophic factor, and 40 ng/mL basic fibroblastic growth factor (all reagents were purchased from Invitrogen, Milan, Italy). Neuronal differentiation was subsequently obtained, and the cells were grown in culture for 15 days in DMEM/FBS with 10 μM retinoic acid.

After the differentiation procedure, the cells presented a typical neuronal morphology showing very thin and long cytoplasmic processes, axon and dendrite presence, and perikaryon (Fig. 2.2A). To evaluate neuronal differentiation, we measured the expression of neuronal markers: neurofilaments light chain (NF-l), neurofilament medium chain (NF-M), microtubule-associated protein 2 (MAP2), and neuronal-specific enolase (NSE) by qRT-PCR assays. In addition to these, we extended the analysis to eight additional genes whose differential expression has been found in neurons from differentiated DPSCs: vimentin (VIM), heme oxygenase 1 (HMOX1), Bradykinin B2 receptor (BDKRB2), matrix metallopeptidase

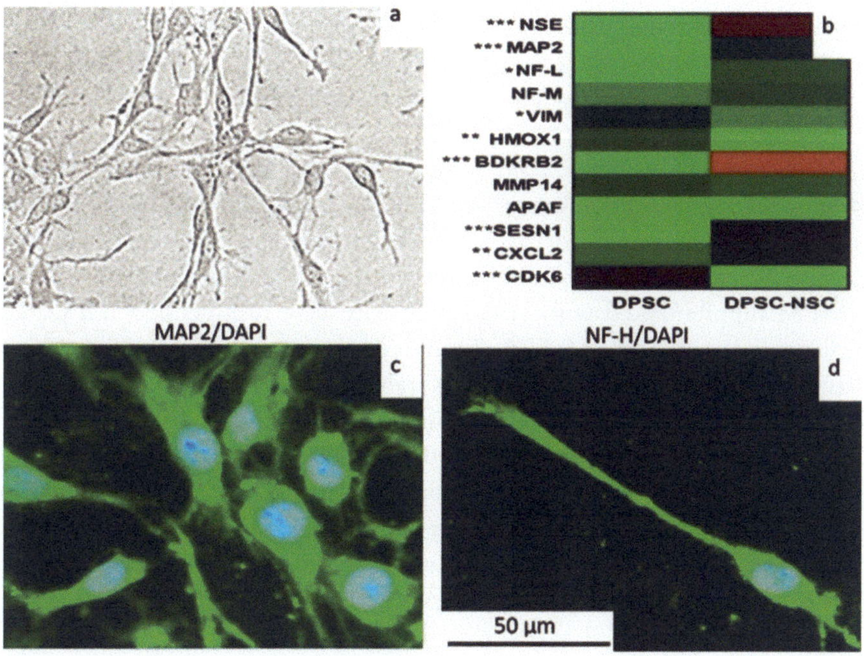

Figure 2.2 Differentiation of dental pulp stem cells into neural stem cells. (A) Representative photomicrograph of neuronal-like stem cells derived from DPSC in the bright field taken from randomly selected slides scanned by a Nikon Ti Eclipse inverted microscope (scale bar 50 μm). (B) Gene expression changes following differentiation. Quantitative real-time PCR assay was performed to assess gene expression changes after 16 days of RA treatment. mRNA levels were normalized to the amount of β-actin mRNA and represented in a heatmap (*$P < .05$ and ***$P < .001$ as determined by two-way ANOVA followed by Sidack post hoc test). (C, D): representative photomicrographs of DP-NSCs show the fluorescent distribution of neuronal marker NF and MAP2. Nuclei were counterstained with DAPI (scale bar 50 μm). MAP2, NF-L, BDRKB2, SESN1, and CXCL2, and a downregulation of VIM, HMOX1, and CDK6 in neuronal cells differentiated from DPSC (Fig. 2.2.C). Moreover, the expression of neuronal markers in DP-NSCs was confirmed by immunostaining of NF—H and MAP2 (Fig. 2.2C and D).

14 (MMP14), apoptotic protease activating factor-1, sestrin 1 (SESN1), C-X-C motif chemokine ligand 2 (CXCL2), and cyclin-dependent kinase 6 (CDK6). These genes are commonly reported to be involved in many biological processes, such as cell cycle progression and regulation (decreased during neural differentiation) or nervous system development and regulation of neurotransmitters (increased during neural differentiation). Our results confirm a significant upregulation of NSE.

2.3 OEC isolation and characterization

OECs were isolated from the olfactory bulbs of 2-day-old mouse pups (P2) (provided by Envigo RMS s.r.l. Italy). All the experimental procedures were carried out according to the Italian Guidelines for Animal Care (D.L. 116/92 and 26/2014), which are in compliance with the European Communities Council Directives (2010/63/EU) and were approved by the Ethical Committee at the University of Catania (Italy). Briefly, the pups were sacked and the bulbs removed and placed in cold (+4°C) Leibowitz L-15 medium (Sigma—Aldrich, Milan, Italy). Then, they were digested in collagenase and trypsin mixture. Trypsinization was stopped by adding DMEM supplemented with 10% FBS. Cells were resuspended and plated in flasks fed with DMEM/FBS. To reduce the number of dividing fibroblasts, the antimitotic agent, cytosine arabinoside (10—5M), was added. In Fig. 2.3A, OECs show an elongated shape with a dense network in bright field. Immunohistochemical analysis of the OECs were performed for the following markers: S-100, Glial Fibrillary Acidic Protein (GFAP), and Nestin. S-100 is a specific marker for OECs (Fig. 2.3B), GFAP highlights the differentiation of OECs toward astroglial phenotype (Fig. 2.3C), while Nestin is a stem cell marker whose expression shows that OECs acquired stem cell features (Fig. 2.3D).

Both DP-NSCs and OECs were grown on 3C—SiC and Si rectangular surfaces at a final density of 0.3×10^3 cells/cm^2 for 48 hours before performing the immunocytochemical procedures and mitochondrial health assay. Control cells were plated on glass coverslips, without Si and 3C—SiC substrates.

2.4 Cell morphology investigation by scanning electron microscopy

Both DP-NSCs and OECs were cultured on 3C—SiC and Si for 48 hours. After incubation, cells were washed with Phosphate Buffer Solution (PBS) and fixed with 2% glutaraldehyde for 1 hour at room temperature. Cells

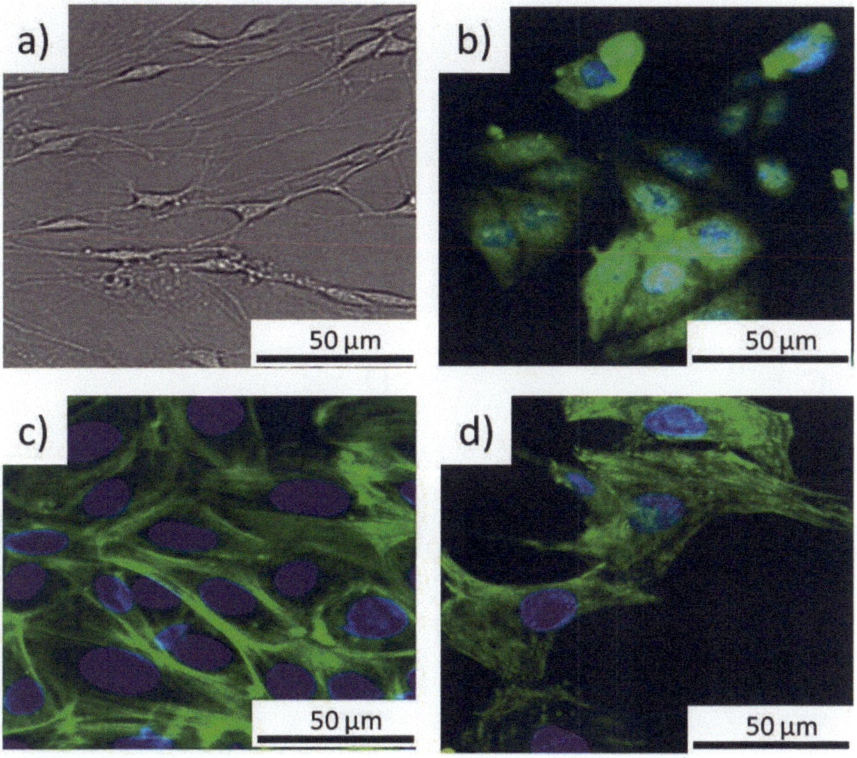

Figure 2.3 Characterization of olfactory ensheathing cells. (A) Representative photomicrograph of OECs in the bright field taken from randomly selected slides scanned by a Nikon Ti Eclipse inverted microscope (scale bar 50 µm). (B–D) Expression and distribution of specific neural markers (S100, (B), GFAP (C), and Nestin (D)) in OECs. Nuclei were counterstained with DAPI (scale bar 50 µm).

were dehydrated in graded ethanol solutions from 50% to 100%. SEM images were obtained by using a Zeiss Supra-55 VP field emission scanning electron microscope (FEG-SEM). Control samples on glass were sputtered with gold. Using SEM, we analyzed morphology and adhesive structures of DP-NSCs and OECs growing on Si and 3C–SiC (Fig. 2.4A). After 48 hours of incubation on glass, both control DP-NSCs and OECs exhibited flatter and well-spread morphology with, in the case of DP-NSCs, numerous adhesive structures (filopodia and lamellipodia). On Si and 3C–SiC, DP-NSCs acquired a rounded form, which is typical of the first phases of substrate adhesion, and large adhesion structures. However, DP-NSCs grown on 3C–SiC exhibited a high number of thin filopodia (arrows in Fig. 2.4B) and large lamellipodia whose ability to form intercellular

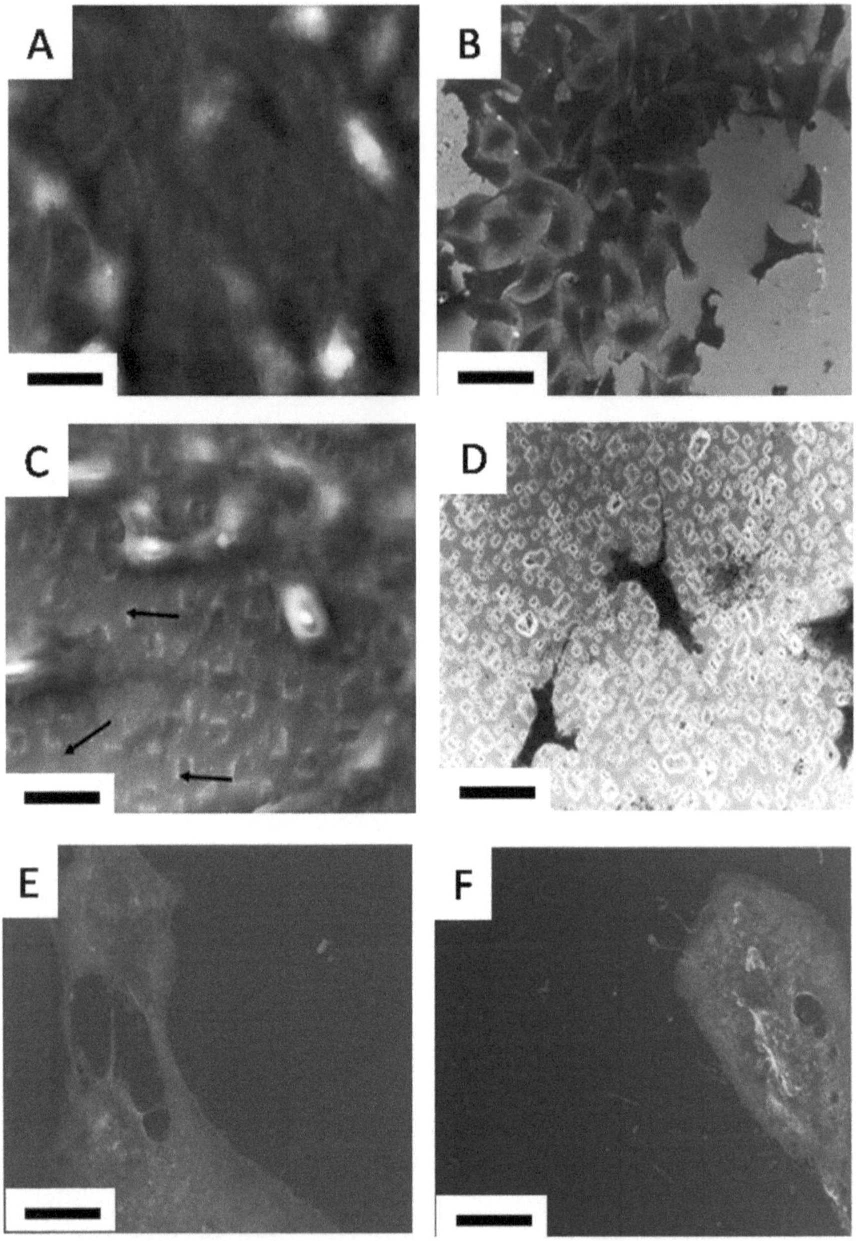

Figure 2.4 Investigation of DP-NSCs and OECs morphology by scanning electron microscopy. (A) and (B) are related to Si substrate with NP-NSCs and OECs, respectively. (C) and (D) are related to SiC substrate with NP-NSCs and OECs, respectively. (E) and (F) are related to Control substrate with NP-NSCs and OECs, respectively. SEM micrograph shows the round morphology of DP-NSCs grown on 3C–SiC (C) and Si (A) compared with flat morphology of those growing on glass (control E). On 3C–SiC, DP-NSCs exhibit a high number of thin filopodia (arrows in C) compared to Si. Compared with flat control cells (A), on 3C–SiC (F) and on Si (D), OECs acquire a rod-shaped morphology with long cellular extensions visible on 3C–SiC compared with Si. Scale bar 10 μm (A,C,E,F) and 20 μm (B,D).

connections did not seem to be influenced by the presence of cubic crystals. On Si and 3C−SiC, OECs acquired a rod-shaped morphology with long cellular extensions when seeded on 3C−SiC compared with those growing on Si (Fig. 2.4F).

3. Si/3C−SiC substrate influence on mitochondrial activity

To investigate the biocompatibility of Si and 3C−SiC on DP-NSCs and OECs, we used a double stain-based commercial kit to simultaneously measure two important cell-health parameters: mitotoxicity and cytotoxicity. In particular, the MitoHealth red stain accumulates in live-cell mitochondria proportionally to the mitochondrial membrane potential, while the Image-iTDEAD $Green_{TM}$ viability stain measures cytotoxicity. Representative images show how the exposure to Si decreased the mitochondria membrane potential and produced cytotoxicity after 48 hours of incubation, while mitotoxicity and cytotoxicity of 3C−SiC-exposed cells were similar to controls for both DP-NSCs (Fig. 2.5A) and OECs (Fig. 2.5A). Fluorescence intensity ratios of red/green channels, normalized by blue channel (DAPI staining), show a reduced compatibility of Si when compared to 3C−SiC (3C−SiC vs. Si, $P < .005$; control group vs. Si, $P < .05$; differences in fluorescence intensity were not significant statistically between 3C−SiC and control group) in both DP-NSCs (Fig. 2.5B) and OECs (Fig. 2.5B). To further confirm the mitotoxicity induced by Si wafers in DP-NSCs and OECs, mitochondrial membrane potential (MMP) reduction was analyzed through the use of JC-1. As shown in Fig. 2.6, 3C−SiC did not impair MMP in DP-NSCs and slightly depolarized the mitochondria in OECs ($^*P < .05$). On the other side, silicon wafer altered the mitochondrial membrane potential both in DP-NSCs and OECs as demonstrated by the increment in the fluorescence emission of JC-1 monomers reported in Fig. 2.6A and B for DP-NSCs and 8C-D for OECs in Fig. 2.7.

4. Summary

Silicon carbide is a biocompatible and hemocompatible material that is attracting increasing scientific interest as a promising material for the manufacture of implantable medical devices. The biocompatibility of 3C−SiC with the neuronal stem cells is the first step in the use of this wide

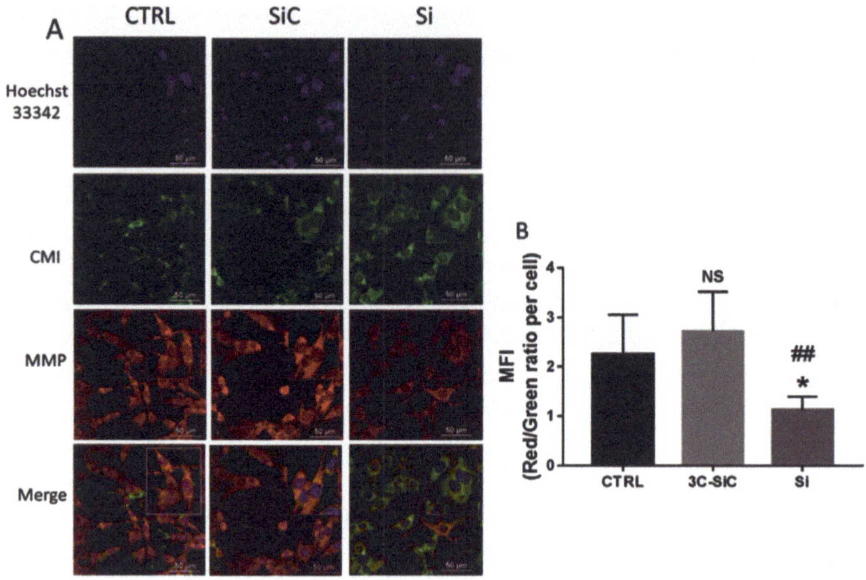

Figure 2.5 (A) Effects of Si and 3C—SiC on mitochondrial membrane potential and cell membrane integrity of DP-NSCs. (A) Representative results were taken from randomly selected slides scanned by a Nikon Ti Eclipse inverted microscope. MitoHealth (red) stains stable mitochondrial membrane potential, DEAD Green (green) stains deadly cells, Hoechst 33342 (blue) stains nuclei. A merged image for all experimental conditions was created with NIS elements software (scale bar 50 μm). (B) Mean fluorescence intensities (MFI) ratio of MitoHealth (red) and DEAD Green (green) per cell. Differences in MFIs were not statistically significant between glass-plated control cells and those plated on 3C—SiC for 48 hours (3C—SiC vs. Si, $P < .005$; control group vs. Si, $P < .05$; differences in fluorescence intensity were not significant statistically between 3C—SiC and control group).

bandgap semiconductor as a clinical tool for lesioned neural areas or in the context of neurodegenerative diseases.

The experiments reported in this chapter were focused to investigate the biocompatibility of Silicon and 3C—SiC with an in vitro model of human neuronal stem cells. These cells were obtained after isolation and differentiation of adult stem cells from dental pulp (DP-NSCs) and mouse OECs, a specific glial cell type exhibiting stem cell properties. Particularly, we examined the effects of 3C—SiC on neural cell morphology, viability, and mitochondrial membrane potential. Data indicate that both DP-NSCs and OECs cells, cultured on 3C—SiC, avoided oxidative stress events and did not exhibit morphological modifications or adverse reactions in the mitochondrial membrane.

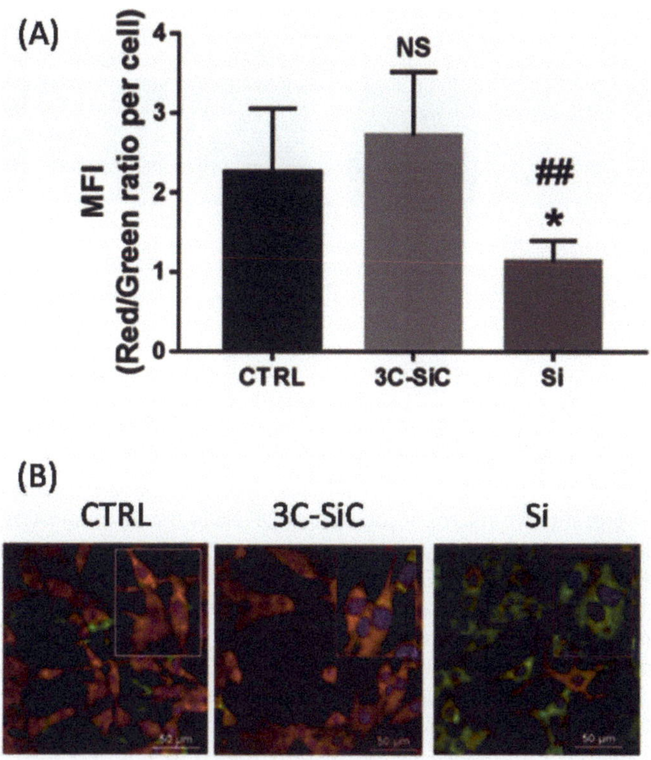

Figure 2.6 Effects of Si and 3C–SiC on mitochondrial membrane potential and cell membrane integrity of OECs. (A) Representative results were taken from randomly selected slides scanned by a Nikon Ti Eclipse inverted microscope. MitoHealth (red) stains stable mitochondrial membrane potential, DEAD Green (green) stains deadly cells, Hoechst 33342 (blue) stains nuclei. A merged image for all experimental conditions was created with NIS Elements software (scale bar 50 μm). (B) Mean fluorescence intensities (MFI) ratio of MitoHealth (red) and DEAD Green (green) per cell. Differences in MFIs were not statistically significant between glass-plated control cells and those plated on 3C–SiC for 48 hours (3C–SiC vs. Si, $P < .005$; control group vs. Si, $P < .05$; differences in fluorescence intensity were not significant statistically between 3C–SiC and control group).

Therefore, the data reported in this chapter indicate that 3C–SiC may be an excellent support in the realization of long-term implantable biochips since it shows a biocompatibility that overlaps with that achieved with other carbon-derived materials. Furthermore, the synergistic effect of stem cell transplantation and biomaterial supports for implantation may prove to be a very promising approach for nerve injury treatment. Continuing research will hopefully demonstrate this to be the case so that medical professionals

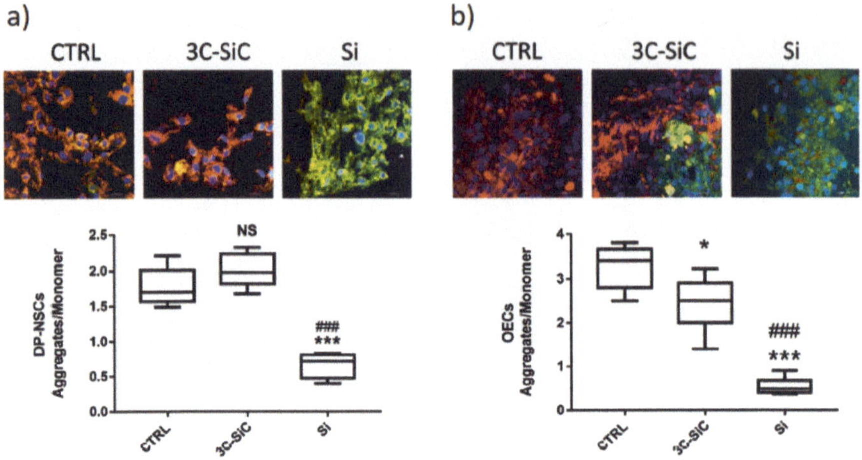

Figure 2.7 Effects of Si and 3C—SiC on mitochondrial membrane potential of DP-NSCs and OECs. Representative microphotograph of DP-NSCs (Panel a) and OECs (Panel c) stained with JC-1 after 48 hours of exposure to 3C—SiC and Si. Mitochondrial J-aggregates in red; cytosolic JC-1 monomers in green; DAPI (blue) stain nuclei. A merged image for all experimental conditions was created with NIS Elements software (scale bar 20 μm). Mean fluorescence intensities (MFI) ratio of J-aggregates (red) and JC-1 monomers (green) per cell were calculated for DP-NSCs (Panel b; $^{***}P < .001$ Si vs. Control and $^{\#\#\#}P < .001$ Si vs. 3C—SiC as determined by one-way ANOVA followed by Tukey post hoc test) and OECs (Panel d; $^{*}P < .05$ 3C—SiC vs. Control, $^{***}P < .001$ Si vs. Control and $^{\#\#\#}P < .001$ Si vs. 3C—SiC as determined by one-way ANOVA followed by Tukey post hoc test).

will have a new treatment pathway with which to treat patients with nervous system disease and/or trauma.

References

[1] E. Fuchs, T. Chen, A matter of life and death: self-renewal in stem cells, EMBO Report 14 (2013) 39—48.

[2] W. Zakrzewski, M. Dobrzyński, M. Szymonowicz, Z. Rybak, Stem cells: past, present, and future, Stem Cell Research Therapy 10 (2019) 1—22.

[3] M.L. Condic, Totipotency: what it is and what it is not, Stem Cells and Development 23 (2014) 796—812.

[4] G. Liu, B.T. David, M. Trawczynski, R.G. Fessler, Advances in pluripotent stem cells: history, mechanisms, technologies, and applications, Stem Cell Reviews and Reports 16 (2020) 3—32.

[5] G. Bonaventura, et al., Different tissue-derived stem cells: a comparison of neural differentiation capability, PloS One 10 (2015) e0140790, https://doi.org/10.1371/journal.pone.0140790.

[6] J.-S. Song, D. Stefanik, M. Damek-Poprawa, F. Alawi, S.O. Akintoye, Differentiation and regenerative capacities of human odontoma-derived mesenchymal cells, Differentiation; Research in Biological Diversity 77 (2009) 29—37.

[7] S. Gronthos, M. Mankani, J. Brahim, P.G. Robey, S. Shi, Postnatal human dental pulp stem cells (DPSCs) in vitro and in vivo, Proceedings of the National Academy of Sciences 97 (25) (2000) 13625–13630.
[8] M. La Noce, et al., Dental pulp stem cells: state of the art and suggestions for a true translation of research into therapy, Journal of Dentistry 42 (2014) 761–768.
[9] K. Dalamagkas, M. Tsintou, A.M. Seifalian, Stem cells for spinal cord injuries bearing translational potential, Neural Regeneration Research 13 (2018) 35–42.
[10] E.S. Rosenzweig, et al., Restorative effects of human neural stem cell grafts on the primate spinal cord, Nature Medicine 24 (2018) 484.
[11] R. Pellitteri, M. Spatuzza, S. Stanzani, D. Zaccheo, Biomarkers expression in rat olfactory ensheathing cells, Frontiers and Bioscience 2 (2010) 289–298.
[12] F. Azarbal, M.J. Price, Newer-generation metallic stents, Updates in Percutaneous Coronary Intervention, an Issue of Interventional Cardiology Clinics, EBook 8 (2019) 95.
[13] S. Mingui, M. Mickle, L. Wei, L. Qiang, R.J. Sclabassi, Data communication between brain implants and computer, IEEE Transactions on Neural Systems and Rehabilitation Engineering 11 (2003) 189–192, https://doi.org/10.1109/TNSRE.2003.814421.
[14] C.L. Frewin, C. Locke, S.E. Saddow, E.J. Weeber, In 2011 Annual International Conference of the IEEE Engineering in Medicine and Biology Society, IEEE, 2018, pp. 2957–2960.
[15] Y. Xing, Z. Xia, J. Rao, Semiconductor quantum dots for biosensing and *in vivo* imaging, IEEE Transactions on NanoBioscience 8 (2009) 4–12, https://doi.org/10.1109/TNB.2009.2017321.
[16] M. Jorfi, J.L. Skousen, C. Weder, J.R. Capadona, Progress towards biocompatible intracortical microelectrodes for neural interfacing applications, Journal of Neural Engineering 12 (2014) 011001.
[17] N.S. Peachey, A.Y. Chow, Subretinal implantation of semiconductor-based photodiodes: progress and challenges, Journal of Rehabilitation Research and Development 36 (1999) 371–376.
[18] A.M. Engebretson, Benefits of digital hearing aids, IEEE Engineering in Medicine and Biology Magazine 13 (1994) 238–248.
[19] M. Anheim, et al., Improvement in Parkinson disease by subthalamic nucleus stimulation based on electrode placement: effects of reimplantation, Archives of Neurology 65 (2008) 612–616.
[20] X. Peng, J.L. Hickman, S.G. Bowles, D.C. Donegan, C.G. Welle, Innovations in electrical stimulation harness neural plasticity to restore motor function, Bioelectronics in Medicine 0, Null (2018), https://doi.org/10.2217/bem-2019-0002.
[21] A. Subramanian, U.M. Krishnan, S. Sethuraman, Development of biomaterial scaffold for nerve tissue engineering: biomaterial mediated neural regeneration, Journal of Biomedical Science 16 (2009) 108.
[22] M.I. GuÃànther, M. GuÃànther, M. Schneiders, R. Rupp, A. Blesch, AngleJ: a new tool for the automated measurement of neurite growth orientation in tissue sections, Journal of Neuroscience Methods 251 (2015) 143–150.
[23] M. Onuma-Ukegawa, et al., Bone marrow stromal cells combined with a honeycomb collagen sponge facilitate neurite elongation in vitro and neural restoration in the hemisected rat spinal cord, Cell Transplantation 24 (2015) 1283–1297, https://doi.org/10.3727/096368914X682134.
[24] A. Hurtado, et al., Robust CNS regeneration after complete spinal cord transection using aligned poly-L-lactic acid microfibers, Biomaterials 32 (2011) 6068–6079.
[25] H.E. Olson, et al., Neural stem cell-and schwann cell-loaded biodegradable polymer scaffolds support axonal regeneration in the transected spinal cord, Tissue Engineering A 15 (2009) 1797–1805.

[26] G. Bozkurt, et al., Chitosan channels containing spinal cord-derived stem/progenitor cells for repair of subacute spinal cord injury in the rat, Neurosurgery 67 (2010) 1733–1744.
[27] H.-s Park, M.-S. Gong, J.C. Knowles, Catalyst-free synthesis of high elongation degradable polyurethanes containing varying ratios of isosorbide and polycaprolactone: physical properties and biocompatibility, Journal of Materials Science: Materials in Medicine 24 (2013) 281–294.
[28] H. Suzuki, et al., Artificial collagen-filament scaffold promotes axon regeneration and long tract reconstruction in a rat model of spinal cord transection, Medical Molecular Morphology 48 (2015) 214–224.
[29] S.E. Saddow, Silicon Carbide Biotechnology: A Biocompatible Semiconductor for Advanced Biomedical Devices and Applications, 2012. Elsevier © 2016.
[30] A. Oliveros, A. Guiseppi-Elie, S.E. Saddow, Silicon carbide: a versatile material for biosensor applications, Biomedical Microdevices 15 (2013) 353–368.
[31] M. Kamble, et al., Synthesis of cubic nanocrystalline silicon carbide (3C-SiC) films by HW-CVD method, Silicon 9 (2017) 421–429, https://doi.org/10.1007/s12633-015-9358-8.
[32] S.N. Gorin, L.M. Ivanova, Cubic silicon carbide (3C-SiC): structure and properties of single crystals grown by thermal decomposition of Methyl trichlorosilane in hydrogen, Physica Status Solidi (B) 202 (1997) 221–245, https://doi.org/10.1002/1521-3951(199707)202:1<221::AID-PSSB221>3.0.CO; 2-L.
[33] S. Afroz, S. Thomas, G. Mumcu, S. Saddow, in: Sensors, IEEE, 2013, 1–4.
[34] C.L. Frewin, S.E. Saddow, Google Patents, 2014.

CHAPTER 3

Graphene on SiC: platform for spinal cord repair studies

Domenica Convertino[1], Laura Marchetti[1,2] and Camilla Coletti[1]
[1]Center for Nanotechnology Innovation@NEST, Istituto Italiano di Tecnologia, Pisa, Italy; [2]Department of Pharmacy, University of Pisa, Pisa, Italy

Contents

1. Introduction

The peripheral nervous system is a complex network of nerve cells that comprises the communication pathway between the central nervous system (CNS) and the periphery of the body. It is divided into two portions: the sensory fibers that transmit sensory signals from the peripheral areas of the body to the CNS and the motor fibers that transmit impulses from the CNS

Silicon Carbide Technology for Advanced Human Healthcare Applications
ISBN 978-0-323-90609-8
https://doi.org/10.1016/B978-0-323-90609-8.00002-8

to the peripheral organs to cause an effect [1]. Following either a traumatic event or a disease, these pathways could be damaged, resulting in the loss of sensory and muscle functions and treatment is needed to restore the original function. A peculiar characteristic of peripheral nerves, compared to central nerves, is their ability to spontaneously regenerate after a traumatic injury, caused by either a trauma or a disease.

In the presence of a significant gap between the proximal and distal nerve stumps, the common surgical approach consists of a direct suture (end-to-end suture) that may not be sufficient due to the substance loss between the stumps, thus additional tissue to bridge the gap is needed to restore the nerve pathway. The most common surgical approaches use nerve conduits (generally, autograft or allograft) as "bridges" between the nerve stumps that physically guide the regrowth of the axons [2] (Fig. 3.1).

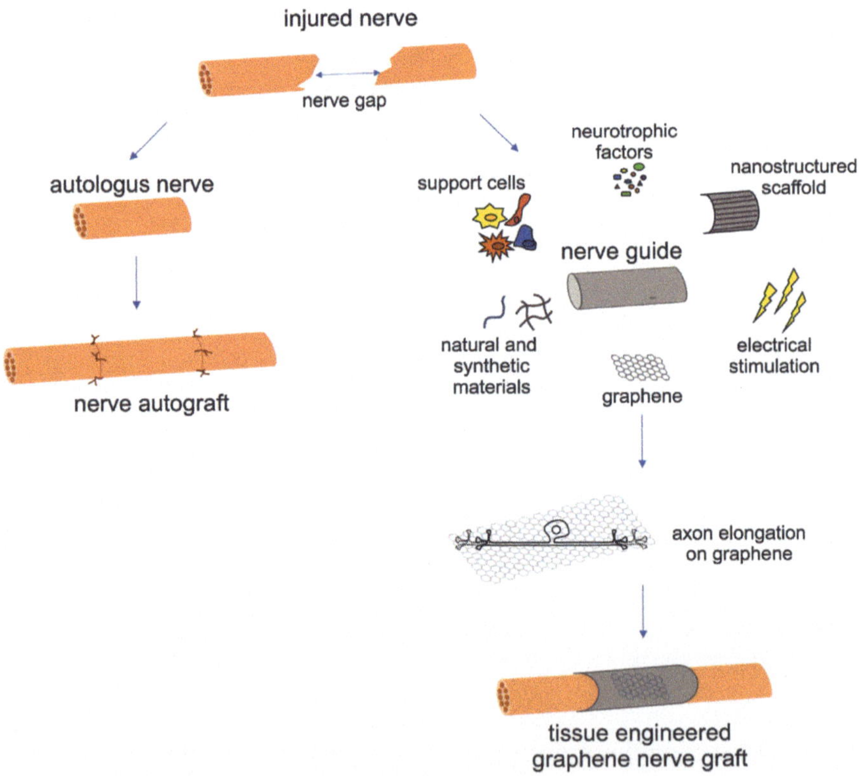

Figure 3.1 Schematic illustrating nerve grafts for nerve repair. Left: autologous nerve graft. Right: engineered natural or synthetic nerve graft, enriched with support cells, neurotrophic factors, and/or carbon-based materials. Graphene-based nerve grafts can be used to accelerate neurite outgrowth.

The current gold standard in nerve injury repair is the autograft; however, it presents some limitations due to the donor site morbidity or low availability of donor nerves. Furthermore, allografts are also limited to filling small gaps and require systemic immunosuppression that limits their usage [1,3,4]. For these reasons, in recent years, new more promising approaches have been proposed to treat nerve injury, including the development of nerve guidance conduits. In fact, the use of tissue-engineered nerve grafts as a bridge connecting two nerve stumps has been shown to improve nerve regeneration and functional recovery. This is accomplished by guiding the regenerating axons across the lesion site, thus reducing scar formation and increasing the concentration of neurotrophic factors [2,5,6]. In addition, the presence of appropriate topographic and biophysical cues helps the process by reducing off-target reinnervation and axonal dispersion, and by promoting neural differentiation and neural network maturation as shown in Fig. 3.1 [7,8].

The nerve guides can be realized with different materials whose properties positively contribute to the nerve regeneration process. Among them, silicon is known to stimulate scar tissue formation due to its nonresorbable nature, thus Si lacks long-term stability. Other natural polymers, such as collagen, alginate, and chitosan, have poor mechanical and electrical properties [4,6]. As a direct consequence of the need to find stable and effective nerve guides, new materials have been proposed as promising candidates for tissue engineering applications. Among them, and due to their peculiar properties (i.e., transparency, flexibility, chemical stability, conductivity, biocompatibility), graphene and other carbon-based materials have been attracting enormous research interest in the biomedical and regenerative medicine fields [9,10]. Graphene was the first two-dimensional (2D) material to be studied: a single layer of sp^2-hybridized carbon atoms arranged in a 2D honeycomb lattice, which was first isolated in 2004 from graphite [11]. It possesses superior electrical and thermal conductivity [12,13], it is 97.7% transparent to visible light [14], exhibits record tribological properties (Young's modulus on the order of 1 TPa and intrinsic strength of 130 GPa [15], while being as flexible as plastic [16,17]). In the past years, a lot of studies have shown graphene's potential as a conductive neural interface, by demonstrating its capability to improve adhesion, differentiation, proliferation, and outgrowth of different cell types [18—24]. Thanks to the latest developments, graphene scaffolds have been proven to support nervous system regeneration, also when applied in vivo [9,25—27].

This chapter discusses the potential of graphene as a conductive peripheral neural interface to realize a biocompatible nerve guide to enhance axon regeneration. We discuss the use of graphene on SiC as an ideal surface for neural interface studies, due to its extreme cleanliness and high crystallinity. At the end of this chapter, we move to a more cost-effective model of chemical vapor deposition (CVD) graphene grown on Cu and transferred to substrates of choice, whose chemical composition and flexibility can be chosen to meet the fundamental requirements for effective nerve tissue regeneration.

2. Graphene as a neural interface

This section addresses the basic properties of graphene and gives an overview of its biomedical applications, focusing in particular on neural regenerative applications. Existing works on graphene neural interfaces are reported, with particular attention on the advantages and disadvantages of using uncoated or polymer-coated graphene.

2.1 Advantages of graphene for neural regenerative medicine

Until recently, most of the studies investigating the potential of graphene-based materials for biomedical applications focused on three different types of graphene obtained with top-down approaches: graphene oxide (a covalently functionalized form), reduced graphene oxide, and liquid phase exfoliated graphene [10,26,28–33]. However, these graphene forms usually lack graphene's unique electrical and tribological properties due to a variable in the ratio of sp^2 and sp^3 carbon fractions that alter the material's electronic and structural properties [34]. Conversely, graphene obtained with bottom-up approaches, such as chemical vapor deposition on metals and thermal decomposition of silicon carbide, can be considered "pristine graphene," as the structural and electrical properties of these materials (when obtained with optimized growth conditions) can be compared to those of exfoliated graphene flakes from graphite [35–37].

Different from those graphene-based (GB) materials, the use of pristine graphene is preferable in those applications that could benefit from its excellent electrical conductivity [35–37]. In particular, the use of a highly conductive material is advantageous for nervous system regeneration applications, where an improved proliferation, differentiation, and axon regeneration has been observed both in the presence of an external electrical stimulation [9,20,38] and endogenous electric signals [39,40]. For these reasons, and knowing the potential of graphene and carbon nanotubes, several studies have been conducted to realize bioactive scaffolds in which carbon-based materials replaced conductive polymers as conductive fillers [4,38,41].

Graphene has several properties suitable for biomedical applications and, in particular, for neural regenerative medicine:

i. Biocompatibility: graphene has the ability to functionally interface with neuronal tissue with a minimal inflammatory response, stimulating cell adhesion, proliferation, and differentiation [42–44].

ii. Chemical stability: thanks to its electronic structure, graphene is chemically inert. It forms a corrosion barrier against environmental and technological agents, improving long-term stability in physiological environments [43,45].

iii. Transparency: graphene is transparent to light [14]. This allows one to directly probe cell–substrate interaction with a label-free approach or to realize transparent electrodes that combine imaging and electrophysiology [46].

iv. Flexibility: graphene can be conformally transferred to any kind of surface and, thanks to its excellent mechanical properties, has been applied to realize flexible and stretchable/wearable devices [47].

v. Electrical conductivity: graphene's excellent electrical conductivity [12,48] could help with the coupling of graphene with neural cells thus providing a high sensitivity pathway for electrical signal changes during stimulation [19,49].

Hence, graphene's properties are ideal to realize a neural scaffold, and this 2D material has been shown to improve cell adhesion, proliferation, differentiation, and outgrowth, thus supporting nervous system regeneration [9,25–27]. However, to date, only a few studies have investigated the interaction of pristine graphene with peripheral neurons [23,24,50]. Most of the existing studies adopting pristine graphene focused on its possible benefits for central nervous system applications [18,51]. Indeed, graphene-based devices for high-resolution neurophysiological recording and brain stimulation have been developed and already tested in vivo [46,52,53]. Until recently, the lack of studies on the adoption of pristine graphene for spinal cord injuries left other carbon-based materials to star in this play [9,26,54,55].

2.2 Interfacing neurons on coated and uncoated graphene: a comparative study

To date, different neural cell types have been interfaced with pristine graphene both in uncoated and coated forms. The first studies used polymer-coated graphene and explored its impact on neural stem cell (NSC) differentiation and neural network formation [19,56]. It was demonstrated that graphene enhances NSC differentiation into neurons [19] and supports the growth of a functional neural network, improving neural performance and electrical signaling [56]. Another study suggested that polymer-coated graphene accelerates NSC differentiation and maturation during development, especially with regard to bioelectric properties, that is, hyperpolarizing the resting membrane potential, upregulating the expression of TREK-1 potassium channels, and increasing the probability of firing action potentials [57]. In addition, coated graphene was found to enhance neurite sprouting and outgrowth [18].

Other studies investigated the interaction of graphene coated with fetal bovine serum (FBS) with peripheral neurons and reported a positive effect on cell proliferation and neurite outgrowth [21,50]. Lee et al. investigated the morphology and proliferation of PC12 cells on FBS-coated graphene. They claimed that graphene promoted neurite outgrowth, but did not quantify the neurite length and they used bare glass as a control without exploring the effect of FBS coating on the controls [50]. Similarly, Hong et al. found an enhanced PC12 cells proliferation on FBS-coated graphene compared to bare glass, but this study also did not investigate the effect of the FBS coating alone, comparing FBS-coated graphene only with bare glass [21]. It should also be mentioned that FBS is not a traditional coating for neural cell culture [58].

Some studies to date have also investigated the survival of specific neurons on uncoated graphene. However, the use of bare graphene was reported to reduce both retinal ganglion cell and dorsal root ganglion (DRG) neuron adhesion and spreading, inducing cell aggregation in clumps and the production of neurite bundles [23,59]. A lower adhesion was also observed for cortical neurons, where a reduced neuronal growth, attachment, and survival were observed when compared with poly-d-lysine (PDL) coated dishes, even if graphene performed better than bare control dishes [60]. A possible explanation of this reduced adhesion was presented in Veliev et al. [61]. They proposed that neural adhesion and cytocompatibility are deeply influenced by graphene quality, as defective graphene was shown to inhibit cell growth.

The use of bare graphene should be preferred whenever possible. In fact, the use of a coating, in short-term cultures, may hide the potential toxicity of the material underneath [59]. The coating could also affect the electrical coupling when graphene is used for stimulation and recording of electrogenic cell signals thereby increasing the background noise and reducing the sensitivity of the recording [61]. However, it is well known that neurons produce their own extracellular matrix (ECM) even in culture conditions [62]. Natural ECM molecules are deposited on the surface of biomaterials and affect cellular response, implying that even if a bare graphene substrate is used, it will soon be coated with natural ECM. Accordingly, the cells will sense graphene under ECM, whether it is previously coated or not. Using uncoated or coated graphene depends on the application, preferring uncoated graphene when interested in the most natural neural development processes possible, and coated graphene when a better neural adhesion to the material in the early stages of cell culture is necessary. In this work, we present results on both coated and uncoated graphene, with a particular focus on graphene morphology and wettability after some commonly used polymeric coatings.

3. Graphene on SiC for nerve regeneration

In this section, we focus on using pristine epitaxial graphene on SiC to assess its effect on axonal sprouting and viability. First, we give a brief overview of the growth of graphene on SiC via thermal decomposition and its characterization (Section 3.2). Then, we analyze how traditional polymeric coatings for neural cultures distribute onto the extremely flat and hydrophobic graphene at the nanometric scale (Section 3.3). Finally, we focus on the effect of polymeric-coated pristine graphene (on SiC) on neurite outgrowth of PC12 and primary sensory neurons (Section 3.4) [23].

3.1 Epitaxial graphene on SiC as ideal neural interface

As discussed in Section 2.1, graphene can be synthesized by various methods, depending on the required properties and targeted application. The two main techniques for wafer-scale synthesis of high-quality graphene are thermal decomposition of SiC [37,63,64] and CVD of graphene on transition metals [65–67]. The use of graphene grown via thermal decomposition of SiC (referred to in this chapter as epitaxial graphene [68]) guarantees an extremely clean material as it does not involve film transfer; however, the lack of flexibility of the SiC substrate and the elevated cost of the SiC crystal (a 4-inch SiC substrate can easily cost thousands of dollars) limits its wide applicability. On the contrary, the use of CVD on copper (Cu) foils [66] has more potential as it is much cheaper and graphene can then be transferred to substrates of choice, which can have different mechanical and electrical properties.

Epitaxial graphene represents an ideal model to study the effect of graphene on peripheral neurons. It is grown directly on a transparent substrate that allows for the examination of cell morphology with a label-free approach using standard transmitted light microscopy; moreover, the transfer-free approach ensures cleanliness and reduces contaminants. However, flexibility and scalability are requirements in neural regeneration that cannot be easily met by using graphene on SiC and, for this reason, it represents a proof-of-concept material that might pave the way to further studies involving other pristine graphene forms.

3.2 Epitaxial graphene on SiC: sample preparation and characterization

In the thermal decomposition process of SiC, the SiC substrates are annealed at high temperature leading to the selective desorption of silicon (Si) atoms and the rearrangement of the carbon (C) atoms left behind to form graphene [63]. Graphene can be grown both on the silicon-terminated (0001) surface and carbon-terminated SiC (000 $\overline{1}$) surface, called the Si- and C-face, respectively. The growth modes are not self-limited and are strongly influenced by the choice of the SiC crystal face, resulting in different graphene films [63]. The graphitization process on the Si-face is characterized by the formation of an interface layer between the SiC substrate and the first graphene layer, known as zero, or buffer, layer, with a periodicity of $(6\sqrt{3}x6\sqrt{3})R30°$. About 30% of the carbon atoms in this buffer layer are covalently bound to the Si atoms of the Si-terminated substrate and are inactive in terms of the typical graphene properties [69]. New graphene layers are formed by releasing the buffer layer from the substrate following Si sublimation. In this way, a new buffer layer is formed and the 30 degrees rotation with respect to the SiC substrate is inherited by the new graphene layer [70]. The buffer layer has a significant electronic influence on graphene, characterized by a reduced carrier mobility and an intrinsic electron doping ($n \approx 10^{13}$ cm^{-2}) [68]. To overcome this issue, a technique has been developed that eliminates the negative impact of the interface layer by decoupling the graphene from the SiC substrate via hydrogen intercalation, thereby increasing graphene carrier mobility and achieving charge neutrality [69,71,72]. Molecular hydrogen eliminates the interface bonding by breaking and saturating the bonds between the C and Si atoms, thus releasing the buffer layer and yielding a quasi-free standing monolayer graphene (QFMLG). Specifically, the buffer layer is turned into a quasi-free standing monolayer graphene (QFSMG) and, in the same way, monolayer graphene turns into a decoupled bilayer [69] (Fig. 3.2). While on the Si-face of SiC it is easier to grow homogeneous graphene with a controlled number of layers, on the C-face the thermal decomposition process is rather quick and it is therefore difficult to control the number of layers, generating multilayer graphene [63,64,73]. Moreover, on the C-face, each graphene layer behaves as an isolated layer electronically decoupled from the neighboring ones. Thus, graphene on the C-face shows remarkable carrier mobilities [74,75].

It is known that thermal decomposition of SiC could be performed both in ultra-high vacuum (UHV) or under Ar atmospheric pressure [37,63,76]. The latter is known to allow for a better control in the silicon sublimation thus yielding larger graphene domains [68]. We optimized a process to grow graphene on the Si-face of SiC by thermal decomposition using a resistively heated commercial cold-wall reactor (HT-BM Aixtron reactor) [23,77,78], to assure uniform graphene coverage of the SiC surface and reduce the formation of defects that could influence cell response. Following SiC annealing, graphene grows not only on the Si face but also in multilayer form on the C-face reducing the substrate transparency. This problem can be solved by growing buffer layer graphene (obtained with a lower annealing temperature that reduces the multilayer formation on the

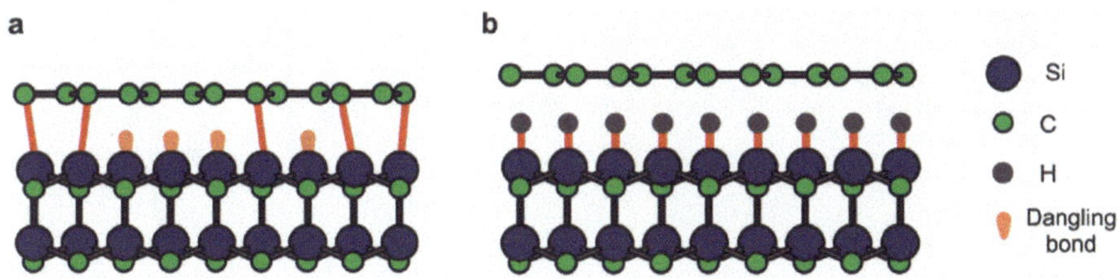

Figure 3.2 Structural model of buffer layer and quasi-free standing graphene (QFSG) graphene. Schematic side view of (A) buffer layer with the carbon layer partially covalently bonded to the Si atoms of the SiC substrate and (B) quasi-free standing monolayer graphene formed after hydrogen intercalation. Hydrogen atoms saturate the Si atoms of the Si-face SiC, releasing the buffer layer into a quasi-free-standing graphene. *(Adapted from Ref. [69].)*

C-face) and by subsequently implementing hydrogen intercalation to obtain QFSMG. In addition, since the graphene crystallinity and uniformity are strongly influenced by the quality of the initial SiC surface, the SiC substrate is previously prepared by using hydrogen etching [37,79,80]. This method reduces crystalline defects, minimizes surface scratches, and produces large atomically flat terraces on the SiC surface. The resulting surface arises from the unintentional miscut of the wafers and is characterized by a regular array of atomically flat terraces separated by steps of half or multiples of the unit cell height [79] (Fig. 3.3).

Substrate preparation for epitaxial graphene growth was performed with the following steps [23,81]:

i. Cutting square die of about $6 \times 6\ mm^2$ from 1 degree off-axis 4H–SiC(0001) wafers (SiCrystal, W4H76N-1-PO-350);

ii. Cleaning in an ultrasonic bath with acetone and isopropanol to remove organic residuals, followed by deionized (DI) water rinsing and drying with nitrogen;

iii. Cleaning in Piranha solution (H_2SO_4:H_2O_2 = 4:1) for 10 min to remove organic contamination, followed by DI water rinsing and drying with nitrogen.

To obtain uniform and high-quality epitaxial graphene growth, the samples were loaded in the HT-BM Aixtron reactor and hydrogen etched to remove polishing scratches and reveal the atomically flat terraces. The samples were annealed under an H_2/Ar gas mixture at a temperature of 1250°C and a pressure of 450 mbar for 5 min. Buffer layer graphene was

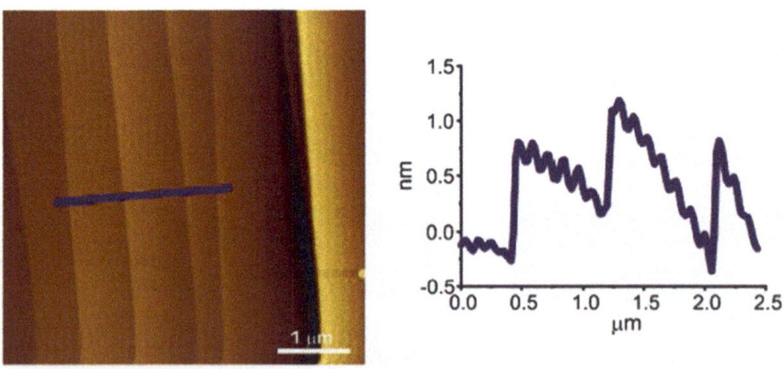

Figure 3.3 AFM images of on-axis 4H–SiC wafer surface morphology after hydrogen etching. The etched Si-face surface with atomically flat with micrometric terraces separated by atomic steps (left). Step profile taken along the step flow direction reveals steps of unit cell height (1 nm) with an average distance of 1 µm (right).

then obtained via thermal decomposition. First, the H-etched sample was annealed in a vacuum at 900°C for 10 min to remove adsorbates, then it was exposed to an Ar atmosphere at around 1250°C for 10 min in the same reactor as described in previous works [23,77,82,83]. Subsequently, the buffer layer was hydrogen intercalated to obtain QFMLG. The process was performed by annealing the samples at 900°C for 10 min in pure hydrogen at atmospheric pressure [23,84].

Assessment of the topography and distribution of the number of layers was conducted via Raman spectroscopy and atomic force microscopy (AFM). Raman characterization was performed using a micro-Raman spectroscope, equipped with a motorized sample stage (inVia Raman, Renishaw) and a 532 nm laser with a spot size of around 0.8 μm in diameter. The laser power was kept at 1 mW with an acquisition time of 2 s.

AFM images of areas up to 10 × 10 μm wide were taken using an AFM+ (Anasys Instruments) operated in tapping-mode using a standard tapping probe (PRE-EX-T125, Anasys Instruments).

The typical morphology of the samples, with the regular arrangement of the terraces and the presence of different graphene thicknesses within the terraces, is shown in Fig. 3.4. The correlation of the two-dimensional spatial distribution of the width of the 2D Raman peak and the ratio of 2D and G peak intensities with the AFM micrographs revealed the mostly monolayer nature of graphene, with bilayer stripes located mostly at the terrace edges [77,85].

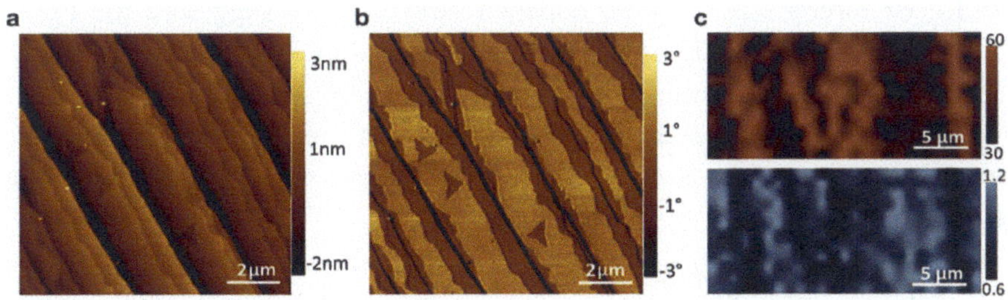

Figure 3.4 Epitaxial graphene characterization via AFM and Raman spectroscopy. (A,B) Tapping mode AFM topography (A) and phase signal (B) of graphene grown on 4H−SiC(0001), showing the terraces arising from hydrogen etching. The contrast in the phase signal is due to monolayer graphene (brighter) or bilayer graphene (darker). (C) 2D Raman peak width (upper image) shows a monolayer character on the terraces (darker areas) and bilayer inclusions in the proximity of the steps (lighter areas). The bilayer inclusions are confirmed by an increase in the ratio of G and 2D Raman peak intensity (lower image).

To assure experimental reproducibility, and deeply understand the effect of graphene on cell viability and morphology, each sample was checked with optical microscopy, AFM, and Raman mapping. This allowed us to exclude samples with macroscopic defects and to select those with a common large-scale morphology and quality to exclude spurious effects on cell cultures.

3.3 ECM-like components distribution on epitaxial graphene on SiC

Polymeric coatings play a critical role in influencing cell response, modulating cell adhesion and morphogenesis and therefore network structure [58,86]. Various types of coating agents can be used, ranging from ECM proteins to polymers, which display different properties able to elicit different cell responses; for example, a more homogeneous and fast neuronal adhesion is prompted by poly-lysine coated surfaces while facilitated neuritogenesis occurs on matrigel and laminin [58].

Given the high hydrophobicity and flatness of graphene, the correct information on coating distribution on graphene at the nanometric scale is crucial to identify the most suitable coatings to adopt for the cell cultures [23].

3.3.1 Surface functionalization

Different surface coatings suggested for the target cell cultures were used to functionalize both graphene and control surfaces to investigate their nanometric morphology. In particular, polymers such as poly-L-lysine (PLL), or biologically derived collagen, are typically suggested for PC12 cells adhesion [87], while a phosphate buffered saline (PBS) solution of PDL alone and PDL with laminin were chosen for DRG neurons.

Graphene on SiC in the form QFMLG was prepared by adopting the procedure reported in Section 3.2. Four different control substrates were used in this study:

i. Hydrogen etched SiC(0001) die, from the same wafer used for graphene growth;

ii. Gold-coated glass coverslips obtained by thermal evaporation of a thin layer of gold (4 nm) using titanium as an adhesive layer. The thin gold layer on glass was deposited to mimic the graphene conductive layer on the SiC substrate;

iii. Bare glass coverslips treated overnight with 65% nitric acid (Sigma—Aldrich);

iv. Polystyrene tissue-culture treated 48-well plates (Corning).

The dimension of all the substrates was about $6 \times 6\ mm^2$. Before surface coating, all substrates were sterilized by 30 min immersion in 96% ethanol, rinsed several times with DI water, and dried under hood.

The graphene and control samples were incubated at 37°C with different coating solutions: 100 μg/mL PLL solution in water (P4832, Sigma–Aldrich), 200 μg/mL Collagene Type I (Sigma–Aldrich) in DI water, 30 μg/mL PDL (P1149, Sigma–Aldrich) in PBS, 30 μg/mL PDL, and 5 μg/mL laminin (Life Technologies) in PBS. After incubation, the samples were rinsed with DI water and dried under a cell culture hood before analyzing their surface via AFM. Three different incubation times were tested, that is, 1, 4, and 12 h to assess the effect of the incubation time on the coating quality, homogeneity, and morphology.

Typically, AFM topography and phase channels were acquired to characterize the substrates and compare coated and uncoated graphene sample morphology with the controls. The AFM micrographs were analyzed using the software Gwyddion 2.45.

3.3.2 Nano-resolved analysis of polymeric coating of graphene and control substrates

Fig. 3.5 shows the AFM topography and phase micrographs for different polymeric coatings at different incubation times on a graphene substrate. The distribution of the PLL coating is fairly homogenous over the graphene surface, independently from the incubation time. PLL tends to form a homogeneous carpet of 1–2 nm spots with no aggregates, while for the Collagen Type I coating network-like aggregates can be detected. Also, in the case of PDL and PDL/laminin-coated graphene, an increased roughness was observed after the coating for all time points and, in particular, the formation of a network-like structure.

The net morphology was independent from the salts in the PBS solution. In fact, even after incubation for 4 h of the same polymeric amount in DI water, a similar morphology and roughness were observed (Fig. 3.6A). Similarly, we excluded that the different molecule arrangements of PLL and PDL were dependent on their concentration (PDL = 30 μg/mL, PLL = 100 μg/mL). We tested a PDL coating solution in DI water with the same concentration used for PLL (100 μg/mL) and observed aggregates similar to the ones observed for the lower PDL concentration, confirming its independence on solution concentration (Fig. 3.6B).

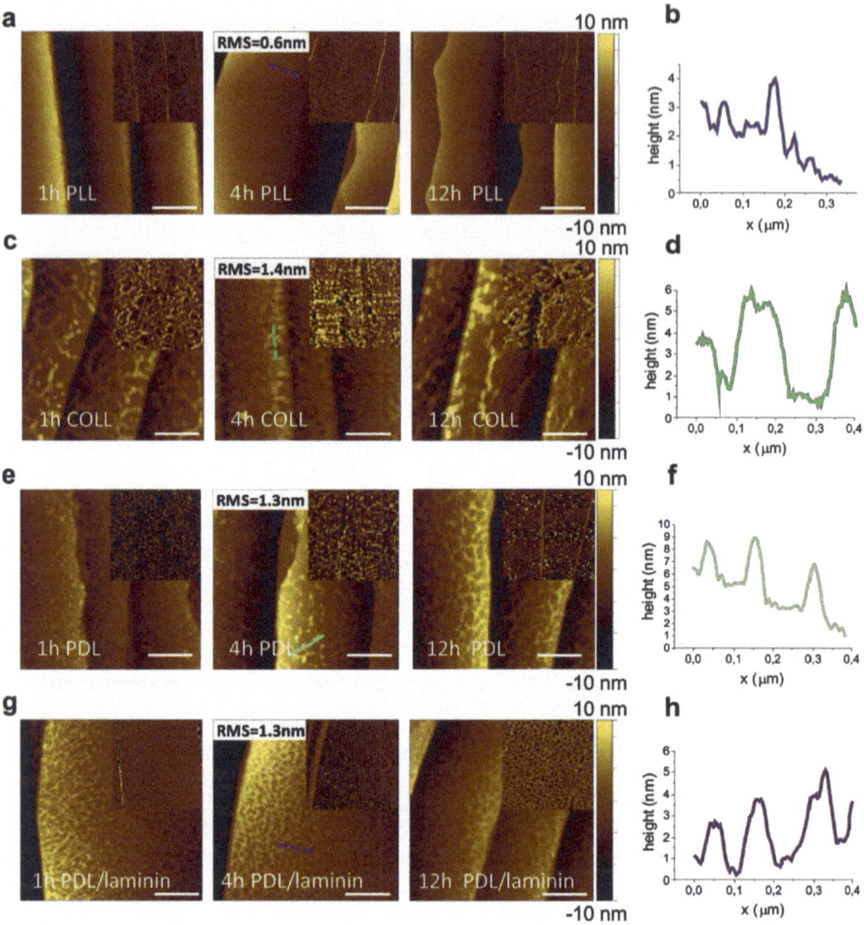

Figure 3.5 AFM micrographs of polymeric coated graphene. AFM topography images of graphene after three different times of incubation (1, 4 and 12 h) with (A) PLL (100 μg/mL in DI water), (C) Collagen Type I coating (200 μg/mL in DI water), (E) PDL (30 μg/mL in PBS) and PDL and laminin coating (30 μg/mL PDL and 5 μg/mLL laminin in PBS) (scale bar: 500 nm). The insets show phase images of the same areas (B, D, F, H) AFM height profile, along the dashed lines with corresponding color in the images, of graphene with each coating after 4 h incubation. The root mean square (RMS) roughness values measured inside a single terrace after 4 h incubation are also reported. *(Adapted from Ref. [23].)*

It is worth noting that, differently from the PLL water solution that was a ready-to-use product, the PDL was supplied as lyophilized powder subsequently dissolved in DI water. Thus, the presence of the network-like structure on graphene could be ascribed to the interaction of the partially undissolved polymer with the highly hydrophobic graphene surface.

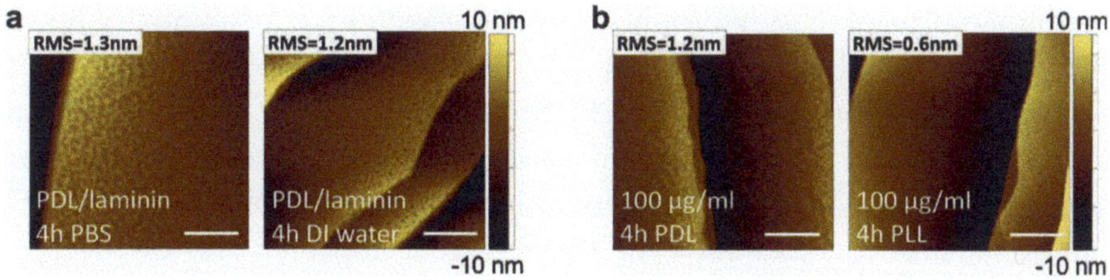

Figure 3.6 AFM micrographs of polymer-coated graphene. (A) AFM topography of graphene samples coated with PDL/laminin (30 µg/mL PDL and 5 µg/mL laminin), dispersed in PBS and DI water after 4h incubation show similar net structures. (B) AFM topography of graphene samples coated with PDL and PLL in water at the same concentration (100 µg/mL) after 4 h incubation have different arrangements, showing that the different morphology is not dependent on the concentration but probably on the molecular weight of the two polypeptides (scale bar: 500 nm). The RMS values measured inside a single terrace are also reported. *(Adapted from Ref. [23].)*

The same characterization was also performed on control substrates (SiC, gold, and glass). SiC was coated with PLL, Collagen Type I, PDL, and PDL with laminin. Both PLL and Collagen distributed evenly on SiC, forming a homogeneous carpet with spots of a few nanometers for all the probed incubation times. The same topography was also observed for PDL with or without laminin. The different coating distribution on graphene and SiC could not be ascribed to surface morphology, as they are both characterized by nanometric terraces and comparable root mean square (rms) roughness. The postcoating morphology is probably related to their different hydrophilicity, that is, graphene was much more hydrophobic than SiC, both before and after coating. The contact angle estimated for graphene was 95.8 ± 1.3 degrees while it was 38.3 ± 7.2 degrees for SiC [23,81,88,89]. This implies that SiC hydrophilicity facilitated a uniform spreading and adhesion of the coating molecules, while the high hydrophobicity of graphene prevented a homogeneous distribution of the molecules that tended to form network-like structures.

The gold and glass surfaces with features of about 1 nm and RMS roughness of about 0.5 nm over 1 μm^2 area before coating, impeded the polymeric features after coating. However, the variation of the hydrophilicity observed with contact angle measurements confirmed the presence of the coating. Noncoated gold was more hydrophobic than noncoated glass, with contact angle values of 83.9 ± 2.3 degrees and 35.0 ± 2.6 degrees, respectively. The coatings had opposite effects on the substrates: increasing hydrophilicity for gold (i.e., contact angles up to 42 degrees after collagen coating) and increasing hydrophobicity for glass (i.e., contact angles up to 46 degrees after PLL coating) [23].

For the experiments reported in Section 3.4, a PLL coating with an incubation time of 4 h was selected for the PC12 cell culture for its higher homogeneity, while a PDL with laminin coating was adopted for the DRG culture experiments to mimic the natural extracellular matrix, ECM.

3.4 Epitaxial graphene on SiC influence on axon elongation

We tested the effect of epitaxial graphene on axon elongation using two cellular models: PC12 cells and DRG sensory neurons. The PC12 cell line is a cell clonal line from rat pheochromocytoma tumor, that is able to form neurite-like processes in response to nerve growth factor (NGF) stimulation and constitutes a well-established model for peripheral neurons [87]. DRG neurons are primary sensory neurons with cell bodies in the dorsal root ganglion. They are considered pseudo-unipolar neurons as they possess one axon that bifurcates in two branches: the peripheral axon innervates the sensory organs and regenerates when injured and the central axon enters the spinal cord and fails to regenerate [90].

3.4.1 PC12 and embryonic DRG neurons cell culture

PC12 cells (ATCC CRL-1721TM) were maintained in a humidified atmosphere at 37°C, 5% CO_2 in Roswell Park Memorial Institute Medium (RPMI) 1640 medium supplemented with 10% horse serum, 5% FBS, 1% penicillin/streptomycin and 1% L-glutamine (Gibco). Cells were plated at ~40%–60% confluency onto the substrates previously coated with 100 μg/mL PLL in water (Sigma–Aldrich). Differentiation was achieved using the following procedure: a 5–6 days priming with 15 ng/mL NGF (Alomone Labs) in complete medium, followed by seeding on the substrates with 50 ng/mL NGF in RPMI medium supplemented with 1% horse serum, 0.5% FBS, 1% penicillin/streptomycin, and 1% L-glutamine. 2/3 of the medium was renewed every 2–3 days.

Rat embryonic dorsal root ganglion neurons (R-EDRG-515 AMP, Lonza) were maintained in a humidified atmosphere at 37°C, 5% CO_2 in Primary Neuron Basal medium (PNBM, Lonza) supplemented with L-glutamine (1%), antibiotics (0.1%), and NSF-1 (2% final concentration). Neurons were plated on the substrates previously coated with a PBS solution of 30 μg/mL PDL (Sigma–Aldrich) and 5 μg/mL laminin (Life Technologies). For the survival of the DRG neurons, 100 ng/mL of NGF

(Alomone Labs) were added to the media. 24 h after seeding, 2.5 μM Cytosine arabinoside (AraC, Sigma—Aldrich) was added for inhibition of glia proliferation. Half of the medium was replaced every 3—4 days.

3.4.1.1 PC12 cell morphometric analysis and viability

The cells were viewed at different time points using an inverted microscope equipped with a 20×/40× magnification objective (Leica DMI4000B microscope). Typically, 10 fields per sample were acquired to perform morphometric analysis of PC12 differentiation.

Three parameters were measured as previously reported in Ref. [91]:

i. the percentage of differentiated cells (diff), determined by counting in each field the number of cells with at least one neurite with a length equal to, or longer than, the cell body diameter, and expressed as percentage of the total number of cells in each field;

ii. the average number of neurites per cell in the field (av. neurites/cell);

iii. the mean neurite length, calculated by measuring the longest neurite of each differentiated cell in the field (length).

PC12 cell viability was assessed with the Cell counting Kit-8 assay (CCK-8, Sigma—Aldrich), based on quantification of WST-8 reduction due to the metabolic activity of viable cells. Samples were prepared according to the manufacturer's instructions and measured at the GloMax Discover multiplate reader (Promega). The results are reported as % over the polystyrene well, which was considered as the control. All experiments were repeated at least twice independently.

3.4.1.2 Statistical analysis

For all experiments, we performed two independent cultures with two biological duplicates each. For the morphometric analysis of the PC12 cells, for each substrate we analyzed at least 200 cells (n_c = number of cells) from selected fields (n_f = number of fields) of the four replicates (two biological duplicates per culture) obtained with a 40× objective (Au: $n_f = 17$, $n_c = 203$; Glass: $n_f = 33$, $n_c = 1106$; G: $n_f = 42$, $n_c = 877$; SiC: $n_f = 35$, $n_c = 1004$; Well: $n_f = 37$, $n_c = 724$). For the DRG neurons, we analyzed n_f fields using a 40× objective for a total of n_c cells for each substrate (day1: Au, $n_f = 13$, $n_c = 67$, Glass: $n_f = 14$, $n_c = 75$; G: $n_f = 13$, $n_c = 29$; SiC: $n_f = 12$, $n_c = 35$; day2: Au, $n_f = 16$, $n_c = 89$, Glass: $n_f = 13$, $n_c = 100$, G: $n_f = 12$, $n_c = 34$, SiC: $n_f = 11$, $n_c = 37$). The number of cells analyzed (n_c) is the total pool of the four experiments. All data are expressed as the average value (mean) ± standard error of the mean (s.e.m.) unless stated otherwise. Data were analyzed by using Origin Software and nonparametric Kruskal–Wallis test with Dunn's multiple comparison tests were used for statistical significance with $*P < .05$, $**P < .01$, and $***P < .001$.

3.4.2 Neurite outgrowth of PC12 cell on epitaxial graphene on SiC

We first investigated graphene cytocompatibility and compared it to that of SiC, glass, gold, and polystyrene (pst) control wells, by morphological observation of differentiated PC12 cells and using the WST-8 viability assay. Fig. 3.7 displays selected optical micrographs of PC12 cells in culture. The first two rows show PC12 cells at day 5 cultured in the absence and presence of NGF treatment, respectively. Note that, unlike the untreated cells where almost no differentiation took place, PC12 cells cultured upon NGF treatment have a neuron-like morphology, exhibiting a significant neurite outgrowth on all of the substrates. This effect is also confirmed after 7 days of culture (third row in Fig. 3.7), where an extensive neurite network is visible for all the substrates.

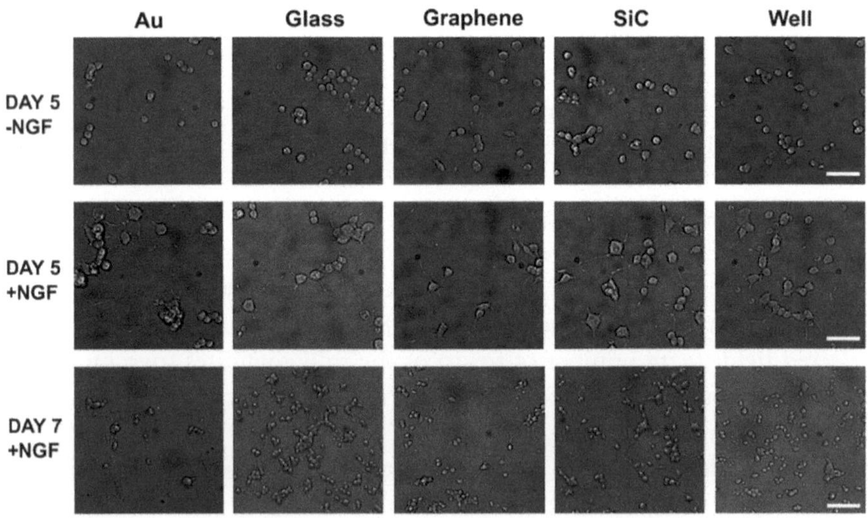

Figure 3.7 PC12 cells cultured on graphene and control substrates. Typical optical micrographs of PC12 cells grown on gold (Au), glass coverslip (Glass), graphene (G), SiC, and polystyrene (Well) coated with PLL (100 μg/mL in DI water, 4 h incubation) in the absence of NGF (first row, scale bar: 50 μm). PC12 cells differentiation upon treatment with NGF at day 5 (second row, scale bar: 50 μm) and day 7 (third row, scale bar: 100 μm). *(Adapted from Ref. [23].)*

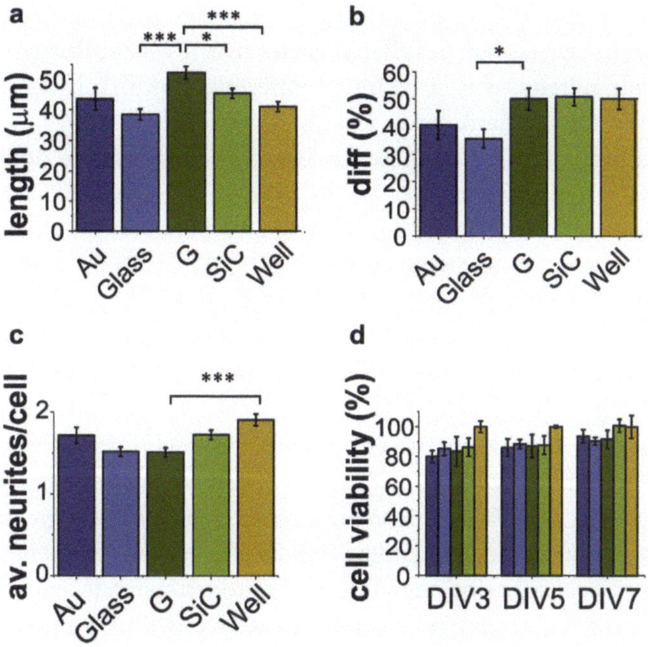

Figure 3.8 Morphometric analysis and cell viability of PC12 cells cultured on graphene and control substrates. Histograms show the quantification of (A) mean neurite length, (B) percentage of differentiated cells, and (C) average number of neurites per cell after 5 days of NGF treatment of two independent experiments per substrate. For each substrate, we analyzed at least 200 cells (n_c) from selected fields (n_f) (Au: $n_f = 17$, $n_c = 203$; Glass: $n_f = 33$, $n_c = 1106$; G: $n_f = 42$, $n_c = 877$; SiC: $n_f = 35$, $n_c = 1004$; Well: $n_f = 37$, $n_c = 724$). (D) Cell viability after 3, 5, and 7 days tested by WST-8. The results are reported as % over the polystyrene control sample. Bars colored as in the other graphs. Data reported as mean ± s.e.m. Nonparametric Kruskal–Wallis test was used for statistical significance, with $^{*}P < .05$, $^{***}P < .001$. *(Adapted from Ref. [23].)*

To better evaluate the differentiation process, selected morphometric parameters were quantified at day 5 and are reported in Fig. 3.8: the percentage of differentiated cells in the fields (diff), the average number of neurites per cell (av. neurites/cell), and the length of the longest neurite per differentiated cell (length). The analysis revealed that after 5 days of culture 50% of the PC12 cells differentiate on graphene. This percentage was better than on glass (*), while it was comparable with SiC and the pst control well, showing that graphene did not affect cell differentiation. The average number of neurites per cell on graphene was lower than on the control well (***). Remarkably, we found that with a mean neurite length of 53.2 µm, graphene induced significantly larger neurite elongation, with neurites longer than on glass (***), the pst well (***), and SiC (*) by 27%, 22%, and 13%, respectively. These results indicate that PC12 cells grow longer neurites on graphene, with a neuronal differentiation that is comparable to that obtained for standard control wells.

The viability of undifferentiated cells was assessed at three different time points (DIV3, DIV5, and DIV7). As visible in Fig. 3.8D, we did not observe significant differences in cell viability between graphene and the control substrates, all showing at least a signal of about 80% over the polystyrene control wells in all the probed times. Moreover, differently from Ref. [21], no increased PC12 cell proliferation on graphene was observed, which could be due to the effect of the FBS coating used in that study.

Our data are in agreement with previous observations of hippocampal neurons, where the neurite sprouting was ascribed to an overexpression of GAP-43 protein [18]. Also, Lee et al. showed a significantly greater neurite outgrowth of human neuroblastoma SH-SY5Y cells on graphene, probably mediated by focal adhesion signaling and mitogen-activated protein kinase signaling cascades and upregulation of genes involved in neurogenesis [92]. Both the studies excluded a neurogenic effect from substrate topography and wettability. Similarly, as epitaxial graphene on SiC has comparable roughness and morphology to the hydrogen etched SiC control, we also exclude that topography influenced cell viability. Thus, we also speculate that for PC12 cells, graphene surface chemistry and electrical conductivity could specifically increase neurite length during differentiation.

3.4.3 DRG primary neurons on epitaxial graphene on SiC

Graphene on SiC was also used to assess its effect on primary DRG neurons. Fig. 3.9 shows selected optical microscopy images of DRG neurons at 1, 4, 9, and 15 days of culture on graphene and controls (SiC, Au, and glass) coated with PDL/laminin. As visible in the first row of Fig. 3.9, after 1 day, neurons adhered uniformly to the underlying substrates.

Starting from day 4, we observed a significant neurite outgrowth and an increase in the axonal length and in the cell body area as shown in Fig. 3.10. Axonal length was quantified at day 1 and day 2, after which the axons started to form complex networks that impeded to further quantify their length with accuracy (see day 9 and 15 in Fig. 3.9). The mean axonal length was higher on graphene than on the controls, confirming the trend reported for PC12 cells, although in this case no statistical significance was

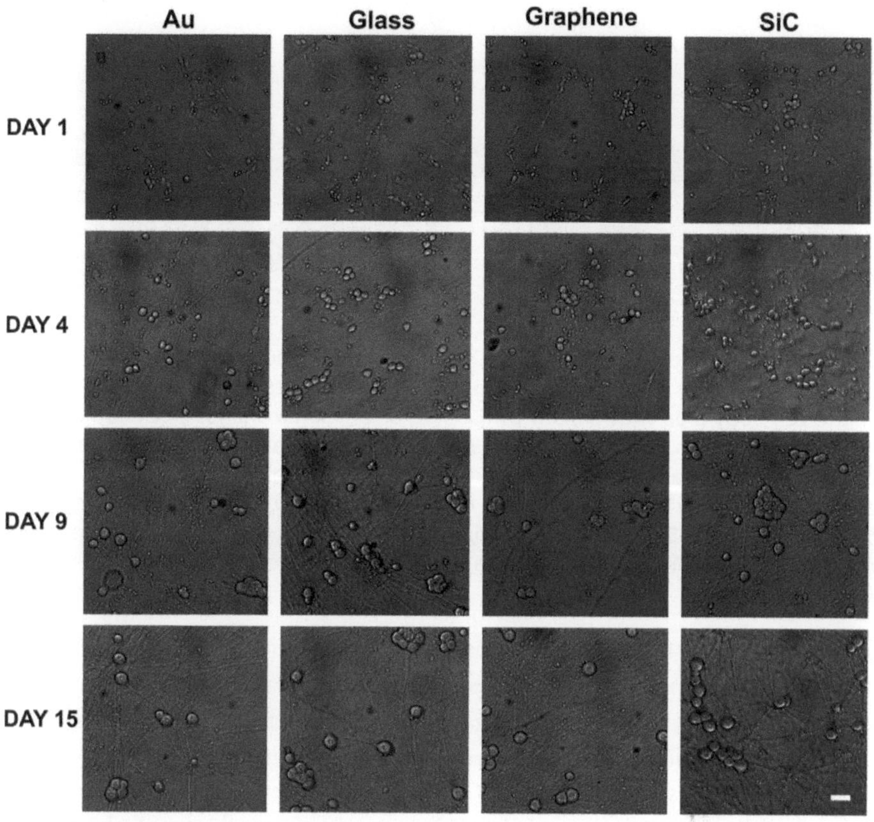

Figure 3.9 DRG neurons cultured on graphene and control substrates. Typical optical micrographs of DRG neurons cultured on gold (Au), glass coverslip, graphene (G), and SiC coated with PDL and laminin (30 μg/mL PDL and 5 μg/mL laminin in PBS, 4 h incubation) at different days of culture. Scale bar: 50 μm. *(Adapted from Ref. [23].)*

observed. This result could be related to an underestimation of the real neurite length, due to the increased neurite network complexity with time, especially on graphene [24].

3.4.4 Peripheral neurons morphology on uncoated epitaxial graphene

We also tested the effect of noncoated epitaxial graphene on primary neurons, knowing that bare substrates have been successfully used for cell growth in numerous studies [30,31,59–61,93,94]. We tested bare graphene using glass and gold as controls. Neuronal growth on glass substrates was observed only if the substrate was coated, on the contrary DRG neurons

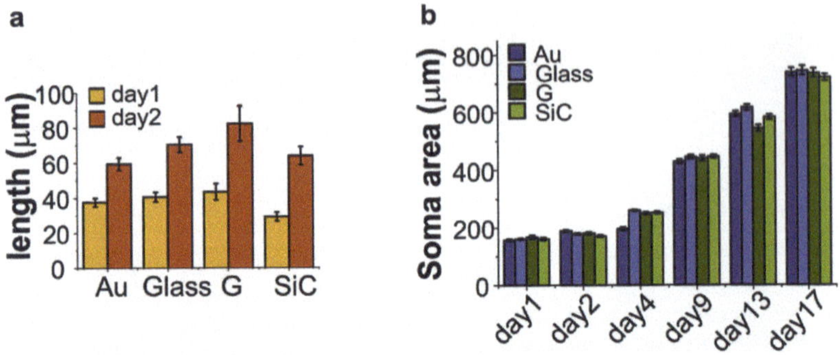

Figure 3.10 Morphometric analysis of DRG neurons cultured on graphene and control substrates. (A) Axon length quantification at 24 and 48 h after cell seeding. (B) Increase of the cell body area with time in DRG cells. For cell soma analyses, cell bodies were approximated to an oval shape and relative areas were evaluated using ImageJ. More than 100 cells per sample were analyzed. We analyzed nf fields for a total of n_c cells for each substrate (day1: Au, $n_f = 13$, $n_c = 67$, Glass: $n_f = 14$, $n_c = 75$; G: $n_f = 13$, $n_c = 29$; SiC: $n_f = 12$, $n_c = 35$; day2: Au, $n_f = 16$, $n_c = 89$, Glass: $n_f = 13$, $n_c = 100$, G: $n_f = 12$, $n_c = 34$, SiC: $n_f = 11$, $n_c = 37$) and data are reported as mean $\pm$ s.e.m. *(Adapted from Ref. [23].)*

survived on both noncoated graphene and gold up to 17 days. On uncoated substrates, neurons already displayed a more complex distribution after 24 h from seeding with neuron aggregates, differently from the coated surface where they distributed homogeneously on the entire sample (Fig. 3.11A).

After 2–3 days of culture, we observed neurites that sprouted radially from the islet, and over longer times the neurons formed a network of small cell body aggregates connected by axonal bundles, which are an indication of poor cellular attachment to the substrates in the absence of a coating. This result resembles the ones previously reported for retinal ganglion cells [59] or cortical neurons [60]. Cell body area on bare graphene was comparable to that on the coated substrate. Higher cell body area on uncoated graphene was observed starting from day 4, but the values did not differ significantly (Fig. 3.12A).

We rarely observed neurite bundles on coated graphene even after long cell culture, while they were already present on uncoated graphene after 2 days of culture and increased in size with time (Fig. 3.12B). This suggests that a surface modification with a hydrophilic coating (i.e., polylysine) turned out to be useful to improve adhesion and neuron homogeneous distribution [18,94], also masking some local structural inhomogeneities and defects in the underlying graphene [61].

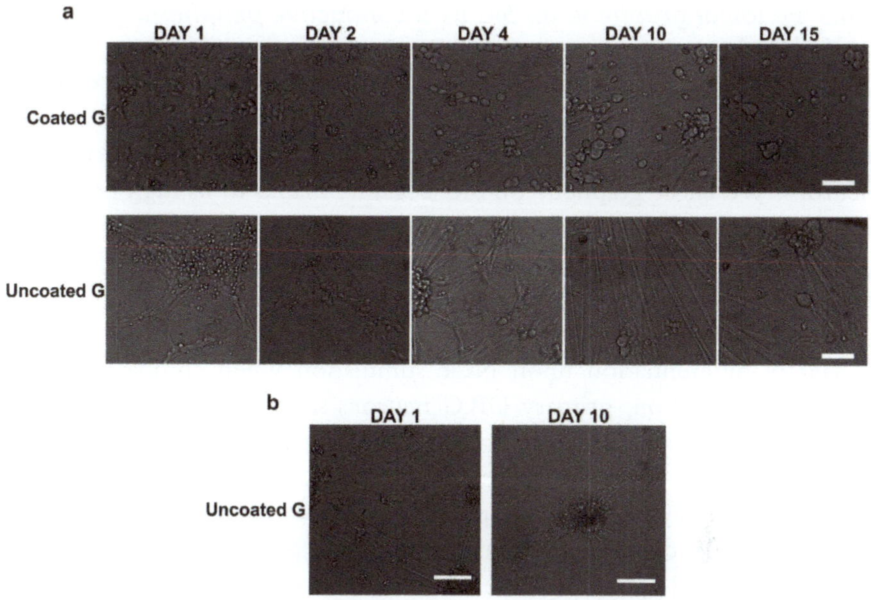

Figure 3.11 DRG neurons cultured on bare substrates. (A) DRG neurons cultured on coated and uncoated graphene versus culture day. Scale bar: 50 μm. (B) Cell body aggregates and neurite bundles on uncoated graphene. Scale bar: 100 μm. *(Adapted from Ref. [23].)*

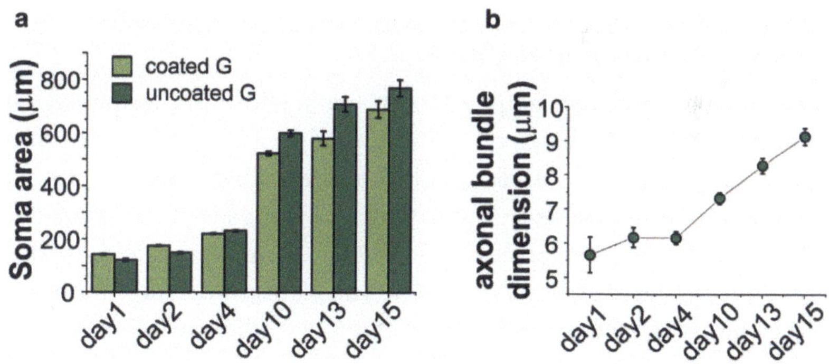

Figure 3.12 DRG neurons cultured on bare substrates. (A) Increase of the cell body area with time of DRG cells on coated and uncoated graphene. (B) Quantification of axonal bundle dimension on uncoated graphene. The diameter of the axonal bundles was evaluated using ImageJ. Data are reported as mean ± s.e.m. *(Adapted from Ref. [23].)*

3.4.5 Epitaxial graphene on SiC as a conductive peripheral neural interface

Aiming at designing graphene-based biocompatible guides to enhance axonal growth, we investigated the survival and differentiation of two established models for peripheral neurons: PC12 cells and DRG primary neurons. We chose graphene on SiC because, thanks to its high crystalline quality and cleanliness, it allowed us to examine the effect of graphene on peripheral neurons while avoiding spurious effects due to contaminations and defects. Indeed, PC12 cells were found to survive equally on graphene and control substrates, with an increased neurite length (up to 27%) at 5 days of differentiation upon NGF stimulation when compared to the controls. In addition, primary DRG neurons survived on peptide-coated and uncoated graphene until day 17, forming a dense axon network, although with a reduced adhesion. The obtained results confirm the potential of highly crystalline graphene as a cytocompatible active material for nerve guidance conduit devices. Indeed, on graphene peripheral neurons survived and grew longer neurites than on control surfaces. However, graphene on SiC could not satisfy the flexibility required for interfacing soft biological tissue. To use graphene as a neural interface, other graphene production methods, such as CVD and transfer to flexible supports, could be more suitable.

3.5 Local stall of NGF signaling endosomes on graphene as a promoter of axon elongation

Despite the potential of graphene for application in peripheral nerve regeneration, the mechanisms governing neurite outgrowth have not been examined in depth. To understand the mechanistic details by which graphene would promote axon outgrowth, previous studies investigated the use of growth-associated protein-43 (GAP-43), a recognized marker of developing and regenerating axons. The mechanisms driving neurogenesis seemed to be shared for central and peripheral neurons on graphene; in fact increased GAP-43 protein levels were reported both in hippocampal neurons grown on CVD graphene [18] and PC12 cells grown on aligned silk-graphene hybrid hydrogels [95]. However, what causes the increased GAP-43, and what is the graphene influence on the structure and dynamics of neuron development, remains unclear. Knowing that graphene is in contact with the extracellular environment surrounding the neural membrane, a recent study investigated how graphene altered neuronal electric activity [51]. They found that graphene altered the distribution of extra-cellular ions at the interface with hippocampal neurons, generating an increased cell firing. Several studies reported that electrical stimulation could modify cellular behavior and promote axonal outgrowth and branching [20,96,97], thus the observed altered cell firing could have an influence on axonal outgrowth. However, since central and peripheral neurons respond differently on nanofabricated biomaterial scaffolds [98,99], this increased neuronal excitability may not necessarily apply to peripheral neurons on graphene [24].

Although the positive effect of graphene on axonal outgrowth was found to be significantly enhanced during the first 2 days after cell seeding [18], all the studies investigating the mechanisms driving neurogenesis on graphene were carried out on mature cultures, from 1 to 3 weeks. Thus, these works did not investigate graphene's influence on the early developmental stage, giving information only on the long-term effects of graphene on neurons.

In our recent work [24], we investigated the molecular mechanisms driving axon elongation in DRG primary neuron cultures on graphene during the early developmental phase, focusing on the correlation between axonal elongation and axonal transport of NGF. We chose NGF as a key player of the time course of axonal elongation of DRG neurons on graphene, as it is the main neurotrophin supporting survival and development of peripheral neurons [100,101]. Actually, the retrograde axonal transport of NGF inside endosomes along microtubules from the axonal tip to the cell soma is the major mechanism sustaining the survival and neurite outgrowth of neurons [102]. Accordingly, we used CVD graphene grown on Cu then transferred to glass, and then performed single-molecule fluorescence microscopy in living DRG neurons to study NGF axonal transport. We classified the NGF vesicles based on the way they moved: stalled (stl) when they did not move; anterograde (ant) and retrograde (ret), when they moved from the cell soma to the axon tip and vice versa; and oscillating (osc) when the movement of the vesicle switched between retrograde and anterograde within a limited space.

We found that in the first 2 days of culture, the axons were longer on graphene than on the glass control by 79% and 73%, respectively (Fig. 3.13A). Remarkably, this axon elongation on graphene correlates with a significant reduction (8.5-fold reduction) of the retrogradely moving vesicles (ret) at DIV2, in favor of a stalled vesicle population (stl) retained locally in the developing axons (Fig. 3.13B).

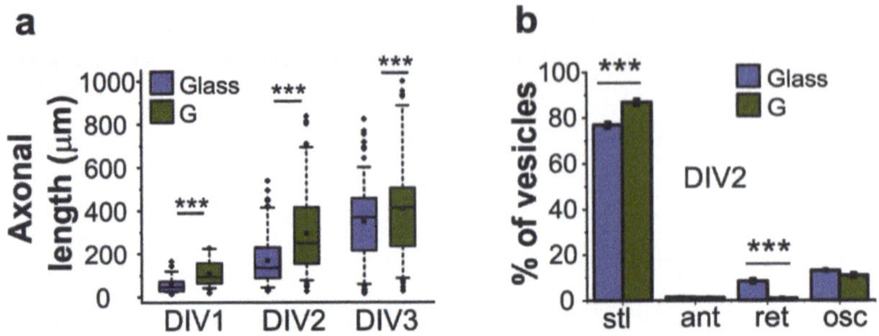

Figure 3.13 Increased axonal elongation and altered axonal transport in DRG neurons grown on graphene. (A) Quantification of the axonal length at different DIV on glass and graphene. A significant difference was found between graphene and control according to Two-way Anova Test. (***P_substrate <0.001, ***P_DIV <0.0001, Two-way Anova). The number of measured axons was as follows: DIV1, glass $n = 42$, graphene $n = 50$; DIV2, glass $n = 109$, graphene $n = 101$; DIV3, glass $n = 147$, graphene $n = 119$; In the box plots, the horizontal line is the median value, boxed area extends from the 25th to 75th percentile, whiskers from the 5th to 95th percentiles, the square is the mean and the circles are outliers. (B) Histograms showing the mean ± s.e.m. of the percentage of vesicles for each population at DIV2 of the independent cultures. Vesicles were classified into four categories: stalled (stl), retrograde (ret), anterograde (ant), and oscillating (osc). The percentage of stalled and retrograde vesicles on graphene at DIV2 were significantly different from the control (***$P < .0001$, One-way Anova, with Bonferroni's Multiple Comparison Test). The number of vesicles at DIV2 in three independent cultures was 3604 for graphene and 5188 for glass. *(Adapted from Ref. [24].)*

We then investigated both the possible electrophysiological and structural changes prompted by graphene to find possible causes for the observed altered NGF trafficking, showing a reduced cell excitability and an altered axon morphology with longer and straighter axonal bundles [24]. Interestingly, all these effects are gradually reduced with time, stabilizing the percentage of increased axonal elongation at lower values already after 3 days of culture (17%), and reaching an excitability and axonal transport comparable to the control after 5 days of culture.

4. Summary

Despite the high potential of graphene for several biomedical applications, including regenerative medicine, only a few studies in the last years have been focusing on interfacing graphene with peripheral neurons. In this chapter, we have discussed the effect of graphene on the adhesion, proliferation, and differentiation of neural cells, focusing in particular on epitaxial graphene. Neurons survived on graphene, both in the uncoated and coated forms. Interestingly, when coated with polymers, graphene prompted a diverse distribution on the polymeric coatings, with different roughness and morphology at the nanometric scale. Epitaxial graphene was able to support the adhesion and growth of two models for peripheral neurons, PC12 cells and DRG primary neurons, inducing an increased neurite length with respect to controls. The increased neurite sprouting and outgrowth makes graphene appealing for applications in peripheral nerve regeneration, as ideal scaffolds should indeed have such beneficial effects. On the other hand, the molecular players behind axon elongation on graphene were analyzed, revealing an altered NGF axonal transport, together with electrophysiological and structural changes prompted by the material—neuron interface. The obtained results indicate a possible avenue for the use of highly crystalline graphene as an active substrate in conduit devices for nerve guidance. Indeed, graphene would also allow for the transmission of electrical signals between neurons and make external electrical stimulation feasible to enhance axon regeneration [103,104]. Undoubtedly, more studies are needed to better understand both the molecular and electrophysiological mechanisms that regulate graphene—neurons interaction and design optimal biocompatible guides to enhance axonal regeneration.

References

[1] G. Hussain, et al., Current status of therapeutic approaches against peripheral nerve injuries: a detailed story from injury to recovery, International Journal of Biological Sciences 16 (1) (2020) 116—134, https://doi.org/10.7150/ijbs.35653.

[2] A. Faroni, S.A. Mobasseri, P.J. Kingham, A.J. Reid, Peripheral nerve regeneration: experimental strategies and future perspectives, Advanced Drug Delivery Reviews 82 (2015) 160—167, https://doi.org/10.1016/j.addr.2014.11.010.

[3] R. Rebowe, A. Rogers, X. Yang, S.C.K. Thomas, L.S. Zhongyu, Nerve Repair with Nerve Conduits : Problems , Solutions , and Future Directions, 2018.

[4] A.C. Pinho, A.C. Fonseca, A.C. Serra, J.D. Santos, J.F.J. Coelho, Peripheral nerve regeneration : current status and new strategies using polymeric materials, Advanced Healthcare Materials 5 (21) (2016) 2732—2744, https://doi.org/10.1002/adhm.201600236.

[5] X. Gu, F. Ding, D.F. Williams, Neural tissue engineering options for peripheral nerve regeneration, Biomaterials 35 (24) (2014) 6143—6156, https://doi.org/10.1016/j.biomaterials.2014.04.064.

[6] R. López-Cebral, J. Silva-Correia, R.L. Reis, T.H. Silva, J.M. Oliveira, Peripheral nerve injury: current challenges, conventional treatment approaches, and new trends in biomaterials-based regenerative strategies, ACS Biomaterials Science and Engineering 3 (12) (2017) 3098—3122, https://doi.org/10.1021/acsbiomaterials.7b00655.

[7] M. Chighizola, T. Dini, C. Lenardi, P. Milani, A. Podestà, C. Schulte, Mechanotransduction in neuronal cell development and functioning, Biophysics Reviews 11 (5) (2019) 701–720, https://doi.org/10.1007/s12551-019-00587-2.
[8] I. Tonazzini, A. Cecchini, Y. Elgersma, M. Cecchini, Interaction of SH-SY5Y cells with nanogratings during neuronal differentiation: comparison with primary neurons, Advanced Healthcare Materials 3 (4) (2014) 581–587, https://doi.org/10.1002/adhm.201300216.
[9] A. Fraczek-Szczypta, Carbon nanomaterials for nerve tissue stimulation and regeneration, Materials Science and Engineering C 34 (1) (2014) 35–49, https://doi.org/10.1016/j.msec.2013.09.038.
[10] D. Bitounis, H. Ali-Boucetta, B.H. Hong, D.H. Min, K. Kostarelos, Prospects and challenges of graphene in biomedical applications, Advanced Materials 25 (16) (2013) 2258–2268, https://doi.org/10.1002/adma.201203700.
[11] K.S. Novoselov, et al., Electric field effect in atomically thin carbon films, Science 306 (5696) (2004) 666–669, https://doi.org/10.1126/science.1102896.
[12] A.H. Castro Neto, F. Guinea, N.M.R. Peres, K.S. Novoselov, A.K. Geim, The electronic properties of graphene, Reviews of Modern Physics 81 (1) (2009) 109–162, https://doi.org/10.1103/RevModPhys.81.109.
[13] A.A. Balandin, Thermal properties of graphene and nanostructured carbon materials, Nature Materials 10 (8) (2011) 569–581, https://doi.org/10.1038/nmat3064.
[14] R.R. Nair, et al., Fine structure constant defines visual transparency of graphene, Science 320 (5881) (2008) 1308, https://doi.org/10.1126/science.1156965.
[15] C. Lee, X. Wei, J.W. Kysar, J. Hone, Measurement of the elastic properties and intrinsic strength of monolayer graphene, Science 321 (5887) (2008) 385–388, https://doi.org/10.1126/science.1157996.
[16] K.S. Novoselov, V.I. Fal'Ko, L. Colombo, P.R. Gellert, M.G. Schwab, K. Kim, A roadmap for graphene, Nature 490 (7419) (2012) 192–200, https://doi.org/10.1038/nature11458.
[17] S.M. Lee, J.H. Kim, J.H. Ahn, Graphene as a flexible electronic material: mechanical limitations by defect formation and efforts to overcome, Materials Today 18 (6) (2015) 336–344, https://doi.org/10.1016/j.mattod.2015.01.017.
[18] N. Li, et al., The promotion of neurite sprouting and outgrowth of mouse hippocampal cells in culture by graphene substrates, Biomaterials 32 (35) (2011) 9374–9382, https://doi.org/10.1016/j.biomaterials.2011.08.065.
[19] S.Y. Park, et al., Enhanced differentiation of human neural stem cells into neurons on graphene, Advanced Materials 23 (36) (2011) 263–267, https://doi.org/10.1002/adma.201101503.
[20] S. Meng, Nerve cell differentiation using constant and programmed electrical stimulation through conductive non-functional graphene nanosheets film, Tissue Engineering and Regenerative Medicine 11 (4) (2014) 274–283, https://doi.org/10.1007/s13770-014-0011-1.
[21] S.W. Hong, et al., Enhanced neural cell adhesion and neurite outgrowth on graphene-based biomimetic substrates, BioMed Research International 2014 (2014), https://doi.org/10.1155/2014/212149.
[22] S.M. Frahs, et al., Prechondrogenic ATDC5 cell attachment and differentiation on graphene foam; modulation by surface functionalization with fibronectin, ACS Applied Materials & Interfaces 11 (45) (Nov. 2019) 41906–41924, https://doi.org/10.1021/acsami.9b14670.
[23] D. Convertino, S. Luin, L. Marchetti, C. Coletti, Peripheral neuron survival and outgrowth on graphene, Frontiers in Neuroscience 12 (2018) 1–8, https://doi.org/10.3389/fnins.2018.00001.

[24] D. Convertino, et al., Graphene promotes axon elongation through local stall of Nerve Growth Factor signaling endosomes, Nano Letters (2020), https://doi.org/10.1021/acs.nanolett.0c00571.

[25] A.E. Jakus, E.B. Secor, A.L. Rutz, S.W. Jordan, M.C. Hersam, R.N. Shah, Three-dimensional printing of high-content graphene scaffolds for electronic and biomedical applications, ACS Nano 9 (4) (2015) 4636–4648, https://doi.org/10.1021/acsnano.5b01179.

[26] X. Liu, et al., Functionalized carbon nanotube and graphene oxide embedded electrically conductive hydrogel synergistically stimulates nerve cell differentiation, ACS Applied Materials & Interfaces 9 (17) (2017) 14677–14690, https://doi.org/10.1021/acsami.7b02072.

[27] Y. Qian, X. Zhao, Q. Han, W. Chen, H. Li, W. Yuan, An integrated multi-layer 3D-fabrication of PDA/RGD coated graphene loaded PCL nanoscaffold for peripheral nerve restoration, Nature Communications 9 (1) (2018), https://doi.org/10.1038/s41467-017-02598-7.

[28] S. Agarwal, et al., Interfacing live cells with nanocarbon substrates, Langmuir 26 (4) (2010) 2244–2247, https://doi.org/10.1021/la9048743.

[29] M. Bramini, et al., Graphene oxide nanosheets disrupt lipid composition, Ca^{2+} homeostasis, and synaptic transmission in primary cortical neurons, ACS Nano 10 (7) (2016) 7154–7171, https://doi.org/10.1021/acsnano.6b03438.

[30] C. Defterali, et al., In vitro evaluation of biocompatibility of uncoated thermally reduced graphene and carbon nanotube-loaded PVDF membranes with adult neural stem cell-derived neurons and glia, Frontiers in Bioengineering and Biotechnology 4 (2016) 1–19, https://doi.org/10.3389/fbioe.2016.00094.

[31] A. Fabbro, et al., Graphene-Based interfaces do not alter target nerve cells, ACS Nano 10 (1) (2016) 615–623, https://doi.org/10.1021/acsnano.5b05647.

[32] R. Rauti, et al., Graphene oxide nanosheets reshape synaptic function in cultured brain networks, ACS Nano 10 (4) (2016) 4459–4471, https://doi.org/10.1021/acsnano.6b00130.

[33] M. Chiacchiaretta, et al., Graphene oxide upregulates the homeostatic functions of primary astrocytes and modulates astrocyte-to-neuron communication, Nano Letters 18 (9) (Sep. 2018) 5827–5838, https://doi.org/10.1021/acs.nanolett.8b02487.

[34] X. Ji, Y. Xu, W. Zhang, L. Cui, J. Liu, Review of functionalization, structure and properties of graphene/polymer composite fibers, Composites Part A: Applied Science and Manufacturing 87 (2016) 29–45, https://doi.org/10.1016/j.compositesa.2016.04.011.

[35] S. Pezzini, et al., High-quality electrical transport using scalable CVD graphene, 2D Materials 7 (4) (2020), https://doi.org/10.1088/2053-1583/aba645.

[36] W.A. de Heer, et al., Large area and structured epitaxial graphene produced by confinement controlled sublimation of silicon carbide, Proceedings of the National Academy of Sciences of the United States of America 108 (41) (2011) 16900–16905, https://doi.org/10.1073/pnas.1105113108.

[37] U. Starke, S. Forti, K. V Emtsev, C. Coletti, Engineering the electronic structure of epitaxial graphene by transfer doping and atomic intercalation, MRS Bulletin 37 (12) (2012) 1177–1186, https://doi.org/10.1557/mrs.2012.272.

[38] C.E. Schmidt, V.R. Shastri, J.P. Vacanti, R. Langer, Stimulation of neurite outgrowth using an electrically conducting polymer, Proceedings of the National Academy of Sciences of the United States of America 94 (17) (1997) 8948–8953, https://doi.org/10.1073/pnas.94.17.8948.

[39] M. Levin, Large-scale biophysics: ion flows and regeneration, Trends in Cell Biology 17 (6) (2007) 261–270, https://doi.org/10.1016/j.tcb.2007.04.007.

[40] S. Sundelacruz, C. Li, Y.J. Choi, M. Levin, D.L. Kaplan, Bioelectric modulation of wound healing in a 3D invitro model of tissue-engineered bone, Biomaterials 34 (28) (2013) 6695–6705, https://doi.org/10.1016/j.biomaterials.2013.05.040.
[41] M. Deng, et al., Electrochemical deposition of polypyrrole/graphene oxide composite on microelectrodes towards tuning the electrochemical properties of neural probes, Sensors & Actuators, B: Chemical 158 (1) (2011) 176–184, https://doi.org/10.1016/j.snb.2011.05.062.
[42] K. Kostarelos, M. Vincent, C. Hebert, J.A. Garrido, Graphene in the design and engineering of next-generation neural interfaces, Advanced Materials 29 (42) (2017) 1–7, https://doi.org/10.1002/adma.201700909.
[43] G. Reina, J.M. González-Domínguez, A. Criado, E. Vázquez, A. Bianco, M. Prato, Promises, Facts and Challenges for Graphene in Biomedical Applications, Chem. Soc. Rev., 2017, pp. 4400–4416, https://doi.org/10.1039/C7CS00363C.
[44] C.J. Bullock, C. Bussy, Biocompatibility considerations in the design of graphene biomedical materials, Advanced Materials Interfaces 6 (11) (2019), https://doi.org/10.1002/admi.201900229.
[45] L. Yan, et al., Chemistry and physics of a single atomic layer: strategies and challenges for functionalization of graphene and graphene-based materials, Chemical Society Reviews 41 (1) (2012) 97–114, https://doi.org/10.1039/c1cs15193b.
[46] D. Kuzum, et al., Transparent and flexible low noise graphene electrodes for simultaneous electrophysiology and neuroimaging, Nature Communications 5 (2014) 1–10, https://doi.org/10.1038/ncomms6259.
[47] T. Das, B.K. Sharma, A.K. Katiyar, J.H. Ahn, Graphene-based flexible and wearable electronics, Journal of Semiconductors 39 (1) (2018), https://doi.org/10.1088/1674-4926/39/1/011007.
[48] P. Bøggild, et al., Mapping the electrical properties of large-area graphene, 2D Materials 4 (4) (2017), https://doi.org/10.1088/2053-1583/aa8683.
[49] C. Heo, et al., The control of neural cell-to-cell interactions through non-contact electrical field stimulation using graphene electrodes, Biomaterials 32 (1) (2011) 19–27, https://doi.org/10.1016/j.biomaterials.2010.08.095.
[50] J.H. Lee, et al., Enhanced neurite outgrowth of PC-12 cells on graphene-monolayer-coated substrates as biomimetic cues, Journal of the Korean Physical Society 61 (10) (2012) 1696–1699, https://doi.org/10.3938/jkps.61.1696.
[51] N.P. Pampaloni, et al., Single-layer graphene modulates neuronal communication and augments membrane ion currents, Nature Nanotechnology 13 (8) (2018) 755–764, https://doi.org/10.1038/s41565-018-0163-6.
[52] D.W. Park, et al., Graphene-based carbon-layered electrode array technology for neural imaging and optogenetic applications, Nature Communications 5 (2014) 1–11, https://doi.org/10.1038/ncomms6258.
[53] C. Hébert, et al., Flexible graphene solution-gated field-effect transistors: efficient transducers for micro-electrocorticography, Advanced Functional Materials 28 (12) (2018) 1–15, https://doi.org/10.1002/adfm.201703976.
[54] S.H. Ku, M. Lee, C.B. Park, Carbon-based nanomaterials for tissue engineering, Advanced Healthcare Materials 2 (2) (2013) 244–260, https://doi.org/10.1002/adhm.201200307.
[55] X. Ding, H. Liu, Y. Fan, Graphene-based materials in regenerative medicine, Advanced Healthcare Materials 4 (10) (2015) 1451–1468, https://doi.org/10.1002/adhm.201500203.
[56] M. Tang, Q. Song, N. Li, Z. Jiang, R. Huang, G. Cheng, Enhancement of electrical signaling in neural networks on graphene films, Biomaterials 34 (27) (2013) 6402–6411, https://doi.org/10.1016/j.biomaterials.2013.05.024.

[57] R. Guo, et al., Accelerating bioelectric functional development of neural stem cells by graphene coupling: implications for neural interfacing with conductive materials, Biomaterials 106 (2016) 193–204, https://doi.org/10.1016/j.biomaterials.2016.08.019.
[58] Y. Sun, et al., Surface coating as a key parameter in engineering neuronal network structures in vitro, Biointerphases 7 (1) (2012) 29, https://doi.org/10.1007/s13758-012-0029-7.
[59] A. Bendali, et al., Purified neurons can survive on peptide-free graphene layers, Advanced Healthcare Materials 2 (7) (2013) 929–933, https://doi.org/10.1002/adhm.201200347.
[60] D. Sahni, et al., Biocompatibility of pristine graphene for neuronal interface, Journal of Neurosurgery: Pediatrics 11 (2013) 575–583.
[61] F. Veliev, A. Briançon-Marjollet, V. Bouchiat, C. Delacour, Impact of crystalline quality on neuronal affinity of pristine graphene, Biomaterials 86 (2016) 33–41, https://doi.org/10.1016/j.biomaterials.2016.01.042.
[62] T. Hoshiba, C.S. Cho, A. Murakawa, Y. Okahata, T. Akaike, The effect of natural extracellular matrix deposited on synthetic polymers on cultured primary hepatocytes, Biomaterials 27 (26) (2006) 4519–4528, https://doi.org/10.1016/j.biomaterials.2006.04.014.
[63] P.N. First, W.A. de Heer, T. Seyller, C. Berger, J.A. Stroscio, J.-S. Moon, Epitaxial graphenes on silicon carbide, MRS Bulletin 35 (4) (2010) 296–305, https://doi.org/10.1557/mrs2010.552.
[64] C. Berger, et al., Electronic confinement and coherence in patterned epitaxial graphene, Science 312 (5777) (2006) 1191–1196, https://doi.org/10.1126/science.1125925.
[65] Q. Yu, J. Lian, S. Siriponglert, H. Li, Y.P. Chen, S.-S. Pei, Graphene segregated on Ni surfaces and transferred to insulators, Applied Physics Letters 93 (2008) 113103, https://doi.org/10.1063/1.2982585.
[66] X. Li, et al., Large area synthesis of high quality and uniform graphene films on copper foils, Science 324 (5932) (2009) 1312–1314, https://doi.org/10.1126/science.1171245.
[67] V. Miseikis, et al., Deterministic patterned growth of high-mobility large-crystal graphene: a path towards wafer scale integration, 2D Materials 4 (2) (2017), https://doi.org/10.1088/2053-1583/aa5481.
[68] K.V. Emtsev, et al., Towards wafer-size graphene layers by atmospheric pressure graphitization of silicon carbide, Nature Materials 8 (3) (2009) 203–207, https://doi.org/10.1038/nmat2382.
[69] C. Riedl, C. Coletti, T. Iwasaki, A.A. Zakharov, U. Starke, Quasi-free-standing epitaxial graphene on SiC obtained by hydrogen intercalation, Physical Review Letters 103 (24) (2009) 1–4, https://doi.org/10.1103/PhysRevLett.103.246804.
[70] K.V. Emtsev, F. Speck, T. Seyller, L. Ley, J.D. Riley, Interaction, growth, and ordering of epitaxial graphene on SiC{0001} surfaces: a comparative photoelectron spectroscopy study, Physical Review B: Condensed Matter and Materials Physics 77 (15) (2008) 1–10, https://doi.org/10.1103/PhysRevB.77.155303.
[71] C. Riedl, C. Coletti, U. Starke, Structural and electronic properties of epitaxial graphene on SiC(0001): a review of growth, characterization, transfer doping and hydrogen intercalation, Journal of Physics D 43 (37) (2010), https://doi.org/10.1088/0022-3727/43/37/374009.
[72] J.A. Robinson, M. Hollander, M. Labella, K.A. Trumbull, R. Cavalero, D.W. Snyder, Epitaxial graphene transistors: enhancing performance via hydrogen intercalation, Nano Letters 11 (9) (2011) 3875–3880, https://doi.org/10.1021/nl2019855.

[73] D. Convertino, A. Rossi, V. Miseikis, V. Piazza, C. Coletti, Thermal decomposition and chemical vapor deposition: a comparative study of multi-layer growth of graphene on SiC(000-1), MRS Advances 1 (55) (2016) 3667–3672, https://doi.org/10.1557/adv.2016.369.

[74] W. Strupinski, et al., Graphene epitaxy by chemical vapor deposition on SiC, Nano Letters 11 (4) (2011) 1786–1791, https://doi.org/10.1021/nl200390e.

[75] C. Berger, et al., Ultrathin epitaxial graphite: 2D electron gas properties and a route toward graphene-based nanoelectronics, Journal of Physical Chemistry B 108 (52) (2004) 19912–19916, https://doi.org/10.1021/jp040650f.

[76] H. Hibino, H. Kageshima, F. Maeda, M. Nagase, Y. Kobayashi, H. Yamaguchi, Microscopic thickness determination of thin graphite films formed on SiC from quantized oscillation in reflectivity of low-energy electrons, Physical Review B: Condensed Matter and Materials Physics 77 (7) (2008) 1–7, https://doi.org/10.1103/PhysRevB.77.075413.

[77] F. Bianco, et al., Terahertz detection by epitaxial-graphene field-effect-transistors on silicon carbide, Applied Physics Letters 107 (13) (2015) 131104, https://doi.org/10.1063/1.4932091.

[78] A. Candini, et al., High photoresponsivity in graphene nanoribbon field-effect transistor devices contacted with graphene electrodes, Journal of Physical Chemistry C 121 (19) (2017) 10620–10625, https://doi.org/10.1021/acs.jpcc.7b03401.

[79] V. Ramachandran, M.F. Brady, a.R. Smith, R.M. Feenstra, D.W. Greve, Preparation of atomically flat surfaces on silicon carbide using hydrogen etching, Journal of Electronic Materials 27 (4) (1998) 308–312, https://doi.org/10.1007/s11664-998-0406-7.

[80] C.L. Frewin, C. Coletti, C. Riedl, U. Starke, S.E. Saddow, A comprehensive study of hydrogen etching on the major SiC polytypes and crystal orientations, Materials Science Forum 615–617 (2009) 589–592, https://doi.org/10.4028/www.scientific.net/MSF.615-617.589, no. July 2015.

[81] C. Coletti, M.J. Jaroszeski, A. Pallaoro, A.M. Hoff, S. Iannotta, S.E. Saddow, Biocompatibility and wettability of crystalline SiC and Si surfaces, Annual International Conference of the IEEE Engineering in Medicine and Biology Society (2007) 5849–5852, https://doi.org/10.1109/IEMBS.2007.4353678.

[82] J.W. Chen, et al., Efficient n-type doping in epitaxial graphene through strong lateral orbital hybridization of Ti adsorbate, Carbon N. Y. 109 (2016) 300–305, https://doi.org/10.1016/j.carbon.2016.08.006.

[83] T. Mashoff, et al., Increasing the active surface of titanium islands on graphene by nitrogen sputtering, Applied Physics Letters 106 (8) (2015), https://doi.org/10.1063/1.4913562.

[84] J. Kang, et al., MBE growth of self-assisted InAs nanowires on graphene, Semiconductor Science and Technology 31 (11) (2016) 115005, https://doi.org/10.1088/0268-1242/31/11/115005.

[85] C. Coletti, et al., Charge neutrality and band-gap tuning of epitaxial graphene on SiC by molecular doping, Physical Review B 81 (23) (2010) 235401, https://doi.org/10.1103/PhysRevB.81.235401.

[86] Y.H. Kim, N.S. Baek, Y.H. Han, M.A. Chung, S.D. Jung, Enhancement of neuronal cell adhesion by covalent binding of poly-d-lysine, Journal of Neuroscience Methods 202 (1) (2011) 38–44, https://doi.org/10.1016/j.jneumeth.2011.08.036.

[87] L.A. Greene, A.S. Tischler, PC12 Pheochromocytoma Cultures in Neurobiological Research, vol. 3, Accademic Press, New York, 1982.

[88] S. Wang, Y. Zhang, N. Abidi, L. Cabrales, Wettability and surface free energy of graphene films, Langmuir 25 (18) (2009) 11078–11081, https://doi.org/10.1021/la901402f.

[89] A. Oliveros, C. Coletti, C.L. Frewin, C. Locke, U. Starke, S.E. Saddow, Cellular interactions on epitaxial graphene on SiC (0001) substrates, Materials Science Forum 679–680 (2011) 831–834, https://doi.org/10.4028/www.scientific.net/MSF.679-680.831.
[90] S. Neumann, C.J. Woolf, Regeneration of dorsal column fibers into and beyond the lesion site following adult spinal cord injury, Neuron 23 (1) (1999) 83–91, https://doi.org/10.1016/S0896-6273(00)80755-2.
[91] L. Marchetti, et al., Site-specific labeling of neurotrophins and their receptors via short and versatile peptide tags, PLoS One 9 (11) (2014) 1–18, https://doi.org/10.1371/journal.pone.0113708.
[92] J.S. Lee, et al., Graphene substrate for inducing neurite outgrowth, Biochemical and Biophysical Research Communications 460 (2) (2015) 267–273, https://doi.org/10.1016/j.bbrc.2015.03.023.
[93] K. Wang, et al., Biocompatibility of graphene oxide, Nanoscale Research Letters 6 (1) (2011) 1–8, https://doi.org/10.1007/s11671-010-9751-6.
[94] S. Keshavan, S. Naskar, A. Diaspro, L. Cancedda, S. Dante, Developmental refinement of synaptic transmission on micropatterned single layer graphene, Acta Biomaterialia 65 (2018) 363–375, https://doi.org/10.1016/j.actbio.2017.11.005.
[95] L. Wang, et al., Silk-graphene hybrid hydrogels with multiple cues to induce nerve cell behavior, ACS Biomaterials Science and Engineering 5 (2) (2019) 613–622, https://doi.org/10.1021/acsbiomaterials.8b01481.
[96] N. Uesaka, S. Hirai, T. Maruyama, E. Ruthazer, Y. Nobuhiko, Activity dependence of cortical axon branch formation: a morphological and electrophysiological study using organotypic slice cultures, The Journal of Neuroscience 25 (1) (2005) 1–9, https://doi.org/10.1523/JNEUROSCI.3855-04.2005.
[97] B. Singh, et al., Accelerated axon outgrowth, guidance, and target reinnervation across nerve transection gaps following a brief electrical stimulation paradigm: laboratory investigation, Journal of Neurosurgery 116 (3) (2012) 498–512, https://doi.org/10.3171/2011.10.JNS11612.
[98] J.Y. Lee, C.A. Bashur, N. Gomez, A.S. Goldstein, C.E. Schmidt, Enhanced polarization of embryonic hippocampal neurons on micron scale electrospun fibers, Journal of Biomedical Materials Research Part A 92 (4) (2010) 1398–1406, https://doi.org/10.1002/jbm.a.32471.
[99] J.L. Bourke, H.A. Coleman, V. Pham, J.S. Forsythe, H.C. Parkington, Neuronal electrophysiological function and control of neurite outgrowth on electrospun polymer nanofibers are cell type dependent, Tissue Engineering, Part A 20 (5–6) (2013) 1089–1095, https://doi.org/10.1089/ten.tea.2013.0295.
[100] W.D. Snider, Dorsal root ganglion neurons require functional neurotrophin receptors for survival during development, Philosophical Transactions of the Royal Society B: Biological Sciences 351 (1338) (1996) 395–403, https://doi.org/10.1098/rstb.1996.0034.
[101] S.I. Lentz, C.M. Knudson, S.J. Korsmeyer, W.D. Snider, Neurotrophins support the development of diverse sensory axon morphologies, The Journal of Neuroscience 19 (3) (1999) 1038–1048.
[102] B. Cui, et al., One at a time, live tracking of NGF axonal transport using quantum dots, Proceedings of the National Academy of Sciences 104 (34) (2007) 13666–13671, https://doi.org/10.1073/pnas.0706192104.
[103] Y. Lu, X. Liu, D. Kuzum, Graphene-based neurotechnologies for advanced neural interfaces, Current Opinion in Biomedical Engineering 6 (2018) 138–147, https://doi.org/10.1016/j.cobme.2018.06.001.
[104] J. Wang, et al., In vitro and in vivo studies of electroactive reduced graphene oxide-modified nanofiber scaffolds for peripheral nerve regeneration, Acta Biomaterialia 84 (2019) 98–113, https://doi.org/10.1016/j.actbio.2018.11.032.

CHAPTER 4

SiC protective coating for photovoltaic retinal prostheses

Xin Lei[1,a], Sheryl Kane[2,b], Stuart Cogan[3], Henri Lorach[4,c], Ludwig Galambos[5], Philip Huie[6,7], Keith Mathieson[8], Theodore Kamins[5], James Harris[5] and Daniel Palanker[6,7]

[1]Department of Electrical Engineering, Stanford University, Stanford, CA, United States; [2]EIC Laboratories, Norwood, MA, United States; [3]University of Texas at Dallas, Richardson, TX, United States; [4]Hansen Experimental Physics Laboratory, Stanford University, Stanford, CA, United States; [5]Department of Electrical Engineering, Stanford University, Stanford, CA, United States; [6]Hansen Experimental Physics Laboratory, Stanford University, Stanford, CA, United States; [7]Department of Ophthalmology, Stanford University, Stanford, CA, United States; [8]Institute of Photonics, University of Strathclyde, Glasgow, Scotland, United Kingdom

Contents

1. Introduction

The spectrum of implantable electro-neural interfaces for the restoration and control of sensory, motor, and other brain functions is rapidly expanding. Examples include cochlear implants [1–3], deep brain stimulators [4–7], cortical motor prostheses [8–10], cortical visual prostheses [11,12], and retinal prostheses [13–17], among others. Retinal degenerative

[a] Present address: Flexcompute, Boston, MA, United States
[b] Present address: Takeda, Boston, MA, United States
[c] Present address: NeuroRestore, Lausanne, Switzerland

Silicon Carbide Technology for Advanced Human Healthcare Applications
ISBN 978-0-323-90609-8
https://doi.org/10.1016/B978-0-323-90609-8.00008-9

diseases lead to loss of photoreceptors, while neurons in the inner retinal layers are largely preserved. Retinal prostheses seek to restore sight by reintroducing visual information via electrical stimulation of the surviving neurons in the retina. Photovoltaic retinal prosthesis consists of silicon photodiodes in each pixel of the subretinal array, which convert pulsed near-infrared illumination projected from video goggles into an electric current to stimulate the nearby neurons.

The majority of electrical implants employ metal or ceramic enclosures with cable feed-throughs to protect the electronics from exposure to body fluids and associated corrosion [10,14,15,18]. This approach results in rather bulky implants and difficult surgeries that involve separate placements for the power supplies and electrode arrays, and routing of interconnecting cables. Our group developed a silicon photodiode array implanted subretinally for restoration of sight to patients blinded by degenerative retinal diseases, such as age-related macular degeneration and retinitis pigmentosa [16,17]. With pulsed near-infrared light providing both power and visual information, the implant is completely wireless, greatly reducing implant size and simplifying surgery.

As this implant is not packaged in a hermetic metal enclosure, it is exposed to body fluids. Without an optimized protective coating, the device remained functional in short term (under 1 year) during both in vitro and in vivo studies, but with detectable degradation. For long-term in vivo use of integrated circuit (IC) and microelectromechanical systems (MEMS)-based biomedical devices, a biocompatible encapsulation layer is necessary to provide stable protection against water and ion ingress.

Dielectric materials deposited by low-pressure chemical vapor deposition (LPCVD) at high temperatures (800–900°C) have exhibited good stability and barrier properties in long-term in vivo studies [19–21]. However, such temperatures are incompatible with the encapsulation of silicon ICs. Development of an encapsulation layer, which can be deposited at temperatures below 400°C, would be tremendously beneficial as it would allow its use for the protection of Si ICs [22]. Low-temperature (395°C) LPCVD silicon oxide (SiO_2) implanted subretinally in rabbits was found to dissolve after 6–12 months [23]. Polymers, such as Parylene, are used in the medical industry for the encapsulation of neural implants [24–26]. Due to its low relative permittivity, high resistivity, biocompatibility, and conformal deposition, Parylene is suitable as an electrical isolation material for implantable devices for short-term implantation. Adhesion of Parylene to inorganic substrates can be improved by the use of an adhesion promoter and thermal treatment [27]. However, Parylene has a relatively high water vapor transmission rate compared to many dielectric materials [26,28]; therefore, Parylene by itself is not sufficient to protect implanted ICs. Atomic layer deposited Al_2O_3 is conformal and hermetic, yet found to dissolve in water [26,29]. An Al_2O_3 and Parylene bilayer structure was proposed to improve its resistance to moisture and the encapsulation lifetime [26]. Diamond-like carbon coatings [30] and ultra-nanocrystalline diamond coatings [31—33] have demonstrated biocompatibility, resistance to corrosion and wear, and are being used in medical implants, with some concerns regarding delamination in an aqueous environment caused by high residual stress, leakage current, pinholes near sharp corners, and a relatively high deposition temperature.

As an alternative, amorphous silicon carbide (*a*-SiC:H) deposited at a low temperature was proposed as a protective coating due to its availability in semiconductor processing, compatibility with IC technology, biocompatibility [34—36], contamination barrier properties [37—40], and low dissolution rate in saline, compared to other commonly used dielectric materials for IC passivation, such as silicon nitride (SiN_x) and low-temperature SiO_2 [41—44].

In this chapter, we review our recent results on a photovoltaic subretinal prosthesis and the evaluation of its *a*-SiC protective coating. We implanted retinal prosthetic devices for up to 1 year and characterized their degradation by optical and scanning electron microscopy (SEM) to assess the device failure mechanisms in vivo. We also measured the dissolution rates of *a*-SiC, SiN_x, and thermal SiO_2 in accelerated soaking tests to compare the stability of those dielectric materials. We revealed and analyzed the defects in *a*-SiC films, and defined the optimal thickness of the *a*-SiC coating for reliable protection of chronic implants.

2. Design and fabrication of a retinal prosthesis

The Stanford retinal prosthetic system consists of three major components: a pair of goggles with a camera, an image processor, and an implanted photodiode array (Fig. 4.1). The head-mounted camera captures the video of the scene, and the optics in the goggles project the processed video stream onto the retina using pulsed near-infrared illumination. The pixels in the subretinally implanted photodiode array convert light into electric current and stimulate the nearby neurons in the retina. Because the only implanted component of the system is the small photodiode array, the

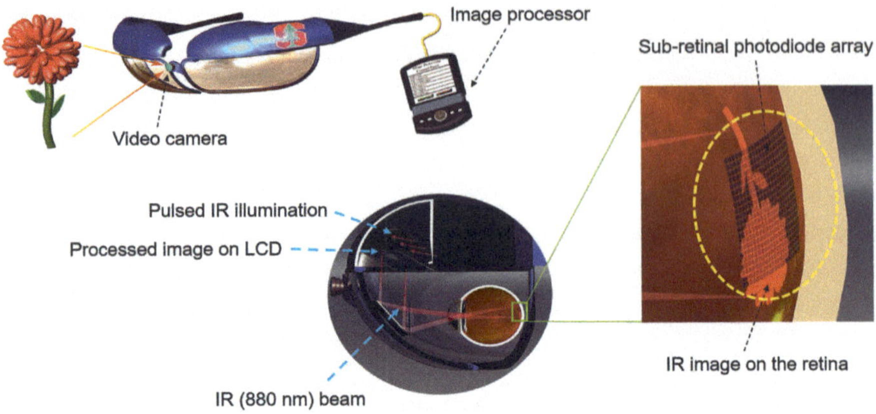

Figure 4.1 Stanford photovoltaic subretinal prosthetic system. The system consists of three major components: goggles with a camera that capture the scene, an image processor that converts the scene to pulsed IR light displayed on the LCD, and an implanted photodiode array that converts the light to electrical current to stimulate neurons in the retina. *(Images from Ref. [16].)*

surgery is greatly simplified in the absence of tethering wires. In addition, as the images are projected onto the photodiode array that is placed under the retina, the link of the visual perception to the natural eye movements is preserved. There are two major reasons to use near-infrared light instead of visible. First, many patients, as in the case of age-related macular degeneration, have remaining vision, therefore the infrared wavelengths will not interfere with the remaining normal vision. This feature enables simultaneous utilization of prosthetic and residual normal vision. From the long end, the near-infrared wavelength range is limited by the silicon material, with its absorption ending near 950 nm.

The prosthetic system is activated by the pulsed near-infrared light (880–915 nm) passing through the transparent neural retina (ganglion cells and the inner nuclear) layer. Light absorbed by the implanted photodiode array generates electric current, which flows from the active to return electrode in each pixel through the inner nuclear layer of the retina. This current stimulates the nearby neurons, which then sends signals to the retinal ganglion cells, and from there signals propagate to the brain through the optic nerve (Fig. 4.2A and B). An equivalent circuit of this system is shown in Fig. 4.2C. The photodiodes (*blue dashed ellipse*) that generate the current are shown at the bottom; the resistor on top (*green dashed ellipse*) describes the electrolyte, and the electrode–electrolyte interface is modeled as a capacitor with parallel and series resistors (*yellow dashed ellipses*). The

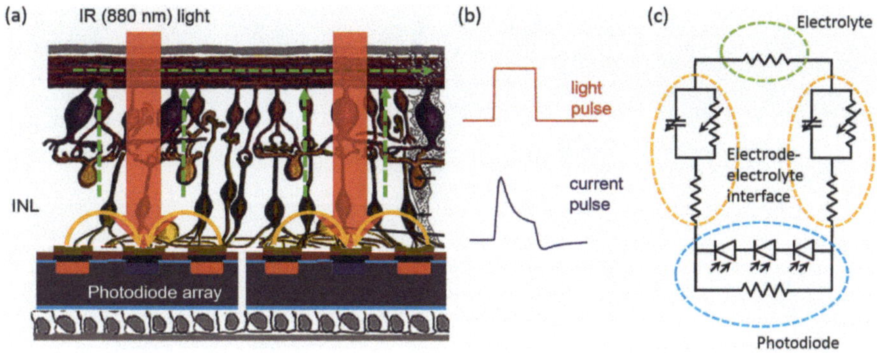

Figure 4.2 Operation of the Stanford photovoltaic subretinal implant. (A) Stimulation mechanism. Incoming near-infrared light is depicted as the downward-pointing *red arrows*. Current generated by the photodiodes is depicted as *orange arrows*. Neural signals are depicted as *green dashed arrows*. (B) Waveforms of the light pulse and the generated current pulse. (C) Equivalent circuitry of the retinal implant in electrolyte. *(Images adapted from Ref. [45].)*

capacitive nature of the electrode—electrolyte interface is a result of the conversion of the electronic current in metal to ionic conduction in the electrolyte. This is also the reason why pulsed rather than continuous light is used for stimulation. During the light pulse, the capacitor of the interface accumulates charge, and it discharges during the dark phase through the reverse current of the photodiode and/or shunt resistor (if it exists), or through the Faradaic resistor (the parallel resistor at the interface). The higher the capacitance of the interface, the more charge can be injected into the electrolyte, thereby enabling more efficient neural stimulation.

Three types of retinal prosthetic implant structures are discussed in this chapter. To minimize confusion, they are denoted as Type I, II, and III, respectively.

Type I structures are retinal prosthetic implants, each consisting of an array of 142 hexagonal pixels, which are 70 μm in width. An individual pixel contains two or three photodiodes connected in series between active and return electrodes. Photodiodes and pixels are isolated by 5 μm-wide trenches filled with undoped polysilicon (Fig. 4.3A). The implants are 1 mm in diameter and 30 μm thick. The main difference in the present devices compared to those previously described [46] is that the electrodes are connected to PN junctions with the opposite polarity—the active electrode connected to the p-type silicon region. This provides anodic-first pulses of current, optimal for subretinal stimulation [18,47].

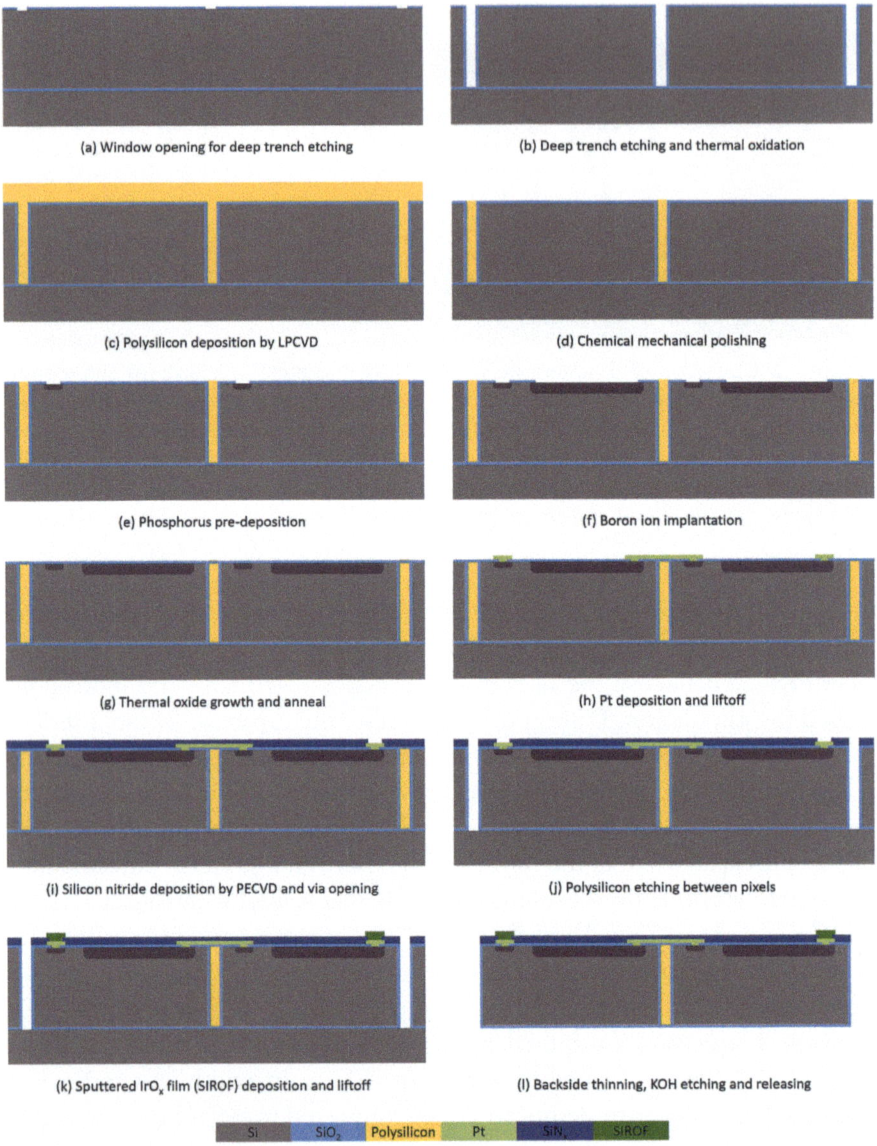

Figure 4.3 Fabrication process of the retinal prosthetic implant (Type I without SiC coating). Fabrication conducted in the SNF using CMOS and MEMS processing methods.

The retinal prosthetic implants were fabricated at Stanford Nanofabrication Facility (SNF) using complementary metal-oxide-semiconductor (CMOS) and MEMS technologies. The fabrication process includes eight lithography steps on silicon-on-insulator wafers with 30 μm silicon device layers, as shown in Fig. 4.3 [48].

To evaluate the effectiveness of the *a*-SiC protective coating, Type I devices were fabricated on two wafers, both having 60 nm of plasma-enhanced chemical vapor deposition (PECVD) SiN_x (Plasma-Therm) on top of 70–80 nm of thermally grown SiO_2 (thermal oxide) on the surface, and one wafer has an additional 240 nm layer of *a*-SiC on the top surface. The backside and sidewalls of all implants were covered with 480 nm of thermally grown SiO_2. Three Type I implants from each wafer were used for in vivo experiments. All of the 142 pixels of each implant were tested.

To facilitate defect analysis of the *a*-SiC coatings, Type II structures were fabricated similarly to Type I devices but on bulk silicon wafers, making the total array thickness ~520 μm. In addition to the 240 nm thick *a*-SiC films, some Type II arrays had thicker *a*-SiC coatings-560 nm. These thick arrays were not used for in vivo experiments.

Type III structures are bulk silicon substrates (520 μm thickness) with 5 μm wide and 33 μm deep trenches etched using the Bosch process (Surface Technology Systems STSetch2) at the SNF. A thermal oxidation at 1000°C for 100 minutes followed the trench etching step to conformally grow 480 nm SiO_2 on the samples. *a*-SiC films of 560 nm thickness were then deposited on the top surface of some samples, and 180 nm-thick *a*-SiC films were deposited on others. Type III structures were used for the defect analysis, but not for in vivo experiments.

3. The degradation of a retinal prosthesis without *a*-SiC coating in vivo

Each of the six Type I retinal prostheses (three with an *a*-SiC coating and three without) were implanted subretinally each in a different rat (six rats in total). The implantation technique was similar to the one previously reported by our group [17,49] and performed in agreement with Stanford University institutional guidelines and the Statement for the Use of Animals in Ophthalmic and Vision Research. After a period of time (from 4 months to 1 year), implants were extracted from the tissue and cleaned in an enzyme solution (Tergazyme, 1%) for 1 day, and then further cleaned with deionized water and isopropyl alcohol. Explanted devices were examined with optical and scanning electron microscopy. Some devices were sputter-coated with a thin layer of metal (~10 nm) to improve the SEM imaging by reducing the charging effects. It was not always possible to compare the same device and the same pixel before and after the implantation due to randomness of the defect locations. However, each optical and SEM image is representative of the type of implant in terms of the device structure and changes after implantation.

Implants without an *a*-SiC coating degraded significantly during the 4-month subretinal implantation period. The SiN_x layer was completely dissolved on all pixels and devices, which was evident from the color change of the devices after implantation (Fig. 4.4C and D compared to region 1 in (B)). Platinum wires connecting the PN junctions to electrodes became exposed (Fig. 4.4D). On one implant, polysilicon in the trench started to degrade (Fig. 4.5C), while on the other implant (Fig. 4.5B), this region did not show any visible changes (Fig. 4.5A). Devices not coated with *a*-SiC not only exhibited considerable degradation after 4 months in vivo, devices with open trenches around each pixel exhibited more erosion than the ones with filled trenches. But regardless of the extent of the degradation, the fact that it is noticeable in all uncoated devices indicates the need for a good protective coating.

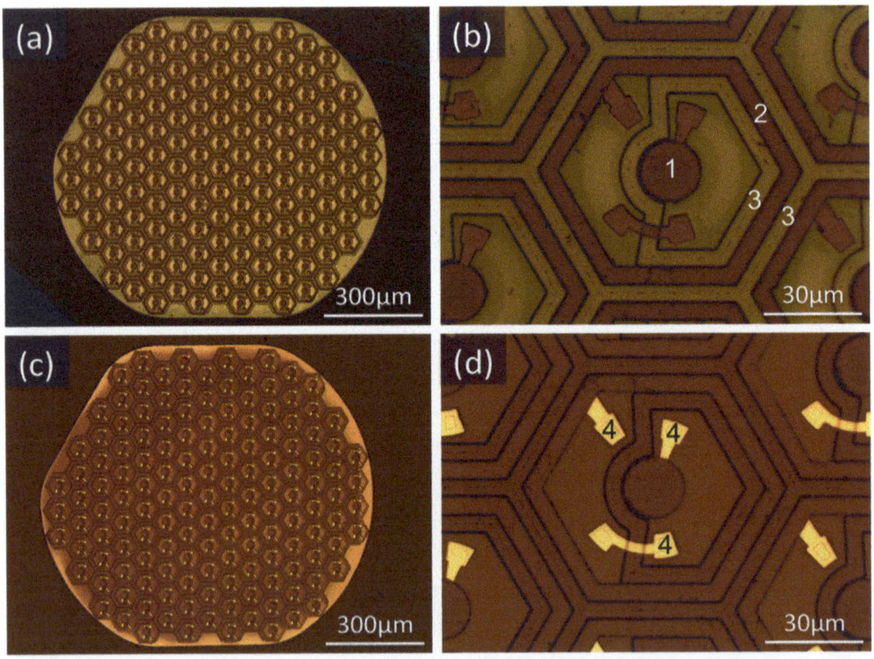

Figure 4.4 Optical microscopy of retinal prostheses (Type I) without *a*-SiC coating. (A) A 2-diode pixel device before implantation. (B) One pixel of the device in (A); 1—active electrode, 2—return electrode, 3—trenches filled with polysilicon. (C, D) 4 months after subretinal implantation in a rat eye. The drastic color change and exposed metal wires (4, bright yellow) indicate the dissolution of SiN_x. *(Reprint from Ref. [50].)*

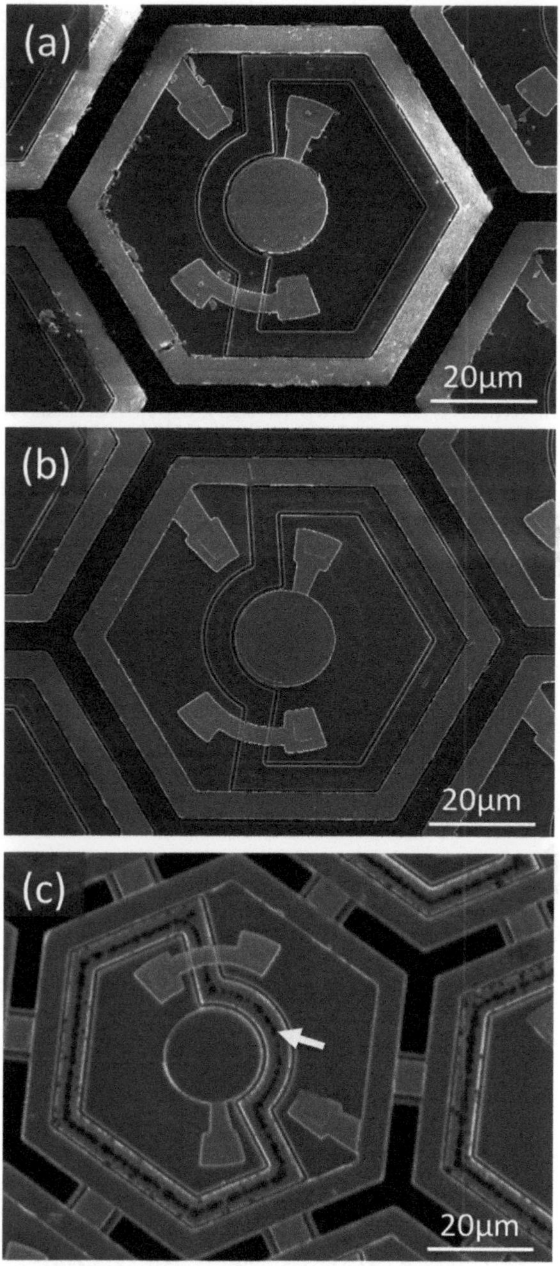

Figure 4.5 Scanning electron microscopy of retinal prostheses (Type I) without *a*-SiC coating. (A) A 2-diode pixel before implantation. (B, C) 4 months after subretinal implantation in a rat eye. The implant in (C) exhibits degradation in the polysilicon trench region (*arrow*), while (B) did not show visible changes compared to (A). All implants shown in this figure are from the same wafer. Only one pixel of each implant is shown, but all pixels on an implant have similar degradation. *(Reprint from Ref. [50].)*

All pixels without *a*-SiC coating implanted for 1 year showed visible degradation. However, the degradation was not uniform across the devices, as shown in Fig. 4.6A; some pixels exhibited more degradation than others. In some of the trenches, the polysilicon was completely dissolved, leaving a thin SiO_2 membrane covering the trench top (Fig. 4.6B, position 1). As a result, the metal wires on top of these empty trenches were mechanically compromised (Fig. 4.6B, position 2, and Fig. 4.6C, positions 2 and 3). Some thin SiO_2 films that originally covered the trench top were displaced after the polysilicon underneath was dissolved (Fig. 4.6C, position 3).

Despite the degradation, the implanted devices continued to function until they were explanted at least 7 months later [17], indicating that the SiO_2 films with metal wires on top of the empty trenches were displaced only during explanation (Fig. 4.6). Prolonged exposure of the implants in vivo will eventually lead to complete dissolution of the polysilicon in the trenches, which is likely to result in the loss of mechanical support, leading to device failure. During very long in vivo exposure, we speculate that the 70 nm of SiO_2 will eventually dissolve as well [51]. Once the active area (single-crystal silicon) of the devices is exposed to physiological environment, the silicon is expected to dissolve rapidly [43], and the devices will eventually stop functioning.

Dissolution of the SiN_x coatings and polysilicon in the trenches was the primary cause of device failure for these retinal prosthetic implants. Eliminating SiN_x and polysilicon should greatly increase the lifetime of the devices.

4. Deposition methods of *a*-SiC

As mentioned in Section 2, one wafer of the Type I devices was coated with an *a*-SiC protective layer. The *a*-SiC was deposited by PECVD at EIC Laboratories, Inc. (Norwood, MA). The precursors were SiH_4 and CH_4 (1:3 ratio of SiH_4/CH_4) in an Ar carrier gas. The deposition temperature was 325°C at a pressure of 800 mTorr and an RF power frequency of 13.56 MHz. The SiN_x used in dissolution rate tests was deposited by PECVD at the SNF using STS PECVD. The precursors were SiH_4 and NH_3 (40:33.5 ratio of SiH_4/NH_3) at a deposition temperature of 350°C and pressure of 650 mTorr. Dual frequency (13.56 MHz and 187.5 kHz) deposition was used. SiN_x was deposited as the top surface coating of retinal prostheses by PECVD at SNF (Plasma-Therm Shuttlelock SLR-730-PECVD). This tool used a capacitive-coupled plasma with 13.56 MHz

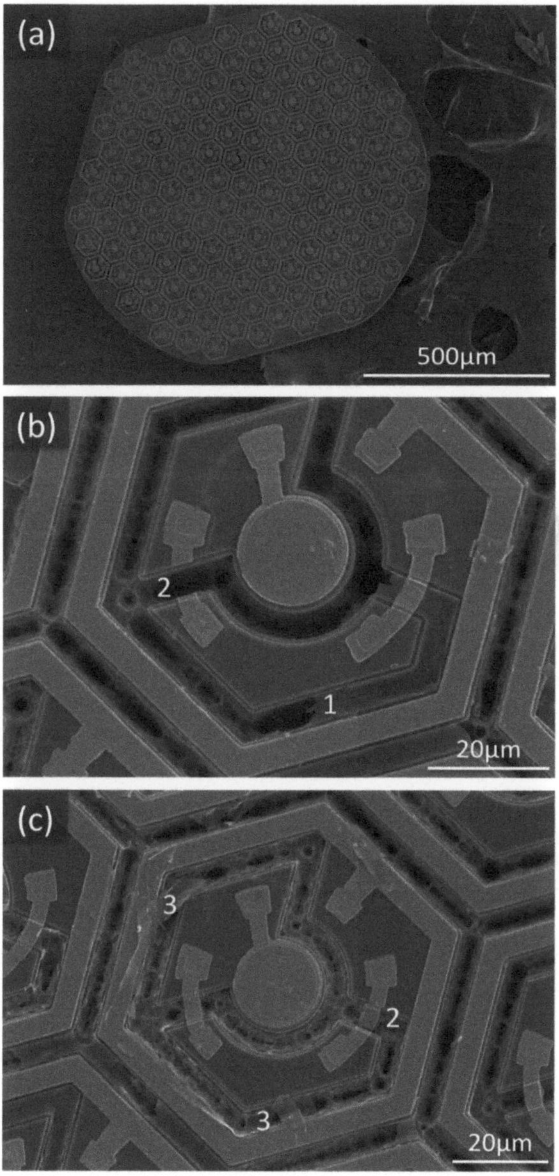

Figure 4.6 Scanning electron microscopy of retinal prostheses (Type I) without *a*-SiC coating after 1-year implantation. (A) All pixels in this device have visible degradation, albeit not uniform across the device. Both 3-diode pixels in (B) and (C) exhibit significant degradation. Polysilicon in some trenches is largely dissolved, leaving only a thin SiO_2 film covering the trench top (B1). Metal wires on top of the dissolved trenches could break (B2, C2). Some SiO_2 films that originally covered the trench top were displaced (C3). *(Reprint from Ref. [50].)*

RF power. Precursors were SiH_4 and NH_3 (5:3 ratio of SiH_4/NH_3), with He and N_2 carrier gases. The deposition temperature was 350°C at a pressure of 950 mTorr. SiO_2 was grown by wet thermal oxidation in a resistance-heated oxidation furnace at 1000°C.

Although not investigated in the current study, *a*-SiC can be used to protect the backside of the retinal prostheses by deposition at a much lower temperature near the end of the fabrication process to be compatible with the sputtered iridium oxide film (SIROF) electrode used in our devices. Amorphous *a*-SiC can be deposited at 175°C by electron cyclotron resonance PECVD [52], at <200°C by PECVD [43,53], and even at room temperature by RF magnetron sputtering [54], although the stability of those films in saline solution needs to be investigated. Therefore, an *a*-SiC coating can be deposited after SIROF deposition and release of the devices. Sidewalls of the devices can also be protected with *a*-SiC by a combination of depositions from the top and bottom. Alternatively, the back and sidewalls of the implant can be coated with metal for protection.

5. Dissolution rates of dielectric coatings using accelerated aging tests

Following the observation of the device degradation and dissolution of SiN_x in vivo, we performed a quantitative analysis of the stability of dielectric coating candidates for retinal prosthetic implants, including *a*-SiC, SiN_x, and SiO_2, by measuring their dissolution rates under accelerated aging test conditions—soaking the devices in saline at 87°C. *a*-SiC, SiN_x, and SiO_2-coated silicon substrates (520 μm thickness) were sealed in glass vials filled with saline, and placed in an oven with the temperature maintained at 87°C for up to 112 days. Samples were periodically taken out of the chamber, rinsed with deionized water, dried, and analyzed. The dissolution rate study at elevated temperature was performed in a low-phosphate saline (LPS), comprising 126 mM NaCl, 5 mM Na_2HPO_4, and 1.4 mM NaH_2PO_4.

Five samples each of the *a*-SiC, SiN_x, and SiO_2 coatings were used in the accelerated aging tests. *a*-SiC and SiN_x were grown on double-side polished silicon substrates. Before the soaking test, the thickness of *a*-SiC and SiN_x films was directly measured by selectively etching away the dielectric materials in a small region and measuring the step using surface profilometry. *a*-SiC films were 694 ± 10 nm thick on each side, and SiN_x films were 520 ± 5 nm thick on each side. SiO_2 was grown on single-side polished silicon substrates. The thickness of SiO_2 films on silicon substrates was measured using spectral reflectometry (Nanometrics Nanospec 210XP), assuming the refractive index of SiO_2 to be 1.45 in the visible range. The five SiO_2 samples were found to be 511±3 nm thick.

During the soaking tests of *a*-SiC and SiN_x, transmission-mode Fourier transform infrared spectroscopy (FTIR, Nicolet 6700) measurements were taken periodically on each sample to monitor changes in the films. The transmission FTIR spectra peaks were fitted, assuming Gaussian peak shapes, near the Si–C (~758 cm^{-1}) or Si–N (~820 cm^{-1}, 930 cm^{-1}) stretch frequencies, and the areas under the peaks were integrated. Before the soaking tests, we calibrated the integrated areas of fitted Gaussian peaks measured by FTIR to the thickness measured by surface profilometry by linear regression on samples of four different thicknesses for both *a*-SiC and SiN_x. All subsequent FTIR peak areas were converted to film thickness using these fitted linear models. Assuming the dissolution rates on both sides of the sample exposed to the same electrolyte are the same, the dissolution rate of a single exposed surface was calculated as half of the observed dissolution rate from two surfaces. For SiO_2 films, spectral reflectometry was performed periodically during the soaking test. The dissolution rate of each film was calculated by plotting the total film thickness versus soaking time.

SiN_x exhibited a highly reproducible and linear dissolution rate of 18.3 ± 0.3 nm/day (single surface) over the course of 28 days at 87°C (Fig. 4.7A). In addition, water penetration and bubbling were visible by day 1, and color changes indicative of thinning occurred throughout the course of soaking. By day 28, white dots appeared, suggesting wafer oxidation. Overnight between days 28 and 29, the remaining silicon nitride on each sample (15–23 nm per side) dissolved, and the wafers oxidized extensively. This result corresponded well with the observations in vivo, where SiN_x films on the retinal prostheses completely dissolved after 4 months.

In contrast, the five samples coated with *a*-SiC exhibited excellent stability. After more than 16 weeks in LPS at 87°C, they showed neither visible degradation nor quantifiable dissolution (Fig. 4.7A). This result is in agreement with the earlier measurement of *a*-SiC dissolution rate over 28 days at 90°C [41] and explains why *a*-SiC-coated devices were much more stable in vivo. The measured film thickness fluctuated within ~2% (standard deviation) over the course of soaking—likely an artifact of the peak fitting procedure. Defects in the *a*-SiC films could also contribute to variation in the measurement, if silicon under the defects oxidizes and dissolves, forming localized corrosion that could scatter light during the FTIR measurements.

Thermally grown SiO_2 dissolved very slowly but steadily at 1.04 ± 0.08 Å/day in saline at 87°C (Fig. 4.7B). Thus, a SiO_2 coating of 70 nm would last for ~700 days under accelerated aging conditions, corresponding to tens of years in vivo. This explains why the single-crystal silicon part of the implant did not degrade in vivo after 1 year, with 70−80 nm of SiO_2 covering it.

Silicon is known to dissolve in saline along preferential crystallographic planes, generating rectangular or square defects [43]. Silicon also reacts actively with many biological enzymes and fluids [55,56] and degrades after interactions with cell cultures [57]. In aqueous media, SiN_x is oxidized to form SiO_2 and NH_3, and SiO_2 hydrolyzes into $Si(OH)_4$ [58−60]. Therefore, a silicon implant with SiO_2 and SiN_x coatings will not survive long enough for chronic human use. *a*-SiC is known to react with O_2 and H_2O at very high temperatures (800−1000°C) [61−63]; however, it is chemically inert under physiological conditions. Except for a possible observation of *a*-SiC surface oxidation [43], no chemical reactions involving *a*-SiC under physiological conditions have been reported.

To estimate the *a*-SiC coating lifetime, we assumed an acceleration factor of $2^{\Delta T/10}$, which has been used for polymers in medical devices and other applications [64], assuming first-order rate kinetics for the dissolution process. Under this scheme, the aging factor at 87°C compared to physiological temperature (37°C) is $2^{(87-37)/10} = 2^5 = 32$, which means that a day of accelerated aging corresponds to about a month at physiological

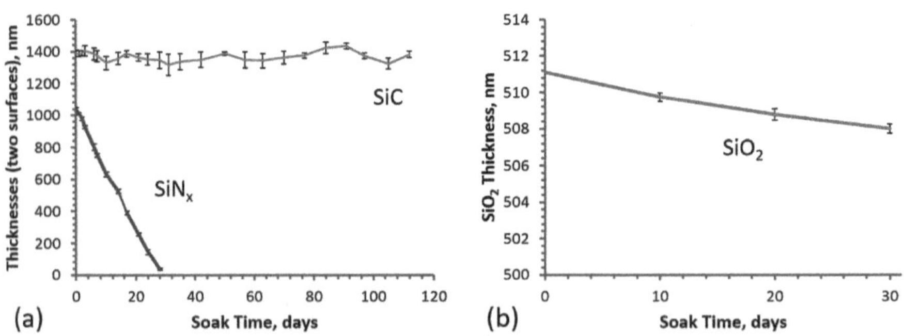

Figure 4.7 Dissolution rate of dielectric materials in saline at 87°C. (A) PECVD SiN_x dissolved at 18.3 nm $\pm$ 0.3 nm/day, while PECVD *a*-SiC showed no quantifiable dissolution up to 112 days. (B) Thermal SiO_2 dissolved at 1.04 ± 0.08 Å/day (data were normalized to the average thickness of SiO_2 on day 0). *(Reprint from Ref. [50].)*

temperature. In this study, the *a*-SiC coatings did not change after 112 days at 87°C, translating to no detectable degradation for roughly 10 years under physiological conditions.

The dissolution rate of *a*-SiC and other dielectric materials might be different with an electric field applied. Further study of the retinal prostheses in vivo with chronic photovoltaic activation will shed more light on this topic.

6. Defect analysis of a retinal prosthesis after chronic implantation in vivo

As mentioned in Section 2, to evaluate the protective properties of *a*-SiC, three devices with 240 nm of *a*-SiC coating were implanted in three different rats for 4 months. One implant did not show any visible degradation under the optical microscope (Fig. 4.8C and D). Two other implants had minor degradation at isolated defect points, visible as small patches of color change near the middle of the polysilicon-filled trenches (Fig. 4.8E and F, *arrows*) compared to the image before implantation (Fig. 4.8A and B). These defects were seen on 51 out of 142 pixels on one device, and 41 out of 142 on another. The patches of color change indicated the presence of defects in the *a*-SiC films near the middle of the polysilicon-filled trenches, which allowed the dissolution of the underlying SiN_x. In summary, unprotected retinal implants degrade during prolonged in vivo exposure, while *a*-SiC films provided effective protection of the implants.

As evident from the in vivo results, continuity of the protective coatings is critical for device longevity. Any defect in the film will expose the underlying materials to a harsh environment. Fig. 4.7 demonstrates a measurable dissolution rate of SiN_x and SiO_2 and will be gradually dissolving during prolonged implantation, while the thickness of *a*-SiC did not change over the course of soaking tests. Therefore, we only performed defect analysis on *a*-SiC films deposited on different structures to find weak points in these films, which may lead to degradation of the devices.

To reveal the defects in the *a*-SiC films, Type II arrays were soaked in buffered oxide etch (BOE) 6:1 (volume ratio of 40% NH_4F in water to 49% HF in water) for 10 minutes to etch SiN_x and SiO_2 through any defects in the *a*-SiC films. After etching, the defects became visible under an optical microscope. Type III structures were analyzed similarly by etching materials underneath the *a*-SiC to reveal defects in the *a*-SiC films. Specifically, samples were soaked in BOE 6:1 for 7 minutes to etch SiO_2. Some samples

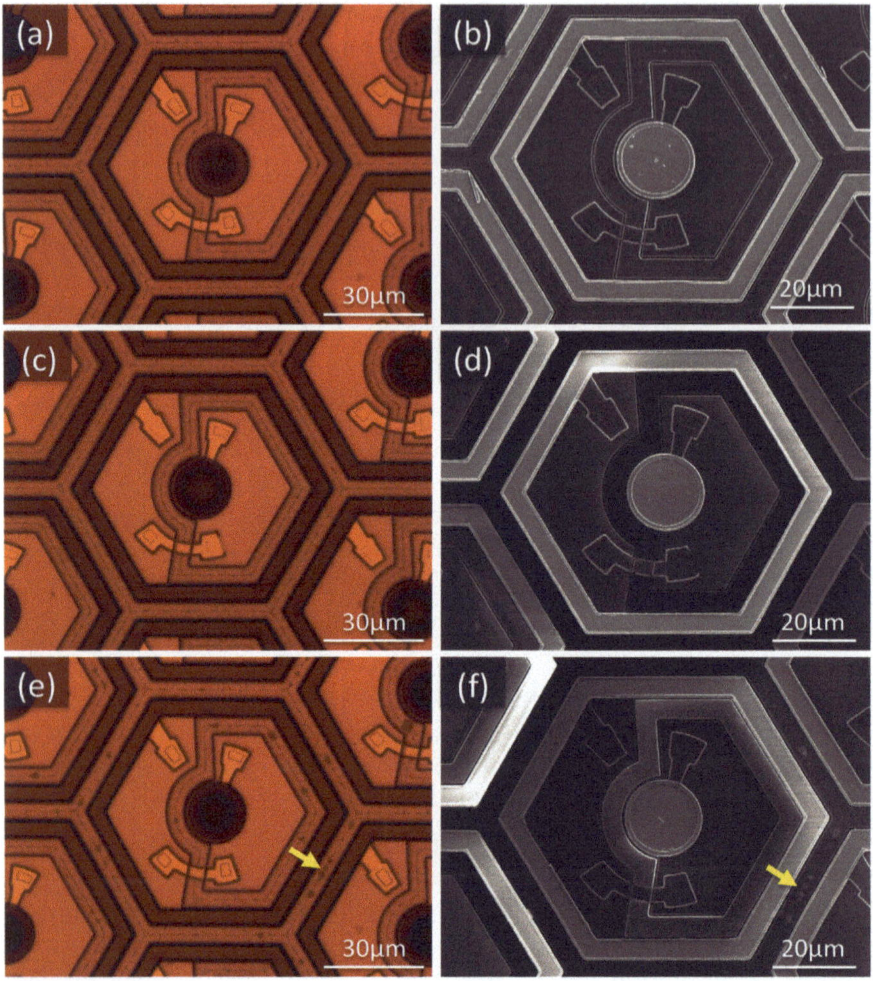

Figure 4.8 Retinal prostheses (Type I) with 240 nm *a*-SiC coating. (A, B) A 2-diode pixel before implantation. (C–F) 4 months after subretinal implantation in a rat eye. (C, D) exhibits no signs of degradation, while (E, F) showed small patches of color change in the middle of the polysilicon-filled trench (*arrows*), indicating defects in the *a*-SiC film. *(Reprint from Ref. [50].)*

were further etched isotropically by xenon difluoride (XeF_2) gas (Xactix e–1) to remove several microns of silicon. For cross-sectional SEM analysis of samples coated with 560 nm *a*-SiC films, an additional SiO_2 etch in BOE 6:1 for 40 seconds was performed after cross-sectioning the sample to recess the oxide and emphasize the *a*-SiC layer.

For 560 nm thick *a*-SiC films, examination of a total area of 11 cm^2 of the top surface of Type III structures showed no defects (Fig. 4.9A). Occasional defects were found on the sidewalls of the trenches covered with *a*-SiC (Fig. 4.9B). The scalloping on the sidewall due to the Bosch process likely increased the defect occurrence. *a*-SiC covered the trench sidewalls and bottoms continuously to the bottom (Fig. 4.10A and B). For 180 nm *a*-SiC films, the trench sidewalls were covered by *a*-SiC only down to ~4.5 μm depth (Fig. 4.10C and E). A thin layer (tens of nanometers) of *a*-SiC covered the bottom of the trenches. Overhanging *a*-SiC films at the corners are visible (Fig. 4.10D) and are emphasized by deliberately etching the underlying SiO_2 layer.

Similar tests on Type II arrays coated with 240 nm thick *a*-SiC films revealed defects exclusively in the middle of the polysilicon-filled trenches (Fig. 4.11B). This result matches well the defects observed after the 4-month in vivo implantation (Fig. 4.8E and F). For samples coated with 560 nm of *a*-SiC, no defects were found anywhere on the structures (Fig. 4.11D). The defect density in the *a*-SiC films depended on both the device topography and the film thickness. The 5 μm-wide trenches were oxidized and filled with polysilicon for electrical isolation and mechanical support (Fig. 4.12A). The middle of the trenches has a small seam where polysilicon grown from the sidewalls joins (indicated by the *arrow* in Fig. 4.12B). The small gaps near the surface are likely to result in defects, if not adequately covered. The 240 nm thick *a*-SiC coating did not cover these gaps (Fig. 4.12C), while a 560 nm layer completely coated the gaps

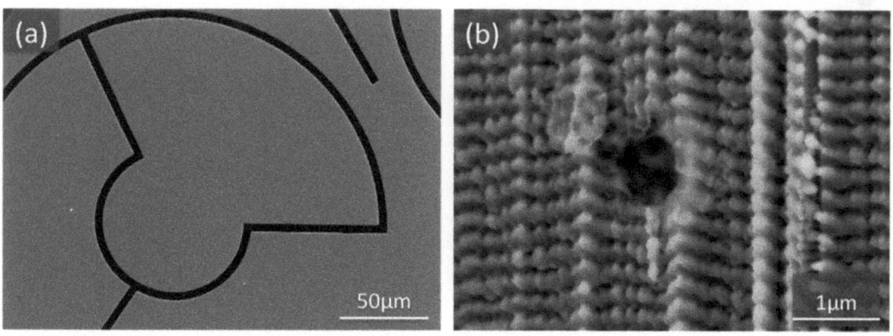

Figure 4.9 Defect characterization of *a*-SiC films (Type III). (A) Top view of 560 nm *a*-SiC film deposited on a smooth surface of 480 nm thermal SiO_2 on a bulk Si substrate with etched and oxidized trenches. No defects were found on 11 cm^2 of the top surface examined. (B) A defect on a trench sidewall. *(Reprint from Ref. [50].)*

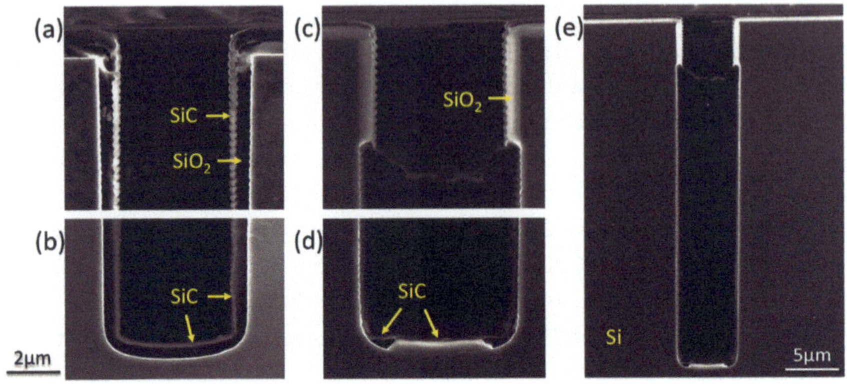

Figure 4.10 Trench coverage of *a*-SiC films (Type III). (A, B) 560 nm *a*-SiC deposited on 480 nm SiO_2 on a bulk Si substrate with etched and oxidized trenches. The continuous *a*-SiC film on the sidewall and bottom is pointed out by the *arrows*. (C, D, E) 180 nm *a*-SiC deposited on 480 nm SiO_2 on Si substrate with etched and oxidized trenches. The *a*-SiC film was continuous only at the top ~4.5 μm of the trench. *(Reprint from Ref. [50].)*

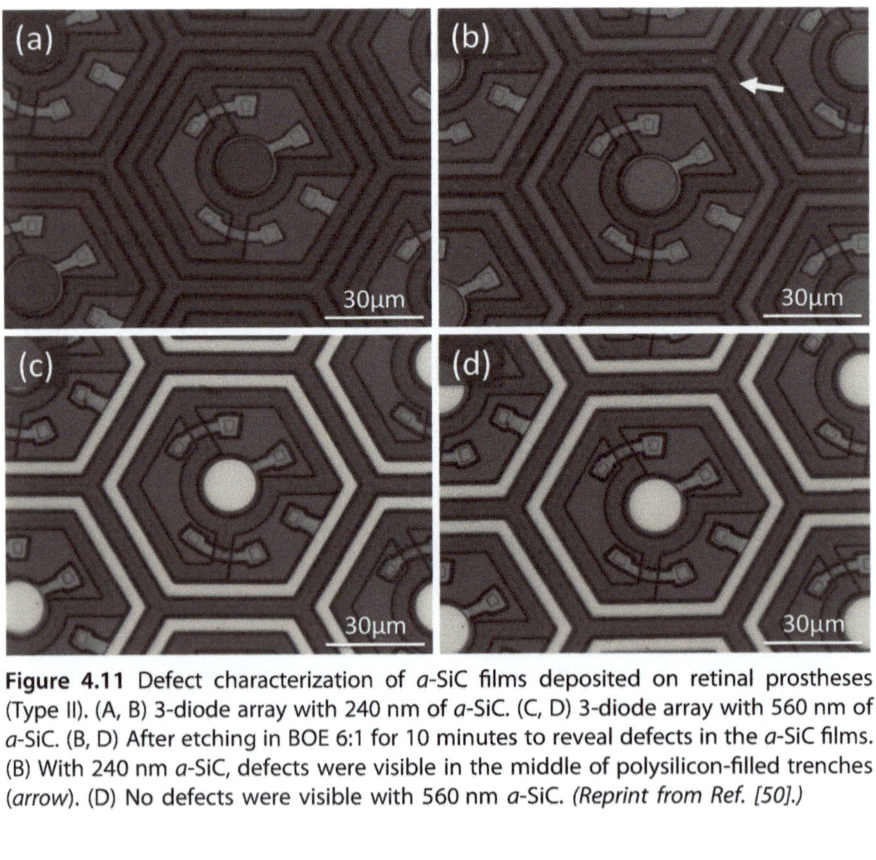

Figure 4.11 Defect characterization of *a*-SiC films deposited on retinal prostheses (Type II). (A, B) 3-diode array with 240 nm of *a*-SiC. (C, D) 3-diode array with 560 nm of *a*-SiC. (B, D) After etching in BOE 6:1 for 10 minutes to reveal defects in the *a*-SiC films. (B) With 240 nm *a*-SiC, defects were visible in the middle of polysilicon-filled trenches (*arrow*). (D) No defects were visible with 560 nm *a*-SiC. *(Reprint from Ref. [50].)*

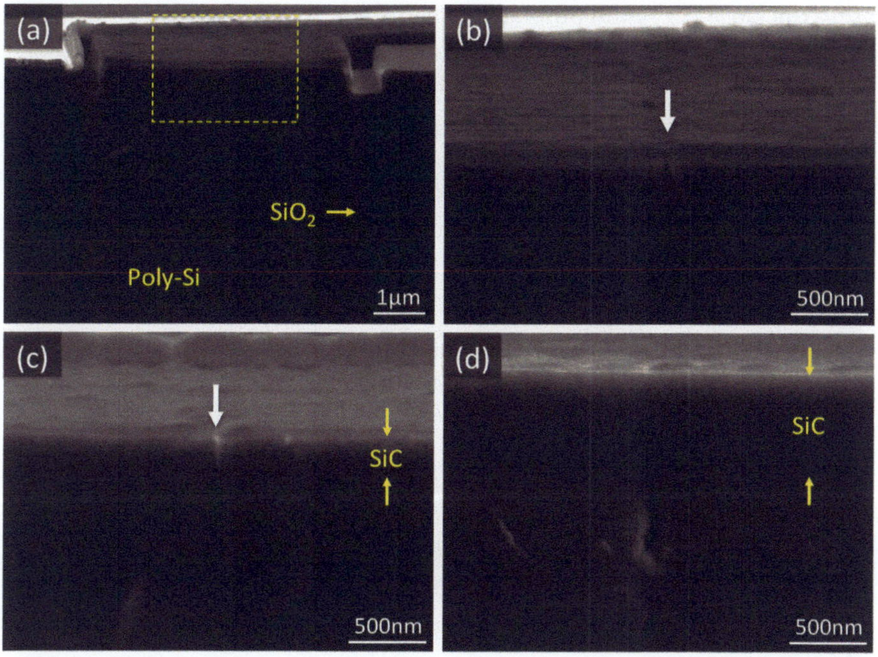

Figure 4.12 Cross-section of retinal prostheses (Type II) in the trench region. (A) Sample with no *a*-SiC coating, showing the top ~5 μm of the polysilicon-filled trench. (A) Zoom-in image of the middle of the trench (*yellow dashed rectangle*) of (A). *White arrow* points to the gap in polysilicon. (C) A sample with 240 nm *a*-SiC coating. A small gap in the middle of the trench was not fully covered by *a*-SiC as indicated by the *white arrow*. (D) Sample with 560 nm *a*-SiC coating completely covering the gap. *(Reprint from Ref. [50].)*

(Fig. 4.12D). Therefore, to properly protect the steps on the surface of the device and eliminate the associated defects in the *a*-SiC films, a minimum thickness of the coating, which depends on the topography of the device, must be used. For our retinal prostheses, an *a*-SiC thickness of 560 nm appears to provide sufficient protection, although this must still be confirmed pending the 1 year in vivo follow-up.

a-SiC films appear to protect the silicon wafers very well: we did not observe dissolution of this coating in accelerated aging, nor any defects in thick (~1 μm) *a*-SiC films deposited on flat surfaces. However, we observed a few defects or weak spots in 200–300 nm thick *a*-SiC films in the middle of the filled trenches (Fig. 4.11B), where the surface of the underlying polysilicon is not smooth (Fig. 4.12C). Eliminating such seams in the trenches would improve the stability of such devices. Alternatively, using thicker *a*-SiC can completely cover these rough features, as shown in Fig. 4.12D with 560 nm coating.

Aside from increasing the *a*-SiC film thickness, the defect density can be reduced by growth interruption during the *a*-SiC deposition. The defects in *a*-SiC films on the trench sidewalls can also be reduced by decreasing the scalloping related to the Bosch process used to etch trenches in the silicon. H_2 annealing at an elevated temperature has been demonstrated to smooth sidewalls [65–67].

7. *a*-SiC as part of the antireflective coating

a-SiC can not only replace SiN_x as the protective coating but also serve as a part of the antireflective coating for the retinal implant, in combination with the underlying SiO_2. Simulation by the transfer matrix method [68,69] (Fig. 4.13) showed that 560 nm of *a*-SiC on top of 310–380 nm of SiO_2 could reduce reflection of 880 nm light below 10% for vertical incidence. SiO_2 and *a*-SiC films of such thickness exhibit low defect densities even in areas of complex topography and, therefore, can provide effective protection.

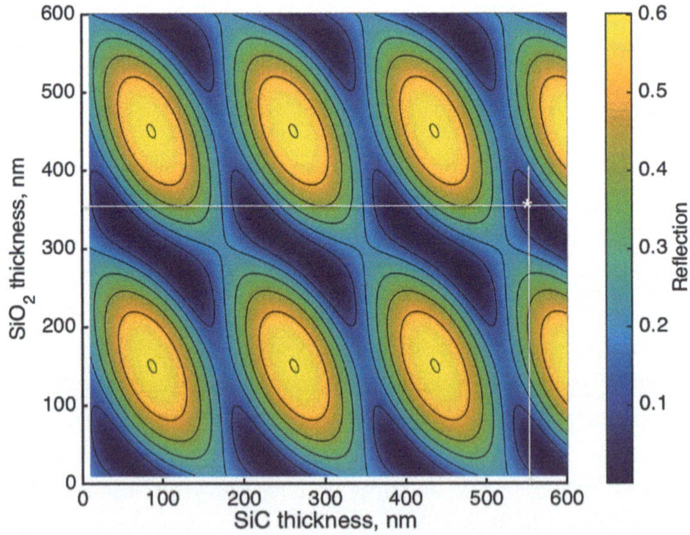

Figure 4.13 Calculated optical reflectivity of the *a*-SiC and thermal SiO_2 stack in saline. 560 nm of *a*-SiC on top of 310–380 nm of SiO_2 could reduce reflection of 880 nm light below 10% for vertical incidence. *(Reprint from Ref. [50].)*

8. Summary

This chapter presented an overview of photovoltaic retinal prostheses and the application of *a*-SiC as the protective coating of these devices. We first introduced the photovoltaic subretinal prosthesis system developed at Stanford University and the design and fabrication of the retinal prosthetic implant device. Significant degradation of unprotected (no *a*-SiC coated) photovoltaic retinal prostheses was found after 4-month implantation, especially in the polysilicon-filled trenches. PECVD *a*-SiC films were much more effective than SiN_x and SiO_2 coatings in protecting the devices in vivo. Accelerated aging tests did not result in a change of the thickness of *a*-SiC films after 112 days in saline at 87°C. The SiN_x coating was much less stable and dissolved at a rate of 18.3 ± 0.3 nm/day at 87°C. Thermal SiO_2 grown at high temperature (1000°C) was more stable but still dissolved very slowly at 1.04 ± 0.08 Å/day at 87°C in saline. *a*-SiC films exhibited some defects on complicated topography and rough surfaces. The defect density could be reduced or eliminated by smoothening the underlying surface or by increasing the *a*-SiC film thickness. Overall, PECVD *a*-SiC films have desirable properties as protective coatings for implantable electronics. A combination of thermal SiO_2 with a PECVD *a*-SiC film should be adequate for providing antireflective coating and protecting retinal prostheses for long-term use.

Acknowledgments

Funding was provided by the US National Institutes of Health (grant R01-EY-018608, D.P.), the Department of Defense (grant W81XWH-15-1-0009, D.P.), and the Stanford Spectrum fund (D.P.). K.M. was supported by an SU2P fellowship as part of an RCUK Science Bridges award. H.L. was supported in part by the Foundation Voir et Entendre (Paris) and Pixium Vision. Fabrication was performed in part at the Stanford Nanofabrication Facility, which is supported by National Science Foundation through the NNIN (grant ECS-9731293). Sample preparation by SEM (FEI XL30 Sirion) was performed at the Stanford Nano Shared Facilities (SNSF). Accelerated *a*-SiC degradation testing at EIC Laboratories was performed partly by Doug Orsi and Chathuri Gunasekharan.

References

[1] P.A. Crosby, C.N. Daly, D.K. Money, J.F. Patrick, P.M. Seligman, J.A. Kuzma, Cochlear implant system for an auditory prosthesis, United States Patent 4 (532) (1985) 930.

[2] H. McDermott, An advanced multiple channel cochlear implant, IEEE Transactions on Biomedical Engineering 36 (1989) 789—797.

[3] B.S. Wilson, C.C. Finley, D.T. Lawson, R.D. Wolford, D.K. Eddington, W.M. Rabinowitz, Better speech recognition with cochlear implants, Nature 352 (1991) 236–238.
[4] A.L. Benabid, P. Pollak, D. Gao, D. Hoffmann, P. Limousin, E. Gay, I. Payen, A. Benazzouz, Chronic electrical stimulation of the ventralis intermedius nucleus of the thalamus as a treatment of movement disorders, Journal of Neurosurgery 84 (1996) 203–214.
[5] P. Limousin, P. Krack, P. Pollak, A. Benazzouz, C. Ardouin, D. Hoffmann, A.L. Benabid, Electrical stimulation of the subthalamic nucleus in advanced Parkinson's disease, New England Journal of Medicine 339 (1998) 1105–1111.
[6] R. Kumar, A.M. Lozano, Y.J. Kim, W.D. Hutchison, E. Sime, E. Halket, A.E. Lang, Double-blind evaluation of subthalamic nucleus deep brain stimulation in advanced Parkinson's disease, Neurology 51 (1998) 850–855.
[7] A. Kupsch, et al., Pallidal deep-brain stimulation in primary generalized or segmental dystonia, New England Journal of Medicine 355 (2006) 1978–1990.
[8] L.R. Hochberg, M.D. Serruya, G.M. Friehs, J.A. Mukand, M. Saleh, A.H. Caplan, A. Branner, D. Chen, R.D. Penn, J.P. Donoghue, Neuronal ensemble control of prosthetic devices by a human with tetraplegia, Nature 442 (2006) 164–171.
[9] L.R. Hochberg, et al., Reach and grasp by people with tetraplegia using a neurally controlled robotic arm, Nature 485 (2012) 372–375.
[10] K.V. Shenoy, M. Sahani, M.M. Churchland, Cortical control of arm movements: a dynamical systems perspective, Annual Review of Neuroscience 36 (2013) 337–359.
[11] P.K. Campbell, K.E. Jones, R.J. Huber, K.W. Horch, R.A. Normann, A silicon-based, three-dimensional neural interface: manufacturing processes for an intracortical electrode array, IEEE Transactions on Biomedical Engineering 38 (1991) 758–768.
[12] R.A. Normann, E.M. Maynard, P.J. Rousche, D.J. Warren, A neural interface for a cortical vision prosthesis, Vision Research 39 (1999) 2577–2587.
[13] E. Zrenner, et al., Subretinal electronic chips allow blind patients to read letters and combine them to words, Proceedings Biological Sciences 278 (2011) 1489–1497.
[14] A.K. Ahuja, J.D. Dorn, A. Caspi, M.J. McMahon, G. Dagnelie, L. Dacruz, P. Stanga, M.S. Humayun, R.J. Greenberg, Argus II Study Group, Blind subjects implanted with the Argus II retinal prosthesis are able to improve performance in a spatial-motor task, British Journal of Ophthalmology 95 (2011) 539–543.
[15] M.S. Humayun, et al., Interim results from the international trial of Second Sight's visual prosthesis, Ophthalmology 119 (2012) 779–788.
[16] K. Mathieson, et al., Photovoltaic retinal prosthesis with high pixel density, Nature Photonics 6 (2012) 391–397.
[17] H. Lorach, et al., Photovoltaic restoration of sight with high visual acuity, Nature Medicine 21 (2015) 476–482.
[18] R.J. Jensen, J.F. Rizzo III, Thresholds for activation of rabbit retinal ganglion cells with a subretinal electrode, Experimental Eye Research 83 (2006) 367–373.
[19] D.J. Anderson, K. Najafi, S.J. Tanghe, D.A. Evans, K.L. Levy, J.F. Hetke, X.L. Xue, J.J. Zappia, K.D. Wise, Batch-fabricated thin-film electrodes for stimulation of the central auditory system, IEEE Transactions on Biomedical Engineering 36 (1989) 693–704.
[20] J.F. Hetke, J.L. Lund, K. Najafi, K.D. Wise, D.J. Anderson, Silicon ribbon cables for chronically implantable microelectrodes arrays, IEEE Transactions on Biomedical Engineering 41 (1994) 314–321.
[21] J.D. Weiland, D.J. Anderson, Chronic neural stimulation with thin-film, iridium oxide electrodes, IEEE Transactions on Biomedical Engineering 47 (2000) 911–918.

[22] J.D. Plummer, M.D. Deal, P.B. Griffin, Silicon VLSI Technology, Prentice Hall, Upper Saddle River, NJ, 2000, p. 725.
[23] H. Hämmerle, K. Kobuch, K. Kohler, W. Nisch, H. Sachs, M. Stelzle, Biostability of micro-photodiode arrays for subretinal implantation, Biomaterials 23 (2002) 797–804.
[24] G.E. Loeb, M.J. Bak, M. Salcman, E.M. Schmidt, Parylene as a chronically stable, reproducible microelectrode insulator, IEEE Transactions on Biomedical Engineering 24 (1977) 121–128.
[25] J.M. Hsu, L. Rieth, R.A. Normann, P. Tathireddy, F. Solzbacher, Encapsulation of an integrated neural interface device with Parylene C, IEEE Transactions on Biomedical Engineering 56 (2009) 23–29.
[26] X. Xie, L. Rieth, L. Williams, S. Negi, R. Bhandari, R. Caldwell, R. Sharma, P. Tathireddy, F. Solzbacher, Long-term reliability of Al_2O_3 and Parylene C bilayer encapsulated Utah electrode array based neural interfaces for chronic implantation, Journal of Neural Engineering 11 (2014) 1–9.
[27] J. Charmet, J. Bitterli, O. Sereda, M. Liley, P. Renaud, H. Keppner, Optimizing Parylene C adhesion for MEMS processes: potassium hydroxide wet etching, Journal of Microelectromechanical Systems 22 (2013) 855–864.
[28] T.N. Chen, D.S. Wuu, C.C. Wu, C.C. Chiang, Y.P. Chen, R.H. Horng, High-performance transparent barrier films of SiO_x/SiN_x stacks on flexible polymer substrates, Journal of the Electrochemical Society 153 (10) (2006) F244–F248.
[29] S.E. Potts, et al., Ultra-thin aluminium oxide films deposited by plasma-enhanced atomic layer deposition for corrosion protection, Journal of the Electrochemical Society 158 (2011) 132–138.
[30] R.K. Roy, K.R. Lee, Biomedical applications of diamond-like carbon coatings: a review, Journal of Biomedical Materials Research Part B: Applied Biomaterials 83 (2007) 72–84.
[31] X. Xiao, J. Birrell, J.E. Gerbi, O. Auciello, J.A. Carlisle, Low temperature growth of ultrananocrystalline diamond, Journal of Applied Physics 96 (2004) 2232–2239.
[32] X. Xiao, et al., In vitro and *in vivo* evaluation of ultrananocrystalline diamond for coating of implantable retinal microchips, Journal of Biomedical Materials Research Part B: Applied Biomaterials 77 (2006) 273–281.
[33] Y.C. Chen, C.Y. Tsai, C.Y. Lee, I.N. Lin, In vitro and in vivo evaluation of ultrananocrystalline diamond as an encapsulation layer for implantable microchips, Acta Biomaterialia 10 (2014) 2187–2199.
[34] A. Bolz, M. Amon, C. Ozbek, B. Heublein, M. Schaldach, Coating of cardiovascular stents with a semiconductor to improve their hemocompatibility, Texas Heart Institute Journal 23 (1996) 162–166.
[35] M. Amon, A. Bolz, M. Schaldach, Improvement of stenting therapy with a silicon carbide coated tantalum stent, Journal of Materials Science: Materials in Medicine 7 (1996) 273–278.
[36] A. Rzany, M. Schaldach, Smart material silicon carbide: reduced activation of cells and proteins on a SiC:H-coated stainless steel, Progress in Biomedical Engineering 4 (2001) 182–194.
[37] C.Y. Chang, Y.K. Fang, C.F. Huang, B.S. Wu, Novel passivation dielectrics — the boron- or phosphorus-doped hydrogenated amorphous silicon carbide films, Journal of the Electrochemical Society 132 (1985) 418–422.
[38] M.J. Loboda, K.W. Michael, Silicon carbide metal diffusion barrier layer, United States Patent 5 (818) (1998) 071.
[39] S.M. Merchant, S. Misra, P.K. Roy, Silicon carbide barrier layers for porous low dielectric constant materials, United States Patent 6 (100) (2000) 587.

[40] S. Nemani, L.Q. Xia, E. Yieh, Dual frequency plasma enhanced chemical vapor deposition of silicon carbide layers, United States Patent 6 (465) (2002) 366 B1.
[41] S.F. Cogan, D.J. Edell, A.A. Guzelian, Y.P. Liu, R. Edell, Plasma-enhanced chemical vapor deposited silicon carbide as an implantable dielectric coating, Journal of Biomedical Materials Research Part A 67 (2003) 856–867.
[42] J.M. Maloney, S.A. Lipka, S.P. Baldwin, In vivo biostability of CVD silicon oxide and silicon nitride films, Materials Research Society Symposium Proceedings 872 (2005) 1–6.
[43] J.M. Hsu, P. Tathireddy, L. Rieth, A.R. Normann, F. Solzbachera, Characterization of a-SiCx:H thin films as an encapsulation material for integrated silicon based neural interface devices, Thin Solid Films 516 (2007) 34–41.
[44] Q. Bai, K.D. Wise, D.J. Anderson, A high-yield microassembly structure for three-dimensional microelectrode arrays, IEEE Transactions on Biomedical Engineering 47 (2000) 281–289.
[45] D. Boinagrov, X. Lei, G. Goetz, T.I. Kamins, K. Mathieson, L. Galambos, J.S. Harris, D. Palanker, Photovoltaic pixels for neural stimulation: circuit models and performance, IEEE Transactions on Biomedical Circuits and Systems 10 (1) (2016) 85–97.
[46] L. Wang, et al., Photovoltaic retinal prosthesis: implant fabrication and performance, Journal of Neural Engineering 9 (2012) 1–11.
[47] D. Boinagrov, S. Pangratz-Fuehrer, G. Goetz, D. Palanker, Selectivity of direct and network-mediated stimulation of the retinal ganglion cells with epi-, sub- and intra-retinal electrodes, Journal of Neural Engineering 11 (2014) 1–11.
[48] X. Lei, High Resolution Photovoltaic Retinal Prosthesis with Three-Dimensional Neural Interface, Dissertation from Stanford University, 2018.
[49] Y. Mandel, et al., Cortical responses elicited by photovoltaic subretinal prostheses exhibit similarities to visually evoked potentials, Nature Communications 4 (2013) 1–9.
[50] X. Lei, et al., SiC protective coating for photovoltaic retinal prosthesis, Journal of Neural Engineering 13 (2016) 046016.
[51] S. Ahn, P.S. Spuhler, M. Chiari, M. Cabodi, M.S. Ünlü, Quantification of surface etching by common buffers and implications on the accuracy of label-free biological assays, Biosensors and Bioelectronics 36 (2012) 222–229.
[52] M.J. Loboda, Low temperature PECVD growth and characterization of a-SiC:H films deposited from silacyclobutane and silane/methane precursor gases, Springer Proceedings in Physics 71 (1992) 271–280.
[53] L. Jiang, X. Chen, X. Wang, L. Xu, F. Stubhan, K. Merkel, a-SiCx-H films deposited by plasma-enhanced chemical vapor deposition at low temperature used for moisture and corrosion resistant applications, Thin Solid Films 352 (1999) 97–101.
[54] N. Ledermann, J. Baborowski, P. Muralt, N. Xantopoulos, J.M. Tellenbach, Sputtered silicon carbide thin films as protective coating for MEMS applications, Surface and Coatings Technology 125 (2000) 246–250.
[55] J.D. Birchall, J.S. Chappell, The chemistry of aluminum and silicon in relation to Alzheimers disease, Clinical Chemistry 34 (1988) 265–267.
[56] S.C. Bayliss, L.D. Buckberry, P.J. Harris, M. Tobin, Nature of the silicon–animal cell interface, Journal of Porous Materials 7 (2000) 191–195.
[57] S.E. Saddow, Silicon Carbide Biotechnology, Elsevier Science, 2012.
[58] J.W. Osenbach, W.R. Knolle, Behavior of a-SiN:H and a-SiON:H films in condensed water, Journal of the Electrochemical Society 139 (1992) 3346–3351.
[59] M. Vogt, R. Hauptmann, Plasma-deposited passivation layers for moisture and water protection, Surface and Coatings Technology 74–75 (1995) 676–681.
[60] G. Schmitt, J.W. Schultze, F. Faßbender, G. Buß, H. Lüth, M.J. Schöning, Passivation and corrosion of microelectrode arrays, Electrochimica Acta 44 (1999) 3865–3883.

[61] R.G. Munro, S.J. Dapkunas, Corrosion characteristics of silicon carbide and silicon nitride, Journal of Research of the National Institute of Standards and Technology 98 (1993) 607–631.
[62] T. Kraft, K.G. Nickel, Y.G. Gogotsi, Hydrothermal degradation of chemical vapour deposited SiC fibres, Journal of Materials Science 33 (1998) 4357–4364.
[63] P. Pastila, V. Helanti, A. Nikkilä, T. Mäntylä, Environmental effects on microstructure and strength of SiC-based hot gas filters, Journal of the European Ceramic Society 21 (2001) 1261–1268.
[64] D.W. Hukins, A. Mahomed, S.N. Kukureka, Accelerated aging for testing polymeric biomaterials and medical devices, Medical Engineering and Physics 30 (2008) 1270–1274.
[65] T. Sato, K. Mitsutake, I. Mizushima, Y. Tsunashima, Micro-structure transformation of silicon: a newly developed transformation technology for patterning silicon surfaces using the surface migration of silicon atoms by hydrogen annealing, Japan Society of Applied Physics 39 (2000) 5033–5038.
[66] H. Kuribayashi, R. Hiruta, R. Shimizu, K. Sudoh, H. Iwasaki, Shape transformation of silicon trenches during hydrogen annealing, Journal of Vacuum Science and Technology A 21 (2003) 1279–1283.
[67] M.C.M. Lee, M.C. Wu, Thermal annealing in hydrogen for 3-D profile transformation on silicon-on-insulator and sidewall roughness reduction, Journal of Microelectromechanical Systems 15 (2006) 338–343.
[68] Z. Knittl, Optics of Thin Films, Wiley, London, 1976.
[69] L.A. Pettersson, L.S. Roman, O. Inganäs, Modeling photocurrent action spectra of photovoltaic devices based on organic thin films, Journal of Applied Physics 86 (1999) 487–496.

CHAPTER 5

A monolithic "all-SiC" neural interface for long-term human applications

Christopher L. Frewin[1], Evans Bernardin[2], Mohammad Beygi[6], Chenyin Feng[3,4] and Stephen E. Saddow[5]

[1]NeuroNexus LLC, Ann Arbor, MI, United States; [2]Department of Medical Engineering, University of South Florida, Tampa, FL, United States; [3]Department of Electrical Engineering, University of South Florida, Tampa, FL, United States; [4]Department of Mechanical Engineering, University of South Florida, Tampa, FL, United States; [5]Departments of Electrical & Medical Engineering, University of South Florida, Tampa, FL, United States; [6]Institute of Electrical and Microengineering, École polytechnique fédérale de Lausanne, Lausanne, Switzerland

Contents

1. Introduction

Investigators in neuroscience have brought the machinations of the nervous system into a clearer view, especially with the initiative called Brain Research through Advancing Innovative Neurotechnologies launched by

Silicon Carbide Technology for Advanced Human Healthcare Applications
ISBN 978-0-323-90609-8
https://doi.org/10.1016/B978-0-323-90609-8.00009-0

former president of the United States, Barack Obama. While this initiative focused on the understanding of how the brain and nervous system work, it also allowed great leaps in technology with which to investigate the nervous system. Not only does this technology continue to help understand and unravel the circuitry of the brain, but it has also allowed many to imagine various therapeutics which could help individuals suffering from neurological disorders or trauma. The brain—machine interface (BMI), also called the brain—computer interface, has become a technology led by neuroscientists, engineers, and computer specialists working in concert to make these therapeutics a reality [1—3]. BMIs integrate solutions by recording from neurons, transporting that information to processors, and calculating an appropriate response from a computer or system to alleviate the issues with the nervous system. Ultimately, the BMI would also be able to send signals into the body, offering the potential of two-way closed-loop communication [2,4]. The potential of bidirectional communication could allow therapeutics bridging damaged areas of the nervous system, restoring function, as in a paralyzed individual, for example. Similar devices can also be used to control external mechanical devices, such as robotic (bionic) limbs, which would contain various sensors that could send information back to the body, such as heat, pressure, and spatial position. This technology could be applied to diseases like Parkinson's or Alzheimer's as well, bridging gaps in the neural network and restoring lost functionality.

Numerous neural interface techniques have been developed for neuroscientific investigations over many years. In this chapter, we will focus on electrically based interactions with the brain to limit the scope of this wide field. Fig. 5.1 illustrates three popular electrical-based neural interfaces and their placement with respect to the human brain. Neural signals can be

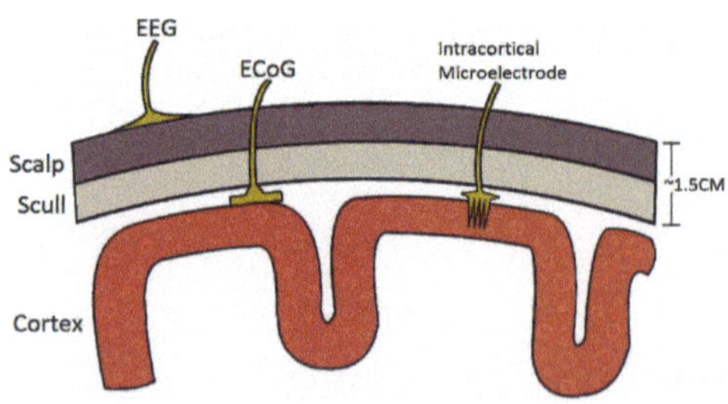

Figure 5.1 Illustration of three popular neural interfaces and their placement with respect to the human brain: EEG (scalp), ECoG (on top of cortical surface and below the skull), and intracortical microelectrode (INI) (implanted in the cortex). Thus, three separate cortical populations interact with the three interfaces.

examined externally and noninvasively, by placing electrodes on top of a patient's head via electroencephalogram (EEG). Electrocorticography (ECoG) (on top of the cortical surface, and below the skull) is more invasive as the electrodes are placed directly on the surface of the brain. Intracortical neural interface (INI) (implanted directly in the cortex) is the most invasive, penetrating the tissue of the brain, but better allows for direct two-way interaction with individual neurons. Thus, these three separate interfaces allow for three, very different cortical interactions: The INI allows the measure electrical action potentials, colloquially referred to as spikes, from individual neurons in the immediate vicinity of the electrode contact, typically less than 50–100 μm away, while also receives local field potentials from neuronal populations [6,7]. ECoG signals can extract local field potential information from neurons within a few hundred micrometers or millimeters from the recording contact [8]. EEG signals contain contributions from large cortical populations even further away, and as a direct consequence, suffer from low signal strength due to electrical signal loss through the scalp and skull [9,10]. For a more detailed explanation of these three methods of interaction, the authors would like to refer the reader to Chapter 7 of the second edition of *Silicon Carbide Biotechnology* [11]. Ultimately, information is key for proper BMI operation, so the choice of interface affects the ability of the BMI to provide therapeutics. For many of the more complex BMI solutions, such as a robotic arm, information from localized field and action potentials are required for proper operation. Therefore, many have looked to devices that have intimate contact with the neuron, that is, the INI, as the interface of choice.

Unfortunately, despite the promises of BMI, the INI has yet to demonstrate the long-term in vivo performance necessary for long-term clinical applications due to either device failure or signal loss within approximately 2 years from implantation. Many state-of-the-art INI devices are simple, constructed of a conductive material that interacts with the extracellular electrolytic solution. Conductive leads connect the electrodes to the outside environment are surrounded by an insulating material. INI devices have been constructed using stacks of multiple materials, with many using silicon derivatives (Si, SiO_2, Si_3N_4), iridium (Ir, IrO_2), titanium nitride (TiN), platinum (Pt), gold (Au), parylene C, and polyimide [3,12–15]. Not only must each material tolerate the biological environment without exacerbating the brain's inflammatory response, but each material must also physically withstand the oxidative and ion-rich aqueous environment, as well as interacting seamlessly with the other device components. Two causes have been attributed to the failure of INI devices: The first is the chronic foreign body response from microglia and astrocytes which extends long beyond the initial implantation and follows a response akin to neural degeneration [16–21]. This foreign body response has often been attributed to the lack of biocompatibility of these devices, where biocompatibility is loosely defined as the ability of a material to interface with the body without causing a negative physical response, as well as the ability of the device to function as designed within acceptable parameters after implantation [22]. Many materials have been previously used in the construction for these devices ranging from ceramics to polymers in combination with various conductive materials. Three materials have been the mainstays used for the device insulation, namely silicon and its derivatives (SiO_2, Si_3N_4), polyimide, and parylene, while platinum derivatives (Pt, Pt Black, Pt–Ir alloys), iridium oxide, titanium oxide, and titanium nitride have been used frequently as electrode interfaces [3,14,15,17]. Numerous investigations have been presented in the literature describing observed neuronal interaction with implanted devices, and all of the previously used materials have significant limitations with respect to long-term reliability [17,23–28].

Abiotic mechanisms have also been attributed as a major failure point for INI technology. Delamination, cracks, and blistering of multilayer structures that constitute these implantable technologies likely contribute to reduced charge delivery and decreased stimulation specificity. Polyimide-insulated tungsten microwire arrays chronically implanted in rats demonstrated insulation damage due to excessive oxidative stress leading to deterioration in the electrode sites [24,29,30]. Recent work by Kozai using implanted NeuroNexus structures identified multiple modes of mechanical failure, which appear to be associated with the inherent strain manifested between microscale material boundaries [31], suggesting that conductor-insulation adhesion is a common site for electrode failure. Chapter 6 of the first edition and Chapter 7 of the second edition of *Silicon Carbide Technology: A Biocompatible Semiconductor for Advanced Biomedical Devices and Applications* investigates the issues of biocompatibility and material stability in much detail and the author refers the reader to these chapters for additional reference [11,32].

One approach to address the biotic and abiotic mechanisms of INI failure has been optimizing the materials required to fabricate the devices. Silicon carbide (SiC) is a physically robust, hemo- and biocompatible, and chemically inert semiconductor. An "all-SiC," or monolithic SiC, device may be the disruptive technology needed in the BMI field to finally achieve long-term and widespread use of this technology in humans [33]. The all-SiC device concept is where SiC serves as all device layers: the base (support), the conducting traces (electrodes), and the surface conformal insulating layer. The monolithic SiC neural probe is realized by forming high-quality pn junctions of heavily doped SiC on a layer of the opposite polarity. Heavily doped semiconductors display semimetallic electrical performance, which allows for efficient electrical conduction in the electrode without the deleterious effects of metal ions interacting with the neural environment. The conformal insulator is realized using amorphous-SiC (*a*-SiC) that can be patterned to open windows to allow electrical conduction to occur between the electrode tips and the brain.

Several generations of monolithic SiC devices have been fabricated, tested, and are reported in this chapter. The devices were fabricated utilizing two polytypes of SiC (4H−SiC [33] and 3C−SiC [34]). The monolithic SiC microelectrodes were fabricated utilizing techniques used in the fabrication of Si-based microelectrodes. Monolithic SiC devices fabricated include planar single-ended microelectrode array (MEAs) (with varying lengths and varying active recording areas), single-ended electrode MEAs for in vitro studies, and 16-electrode Michigan style neural probes for in vivo studies.

All studies and data collected thus far indicate that the monolithic SiC neural device concept can aid in the advancement of chronic INI use in clinical settings. These devices rely on the integration of only robust and highly compatible SiC material, and they may offer a promising solution to probe delamination and biological rejection associated with the use of multiple materials used in many current INI devices. Follow-on work is planned to prove this assertion via in vivo studies.

2. Monolithic 4H−SiC neural interfaces

INIs have made impressive progress in recent years but still display questionable long-term reliability. In this section, we report on the development and characterization of highly resilient monolithic silicon carbide (4H−SiC) neural devices. SiC is a physically robust, biocompatible, and chemically inert semiconductor. The device support was micromachined from p-type 4H−SiC, with conductors created from n-type 4H−SiC that simultaneously provides electrical isolation through the resulting pn junction. *a*-SiC was utilized as the top side insulation, preventing shorting of the pn diode by the electrochemical environment. Electrodes were designed with a geometric surface area (GSA) varying from 496 to 500 k μm^2. Electrical characterization showed high-performance pn diode behavior, with typical turn-on voltages of ~2.3 V and reverse bias leakage below 1 nA_{rms}. Current leakage between adjacent electrodes was ~7.5 nA_{rms} over a voltage range of −50 to 50 V. The devices interacted electrochemically with a purely capacitive relationship at frequencies less than 10 kHz. Electrode impedance ranged from 675 ± 130 kΩ (GSA = 496 μm^2) to 46.5 ± 4.80 kΩ (GSA = 500k μm^2). As the monolithic SiC devices rely on the integration of only robust and highly compatible SiC material, they offer a promising solution to probe delamination and biological rejection often associated with the use of multiple materials used in many current INI devices.

As described in previous sections, there are many failure mechanisms associated with present-day INI devices. The materials used play a vital role in a devices' longevity. It has become increasingly clear that for INI technology to reach a level where it can impact the medical community, a strategy that incorporates solutions to all these failure mechanisms must be developed to reliably acquire high-quality neural recordings. To improve present-day neural probes a material, or materials, which address the previously described modes of failure must be utilized. It is the hypothesis of the monolithic SiC INI that by reducing the heterogeneity of the materials comprising MEAs, the reliability of these devices can be improved. One such material that may prove to be an effective solution is SiC. SiC is a semiconductor material like Si and, due to its semiconductor properties, it is possible to produce both insulating and conducting material forms. This section explores the properties of 4H−SiC that make it a viable material for the advancement of INI technology.

Based on previous in vivo and in vitro results in Chapter 10 of the first edition of *Silicon Carbide Technology: A Biocompatible Semiconductor for Advanced Biomedical Devices and Applications* [32], it was decided to produce all-SiC neural probes capable of active recoding and stimulation within the cortex. The fabricated arrays reported in this chapter are composed completely of a single material, SiC. Devices fabricated from 4H−SiC and 3C−SiC will be reported, with the first demonstration of an "all-SiC" neural interface demonstrated in 4H−SiC first (this section) and a 3C−SiC version, which is preferred, in the next section. In both cases, monocrystalline SiC served as both the substrate and conductive electrode elements of the devices. Taking advantage of the semiconductor properties of SiC the devices use alternatively doped polarity SiC (i.e., n-type on p-type epitaxial layers) to create a pn diode to provide isolation between adjacent electrodes through the substrate. *a*-SiC served as a conformal, top-side insulator coating to prevent the electrochemical environment from shorting the pn diode.

2.1 Device design

Utilizing the knowledge and information accumulated from the previous research summarized in Chapter 1 of this book, it becomes apparent that implantable all-SiC neural devices can be fabricated. Electrodes displaying semimetallic charge transport can be fabricated by degenerately doping the SiC epilayer during the epitaxial growth process. The use of alternate polarity SiC, heavily doped n-type grown on p-type SiC, creates a pn diode that provides isolation between adjacent electrodes. Amorphous SiC (*a*-SiC) can then serve as a conformal, top-side insulating coating to prevent the electrochemical environment from shorting the pn diode. A high-quality 4H–SiC epiwafer was grown and delivered to the University of South Florida (USF) SiC group by researchers at Linköping University (Linköping, Sweden). Once received all-SiC INI development began with the fabrication of devices on 4H–SiC.

Fig. 5.2 demonstrates a cross-sectional view of the developed monolithic-SiC neural probe:

2.1.1 Planar MEA design for electrode testing

The all-SiC neural devices reported here were developed using standard semiconductor device fabrication processes. SiC epitaxial wafers were grown at Linköping University (Linköping, Sweden) via hot-wall chemical

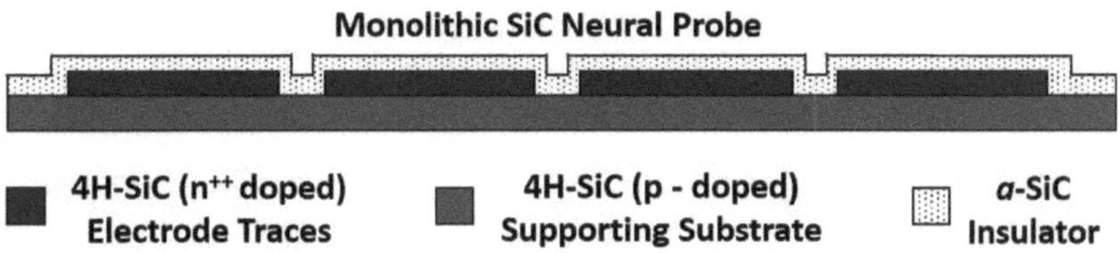

Figure 5.2 Cross-sectional view of an all-SiC neural device probe made using 4H–SiC. Shown for illustration are 4 semimetallic electrode mesas sharing the same probe shank. Degenerately doped SiC electrodes have semimetallic properties. The integral PN junctions create isolation between adjacent electrodes while *a*-SiC is utilized as a conformal top-side insulator preventing the shorting of the pn junctions in liquid environments such as the brain.

vapor deposition [35,36]. A ~5 μm thick, low-doped (aluminum) p-type epitaxial layer of 4H–SiC was homoepitaxially grown on a quarter wafer of 4 degrees off-axis 4H–SiC (0001) [37]. The doping density of the p-type base epitaxial layer was $\sim 1 \times 10^{16}\ \mathrm{cm}^{-3}$. This was followed by the deposition of an opposite polarity 2.5 μm thick, heavily doped (nitrogen) n^+ film that is known to display semimetallic conduction [38]. The two layers formed a pn junction diode, which provided electrical isolation between adjacent electrode mesa traces and offered minimal leakage current.

An insulating *a*-SiC film providing conformal surface insulation was deposited using a PlasmaTherm model 730 plasma-enhanced chemical vapor deposition (PECVD) system. The plasma field frequency was set to 13.56 MHz, substrate temperature to 250°C, and pressure to 900 mTorr. Silane (SiH_4) and methane (CH_4) were used as the reactive gas species at flow rates of 360 and 12 sccm, respectively [39]. Argon (Ar) was used as the carrier gas with a flow rate of 500 sccm. Kapton tape was placed on a blank Silicon (Si) companion wafer before *a*-SiC deposition for thickness measurement of the deposited film using a Dektak D150 profilometer.

Fig. 5.3A shows an image of the microelectrode array (MEA) mask design used to produce planar all-SiC electrodes. Fig. 5.3B shows an optical microscope image of one set of single-ended electrodes with 100 μm diameter active recording area of varying lengths (4, 6, 8, and 10 mm). Fig. 5.3C shows one side of an interdigitated electrode (IDE) device used to measure the isolation between an n^+ mesa and *p* base material. Excellent isolation between the electrodes mesas was observed as will be reported in the next section (Fig. 5.5C).

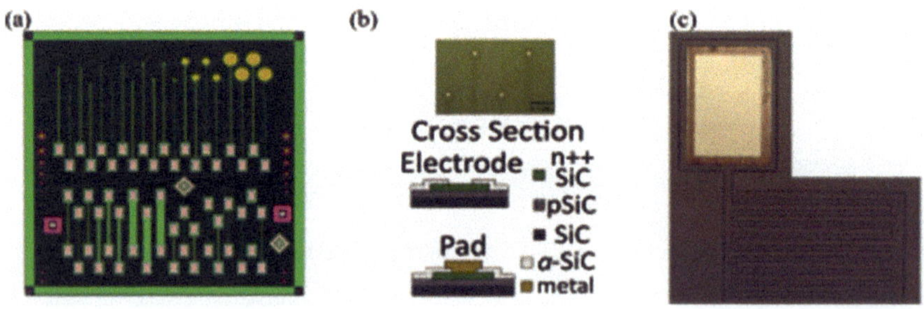

Figure 5.3 All-SiC planar device used for electrical and electrochemical testing. (A) planar MEA mask with single-ended electrodes (top) with recording tip diameters of 25, 50, 100, 400, and 800 μm and test structures (bottom). (B) An optical micrograph of fabricated all-SiC single-ended electrodes (100 μm diameter recording sites). (C) One end of an all-SiC interdigitated electrode (IDE) showing a metal contact pad (top) and a portion of the two interdigitated 50 μm wide mesas of n^+ on *p* base layer with a pitch of 25 μm.

2.1.2 *Implantable probe design for in vivo testing*

The implantable neural probes have been partially fabricated and consist of 16 n^+-doped traces of varying lengths, each of the traces is 10 μm wide and has an active recording tip diameter of 15 μm (Fig. 5.4). Additional fabrication steps are pending to create the free-standing neural devices. First, a deep-reactive ion etching (DRIE) step will be used to define the geometry of the probes by etching through the p^+-doped base layer and the underlying undoped layer. The additional DRIE step will utilize a Ni hard, which allows for a longer etch process. The process to develop the Ni hardmask follows steps utilized for previous metal liftoff processes. A thick layer of Ni (~1 μm) will be deposited. The DRIE etch rate is ~1 μm per minute with a 23:1 selectivity (i.e., for every 23 μm of SiC removed 1.0 μm of the Ni mask will be consumed). To further thin down the SiC substrate, the backside of the material will be thinned (lapped) down until the wafer is ~50 um thick. To free the neural devices from the thinned-down wafer, a DRIE etch will be implemented to blanket etch the remaining backside of the wafer.

2.2 Electrical performance

Capacitance versus voltage measurements of Schottky contacts to the n^+ conductor layer verified that the doping on the n^+ epi layer was on the order of $3.45 \times 10^{18}\ cm^{-3}$ that was consistent with our epi-doping estimates of $\sim 3 \times 10^{18}\ cm^{-3}$ from prior growth runs using the same level of intentional nitrogen doping [40]. Typical doping of the p-type base

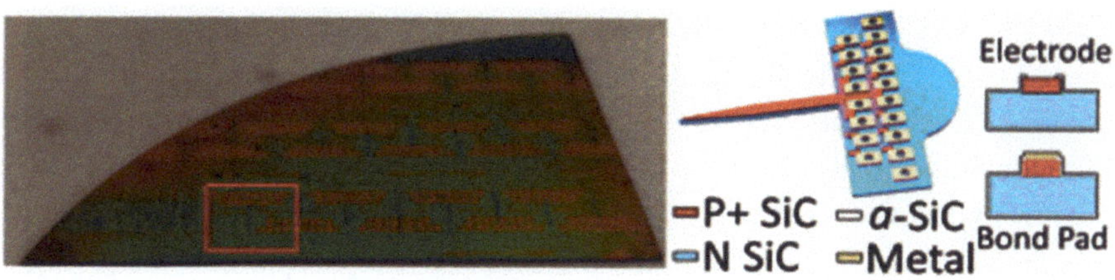

Figure 5.4 Photograph of partially fabricated all-SiC neural implants on a 4H–SiC wafer (Left). Due to the processing challenges of thinning the bulk 4H–SiC substrate (~400 μm), the probe definition etch was not performed thus the individual probes have yet to be separated from the wafer. A single probe (outlined in red) is a 16-channel Michigan Style all-SiC neural probe with holes through the contact pads that allow for connection to an 18-pin Omnetics connector (Omnetics Connector Corp., Minneapolis MN). A graphic representation of the probes is shown on the right. The probe contains 16 n^+-doped traces of varying length and 10 μm width. Each electrode has an active recording tip with a 15 μm diameter.

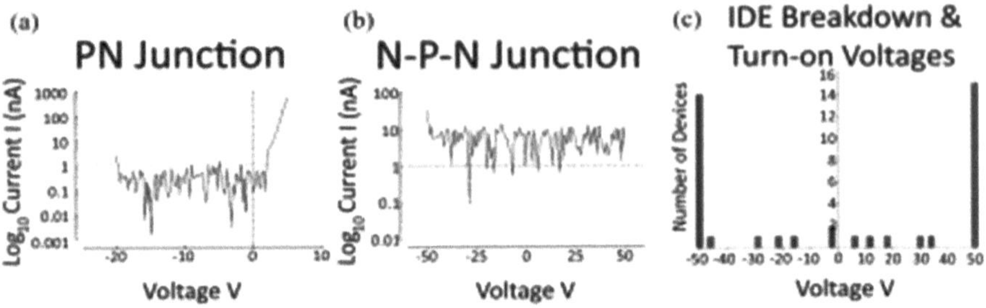

Figure 5.5 4H- All-SiC device electrical characterization. (A) IV measurements from −20 to +5 V on the p−n diodes demonstrate typical forward-biased turn-on voltage ~2.3 V and a leakage current well below 1 nA. (B) Conductive mesa isolation measurement via IV sweep from −50 to +50 V in air. Note long p−n junctions provided excellent isolation with a slight current leakage of less than 7.5 nA_{rms}. (C) Histogram from insulation/isolation measurements on 20 IDE devices from −50 to +50 V. Of 20 devices, only two showed measurable current flow at the p−n diode turn-on voltage (+2.3 V), while 4 IDEs showed current flow at cathodic potentials between −16 and −50 V and the remaining 14 continued to block to at least ±50 V. Under reverse bias, five IDEs experienced leakage current between +6 and +35 V, while the remaining 15 continued to block up to +50 V.

epitaxial layer was $\sim 1 \times 10^{16}\ cm^{-3}$. Fig. 5.5A displays a semi-log IV plot from a selected p−n junction diode. The p−n diode measurements showed a high-performing p−n diode with a typical turn-on voltage of ~2.3 V and a reverse bias leakage that was below our equipment limit of 1 nA. The turn-on voltage value is comparable to values reported in the literature [37,39,41].

The n^+−p−n^+ junction, which isolate adjacent leads through the substrate, was also tested by repeating the IV measurements using the contact pad of one device to the contact pad of its neighboring device. This test helped demonstrate the effectiveness of the n−p−n junction in isolating individual electrodes (and devices) from one another. These measurements were performed under dry (air) conditions at a voltage range of −50 to +50 V. Fig. 5.5B shows that the n−p−n diode has a slight current leakage of less than 7.5 nA_{rms} over the measured this voltage range.

IDE devices were fabricated to test the isolation of both the pn junction and the conformal *a*-SiC top-side insulator (Fig. 5.3C). Of 20 IDE devices tested (Fig. 5.5C), only two demonstrated a significant current flow at the turn-on potential for the junction diodes (+2.3 V) and 4 IDEs showed current flow at cathodic potentials between −16 and −50 V. The remaining 14 forward-biased electrodes continued to block currents to at least −50. Under reverse bias, five IDEs experienced leakage currents of more than 1 nA between 6 and 35 V, while the remaining 15 continued to block up to +50 V.

2.2.1 Electrochemical performance

Electrochemical impedance spectroscopy (EIS) measurements were performed on planar 4H−SiC electrodes in 7.4 pH aerated phosphate-buffered saline (PBS). The results established that trace length did not significantly affect the overall electrical impedance of the SiC electrodes. Devices were fabricated to test the effect that the GSA had on the overall electrode impedance. The results from the EIS measurements performed on 4H−SiC electrodes are shown in Fig. 5.6A. The electrode interaction with the electrolyte displayed a nearly purely capacitive characteristic at frequencies less than 10 kHz, as is displayed by the phase angle of ~80degrees for the

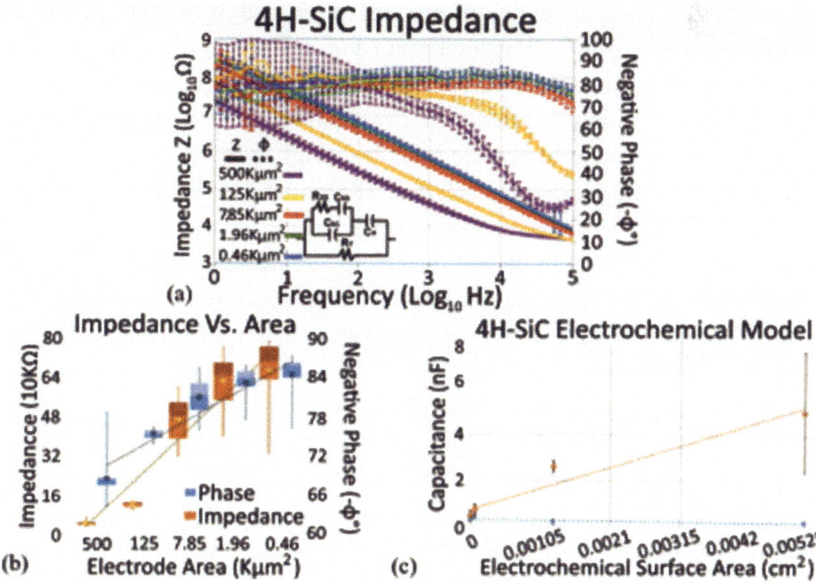

Figure 5.6 (A) Electrochemical impedance spectroscopy (EIS) performed on 4H−SiC electrodes versus geometrical surface area. Error bars represent the standard deviation. Inset shows a basic circuit model that produced an impedance profile similar to the experimental data. (B) A box and whiskers plot for the impedance and phase at the frequency of 1 kHz versus area. Mean impedance and phase are represented with a dot. (C) Charge storage capacity (CSC) obtained via electrochemical modeling of EIS data normalized by the geometric surface area of each electrode. All tests were performed in PBS that was naturally aerated (i.e., no N_2/Ar gas bubbling to remove dissolved O_2) with a pH of 7.4.

electrodes with less than 7.85 k μm^2 geometrical surface area. Another notable trend was that the impedance decreased with an increase in electrode area. Fig. 5.6B displays the impedance and phase angle obtained from the electrodes when measured at 1 kHz, which is the frequency associated with the action potential associated with cortical neural processes. The smallest electrode (496 μm^2) had an average impedance of 675 ± 130 kΩ, which decreased to 46.5 ± 4.80 kΩ for the largest, 500k μm^2 area electrodes. The trend lines added to the graph show a relative linearity associated with all the electrodes.

The inset in Fig. 5.6A shows the circuit model which was used in the ZSimpWin software to predict the impedance response similar to the data obtained from our actual electrodes. The circuit model consists of the Helmholtz double-layer capacitance (C_H) and Faradaic resistance (R_F), normally seen in a Randles circuit model, but includes an additional component exclusive to semiconductors [42,43]. The additional component models the capacitance of the space charge region (C) and the accompanying charging component corresponding to the speed of the change in surface state (R_{SS} and C_{SS}). These components are directly derived from the metal/semiconductor junction. The interaction of the electrolyte and semiconductor leads to pinning of the Fermi level and a bending of the conduction and valence energy bands which, in turn, drive the semiconductor surface into depletion. The Faradaic impedance (R_F) started near 1 GΩ for the largest electrode, increasing to approximately 6 GΩ for the smallest electrodes. The Helmholtz double capacitance (C_H) was on the order of 3 nC for the large-scale electrodes and approached 0.5 nC for the smallest electrodes tested. The surface state resistance (R_{SS}) was in the hundreds of kΩ for the smallest electrodes and only in the tens of kΩ for the largest electrodes.

Fig. 5.7A displays representative cyclic voltammetry (CV) curves for each of the electrodes reported in this study taken across the potential water limit for Pt (−0.6–0.8 V). Fig. 5.7B, on the other hand, shows representative curves using the extended water window (−2.0–2.8 V) from the all-SiC electrodes. Both micrographs demonstrate a decrease in the maximum capacitive current corresponding to a decrease in surface area. Once again, CV data support a dominant capacitive interaction mechanism with the electrolytic ions. The current remains constant for the CV sweep until it nears the potential limit on either side of the voltage sweep. At this point, the charge potential is reversed, leading to a large influx of current

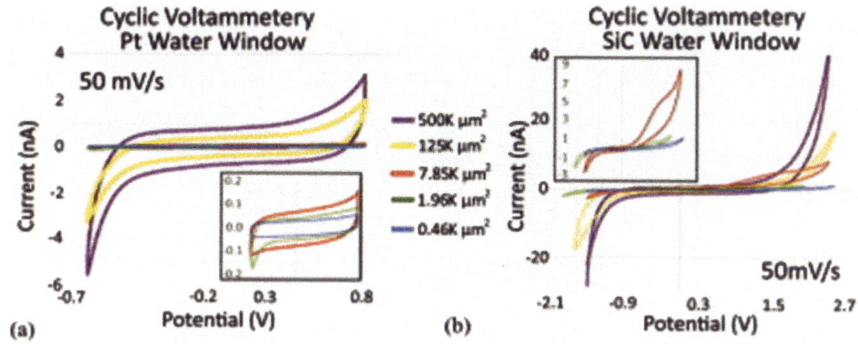

Figure 5.7 (A) CV plot showing a single curve from cyclic voltammetry evaluation of a select 4H–SiC electrode. Curves bounded at the potentials typically used for platinum or iridium electrodes of −0.6 and +0.8 V. Inset shows detail for the three smallest electrodes. (B) Plot of second CV curve from a select electrode. Ramp rate same as for (A), but potential limits were extended until the onset of a large current flux. All tests performed in PBS naturally aerated (i.e., no application of gas bubbling) with a pH of 7.4.

that follows the resistor–capacitor (RC) charging process. After the charging, the current once again remains constant until the next potential ramp shift.

While many of the devices produced curves that were strictly capacitive, a few of the larger area electrodes show increased Faradaic oxidation currents. These oxidation reactions were noticed exclusively on the tests where the potential limits were being evaluated, and an example can be seen in Fig. 5.7B on the 7.85 k μm^2 area electrode. A second observation was that the coupled reduction current was not present on the same electrodes. While these electrodes posed an electrochemical difference, the overall interaction was relatively consistent. This is seen in the variability lower than 5% for the potential limits. The cathodic potential limit was observed to be -1.98 ± 0.08 V while the anodic limit was 2.77 ± 0.07 V.

The difference between the electrodes is more apparent when evaluating the overall CSC and charge delivered per phase. Table 5.1 displays the mean and standard deviation (in parenthesis) of the mean for all the tested electrodes. The table displays CSC for both the standard platinum water window and the expanded SiC water window. The electrodes once again demonstrate a simple area relationship. The smaller electrodes have the largest values for CSC, which decreases with the increase in area. The largest electrodes deliver the largest amount of charge per phase, which decreases with a decrease in area.

Table 5.1 Cathodic and anodic charge storage capacity and charge per phase[a].

GSA (μm^2)	Cathodic				Anodic			
	Charge storage capacity (mC/cm^2)		Charge per phase (nC)		Charge storage capacity (mC/cm^2)		Charge per phase (nC)	
	−0.6–0.8 V	−2.0–2.8 V	−0.6–0.8 V	−2.0–2.8 V	−0.6–0.8 V	−2.0–2.8 V	−0.6–0.8 V	−2.0–2.8 V
502k	4.38×10^{-3} (1.24×10^{-4})	8.00×10^{-2} (0.644)	22 (0.625)	380 (0.642)	3.70×10^{-3} (4.81×10^{-5})	0.257 (0.52)	18.4 (0.242)	1340 (0.520)
125k	1.18×10^{-2} (1.42×10^{-3})	8.61×10^{-2} (1.60×10^{-2})	14.8 (1.78)	108 (20.1)	7.02×10^{-3} (2.9×10^{-4})	0.115 (2.28×10^{-2})	8.82 (0.369)	144 (28.7)
7.8k	2.98×10^{-2} (2.60×10^{-3})	1.01 (0.185)	2.34 (0.204)	79.5 (14.5)	6.22×10^{-2} (3.10×10^{-3})	1.29 (0.113)	4.89 (0.244)	102 (8.87)
1.9k	6.46×10^{-2} (2.07×10^{-3})	1.51 (0.167)	1.27 (4.06×10^{-2})	29.6 (3.27)	0.177 (9.22×10^{-3})	1.37 (0.187)	3.48 (0.181)	27 (3.66)
491	0.194 (5.67×10^{-3})	5.53 (1.38)	0.953 (2.78×10^{-2})	30.4 (6.63)	0.406 (2.22×10^{-2})	5.42 (0.666)	2.00 (0.109)	41.7 (3.81)

[a]Data displayed for both the standard Pt water window as well as for the water window empirically derived for SiC. Standard deviation of the mean is shown in parentheses.

3. Monolithic 3C–SiC neural interfaces

In this section, the design and fabrication of a planar 3C–SiC neural probe on silicon (100) and silicon-on-insulator (SOI) wafers, for ease of manufacture, is reported. Two generations of these all-SiC devices have been fabricated and are reported. The probe is composed of 3C–SiC, which was epitaxially grown on an SOI wafer. A heavily doped n-type (n^+) 3C–SiC film was grown on a moderately doped p-type 3C–SiC layer, forming a p–n junction. The n^+ layer was used to form the electrode traces and recording sites, eliminating the need for metallic conductive traces, as well as for the recording sites that are in direct contact with the extracellular physiological environment. The p–n junction structure provides substrate isolation between conductive traces. A thin film of *a*-SiC was deposited via PECVD on the probe to provide insulation from the external environment. The oxide buried in the SOI wafer served as a sacrificial layer, allowing the SiC probe to be released from the wafer with a selective wet etch (HF) process. This new fabrication approach, based on the demonstrated all-SiC probe design, eliminates residual stresses typically found in similar devices consisting of stacks of heterogeneous films. It is expected that this approach will enhance the long-term material stability of implantable neural probes in the CNS, therefore increasing device reliability over many years. However, now that the manufacture of the probes has been demonstrated, follow-on studies in laboratory animals is required to support this hypothesis.

3.1 First generation 3C–SiC on SOI

The 3C–SiC all-SiC neural probe was developed using variations of standard silicon semiconductor micromachining processes. This started with the epitaxial growth of a 3C–SiC film on an SOI wafer [34], followed by patterning of the 3C–SiC epitaxial films via thin-film contact photolithography techniques. This was followed by the subsequent etching of the electrode traces and recording sites using a DRIE process, deposition of a conformal *a*-SiC film via PECVD, the opening of windows in the *a*-SiC film via RIE (recording and wire-bonding sites), and a final probe definition etch through the buried oxide layer via another DRIE process. The final step was the release of the finished device from the substrate SOI wafer by wet etching the buried oxide layer. The fabrication steps and the details of each step may be found in Ref. [6].

The thickness of the doped epitaxial films was measured using cross-section scanning electron microscopy (SEM) and the composition was verified through energy-dispersive X-ray spectroscopy (EDS). No sulfur-peak was observed in the EDS spectrum, indicating that the device surface was free of chemical residue from the etch processes. Raman spectroscopy and X-ray photoelectron spectroscopy were utilized to assess the 3C−SiC and *a*-SiC film quality, respectively. A commercial connector (Nano Strip, Omnetics Connector Corporation, Minneapolis, MN, USA) was used to make the electrical connections to the probe. Planar single-ended test microelectrodes were fabricated from the same epiwafer material as the implants for ease of electrical testing. CV and EIS in a PBS solution, as well as p−n junction isolation and leakage current tests, were conducted on the test microelectrodes to electrically characterize the fabricated probes.

A 100 mm diameter SOI ((100) Si-oriented) wafer, with an ~27 μm silicon film on top of an ~2 μm buried thermal oxide layer, was used for fabrication of the all-SiC neural probes reported here. The growth process started with epitaxial growth of an ~8 μm thick p-type 3C−SiC film on the SOI wafer, followed by an ~2 μm heavily n-type (n^+) film, using a hot-wall reactor (LPE Epitaxial Technology, Baranzate, Italy) [44]. Heavy doping of semiconductors results in semimetallic performance, which is the case for the n^+ 3C−SiC layer. For this to be achieved, a n^+ doping density of $\sim 10^{19}$ dopants/cm^3 is required. Hydrogen (H_2) was used as a carrier gas, ethylene (C_2H_4) as the carbon precursor, and trichlorosilane ($SiHCl_3$) as the silicon precursor gas [45]. The epitaxial growth temperature was set to ~1370°C with a process pressure of ~75 Torr. The C:Si ratio was kept between 0.8 and 1.2 throughout the epitaxial growth process. Aluminum and nitrogen were the p and n dopants, respectively, and were introduced during the epitaxial growth process [46]. The doping level of the top n^+ 3C−SiC film was measured with a LEI 2017b Mercury (Hg) Probe (Lehighton Electronics, Inc., Lehighton, PA, USA).

3.1.1 Device design

An illustration of the final implant and the associated processing steps is shown in Fig. 5.8. A cross-sectional SEM view of the wafer, which allows for accurate estimation of film thickness (n^+ and p-SiC, Si device film, and buried oxide), is shown in Fig. 5.9A. This figure highlights the various layers and the approximate thickness of each layer on the wafer used for the fabrication.

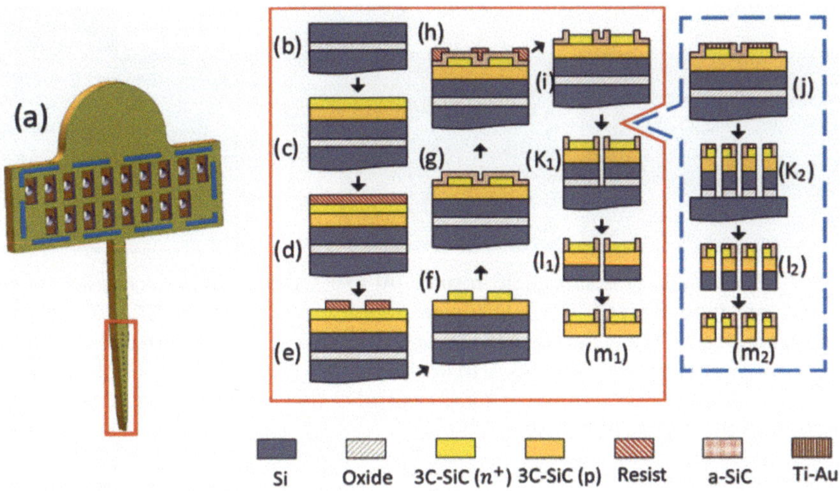

Figure 5.8 The all-SiC fabrication process flow. (A) A rendering of the Michigan-style 3C—SiC probe. Red rectangle shows cross-section at electrode sites while blue rectangle provides the cross-section at the contact pads on the tab. (B) Starting SOI wafer, (C) ~8 μm of p-type 3C—SiC was grown on top, followed by ~2 μm of heavily n-type (n^+) 3C—SiC. (D) The wafer was coated with photoresist and (E) patterned via photolithography. (F) DRIE process was used to form the conductive n^+ mesas and (G) a thin *a*-SiC insulating layer was deposited on top via PECVD. (H) Photoresist was then patterned with photolithography and (I) the *a*-SiC was etched to form windows for the electrode sites using an RIE process. (J) After the *a*-SiC windows were opened, a layer of titanium, followed by gold, was deposited on the contact pads and thermally annealed. A deep DRIE etch through both epilayers and the oxide was performed to (k1) define the probes and (k2) form through-holes in the contact pads. (l_1, l_2) The oxide layer was etched in HF (49%) to release the probes. (m_1, m_2). The probes were soaked inside the KOH solution to remove the residual silicon from the SOI device layer [34].

The two epitaxial 3C—SiC films were measured, and their combined thickness was determined to be ~10 μm. The SOI Si device layer (~27 μm), as well as the thin (~2 μm) buried oxide layer, are also visible in this figure. The epitaxial n^+ film in the center of the wafer was quite rough with a mean surface roughness of ~244 nm and smoother near the wafer edge with a mean surface roughness of ~21 nm. Fig. 5.9B shows the surface morphology of the smooth n^+ layer, which was taken using a DI AFM (Dimension 3100). Although rough in the wafer center (Fig. 5.9C), the surface roughness was low enough for thick layers of photoresist to properly cover the entire surface for the subsequent fabrication steps. However, this roughness would be expected to impact device electrical performance, particularly p—n diode leakage current.

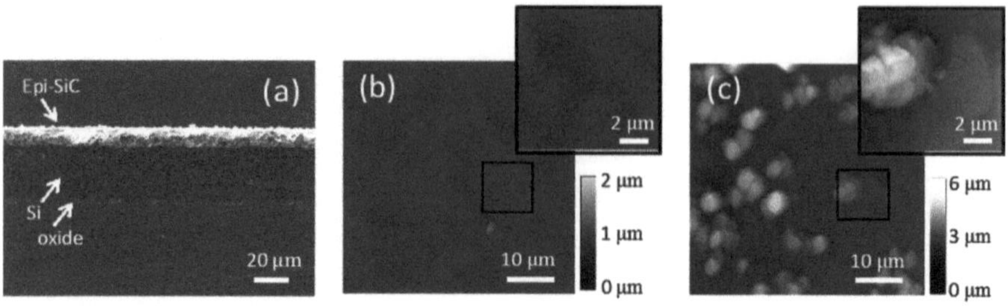

Figure 5.9 Analysis of epitaxial SiC results. (A) Cross-section SEM micrograph of the 3C−SiC epi films on SOI. (B) AFM image (tapping mode) of the 3C−SiC epiwafer specular region on the wafer periphery that shows typical 3C−SiC surface morphology (mean roughness of ~21 nm). (C) AFM image (tapping mode) of the rough surface of the same epiwafer (center) (mean roughness of ~244 nm). The devices were fabricated from the center of the wafer [34].

3.1.2 Electrochemical performance

The doping density of the top n^+ 3C−SiC film was determined by measuring the capacitance-voltage profile of the Schottky contact at 1 MHz and the net charge concentration, N_D-N_A, was estimated to be $\sim 10^{19}\ cm^{-3}$. A similar measurement was also performed on the p-type epitaxial film exposed after DRIE processing and N_A-$-N_D$ was estimated to be $\sim 10^{16}\ cm^{-3}$. These measurements indicate the feasibility of p−n junction formation between two epi films and high electrical conductivity of the top semimetallic n^+ film that formed the traces and electrode sites. EIS was performed to confirm this expectation.

As shown in Fig. 5.10A, current−voltage ($I-V$) measurements on individual diode structures had a rectifying effect due to the diode formed between the n^+- and p-type epitaxial films. To measure turn-on and breakdown voltages and the reverse leakage current, the $I-V$ plot for four diodes on the same wafer was measured. The averaged turn-on voltage for these four diodes was determined to be ~1.4 V, with an average leakage current less than 8 μA_{rms}. In addition, Fig. 5.10A also contains a current-voltage curve, obtained from measurements on one of the IDEs, showing isolation between adjacent traces.

CV curves for four test microelectrodes of the same surface area (491 μm^2) in 7.4 pH PBS are shown in Fig. 5.10B. The upper (+800 mV) and lower (−600 mV) boundaries for the potential were based on the electrochemical window for Pt in water. The shape of the hysteresis cycle showed that the anodic and cathodic currents were charge balanced, with

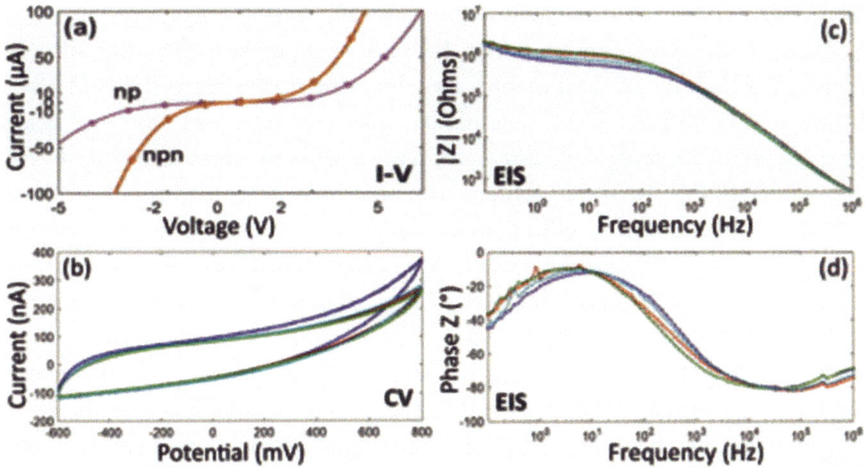

Figure 5.10 All-SiC p–n diode and n–p–n junction characterization and electrochemistry for four test microelectrodes with an area of 491 μm². (A) *I–V* measured from a p–n diode and an n–p–n junction between adjacent traces fabricated on the same wafer used for probe fabrication. (B) The cyclic voltammetry curves swept between +800 and −600 mV with a scan rate of 50 mV/s (C) EIS impedance (*Z*) magnitude (~165 kΩ @1 kHz) and (D) impedance phase angles. The curve for each microelectrode (B–D) is the average of three replicates [34].

no indication of Faradaic current resulting from oxidation or reduction reactions between +800 and −600 mV. However, the phase behavior of the electrode–electrolyte interface (Fig. 5.10D) only supports a capacitive-dominant mechanism at higher frequencies (e.g., −61.2 ± 3.7 degrees at 1 kHz), while at lower frequencies the phase indicates a Faradaic current (e.g., −30.3 ± 4.9 degrees at 100 Hz), which contrasts with earlier results from 4H–SiC microelectrodes reported in the last section [16]. The average anodic CSC was 15.4 ± 1.46 mC/cm^2 (mean ± standard deviation), and the cathodic CSC was 15.2 ± 1.03 mC/cm^2. The average anodic charge per phase was 75.4 ± 5.06 nC, and the average cathodic charge per phase was 74.8 ± 5.06 nC.

Fig. 5.10C and D show the EIS results for the same four test microelectrodes. As expected, the impedance magnitude was found to increase with decreasing frequency. At a frequency of 1 kHz, the impedance was 165 ± 14.7 kΩ (mean ± standard deviation). The electrode–electrolyte interface was determined to be predominately capacitive, as indicated by the negative phase angles for higher frequencies (i.e., >1 kHz).

3.1.3 Fabrication of an implantable 3C–SiC neural interface

A major issue with the previous 4H–SiC probes was the difficulty in releasing a probe of acceptable implant thickness from the 4H–SiC substrate (~400 μm) [33]. Essentially, much of the 4H–SiC substrate would have to be removed, and there was no effective etch stop to prevent over-etching into the device layers. To effectively solve this issue, we used SOI wafers to provide an effective release layer by the simple process of wet etch removal of the buried oxide. However, the SOI wafer used here possessed a relatively thick layer (~27 μm) of silicon that remained on the backside of the probes, which was removed later via KOH soaking. This thick silicon layer can cause residual stress, due to mismatches in the coefficients of thermal expansion and lattice parameters [47] at the interface between the SiC films and silicon, resulting in bowing or bending of the probes. The SOI wafer used in this work had an ~27 μm thick top silicon layer and this may have been the cause of the bowing of the shank and some warping in the connector tab. The shank should be straight for a proper insertion trajectory into the neural tissue. Also, to maximize contact at the connector interface, the tab containing the contact pads should be as planar as possible. Using an SOI wafer with a thin silicon device layer may resolve this deformation problem and will be used in future all-SiC devices.

The two epitaxial 3C–SiC films were measured, and their combined thickness was determined to be ~10 μm. The SOI Si device layer (~27 μm), as well as the thin (~2 μm) buried oxide layer, is also visible in this figure. The epitaxial n^+ film in the center of the wafer was quite rough with a mean surface roughness of ~244 nm and smoother near the wafer edge with a mean surface roughness of ~21 nm. Fig. 5.9B shows the surface morphology of the smooth n^+ layer, which was taken using a DI AFM (Dimension 3100). Although rough in the wafer center (Fig. 5.9C), the surface roughness was low enough for thick layers of photoresist to properly cover the entire surface for the subsequent fabrication steps. However, this roughness would be expected to impact device electrical performance, particularly p–n diode leakage current.

3.1.4 Fabricated 3C-all-SiC neural probe

Epitaxial growth of single-crystalline 3C–SiC with different types of doping enables the realization of a nearly monolithic probe from homogeneous SiC material. The all-SiC probe is a planar neural probe with 16 electrodes for recording and stimulating neurons. The connector tab has 18 metallic pads (approximately 0.8 mm by 0.4 mm) with through holes to

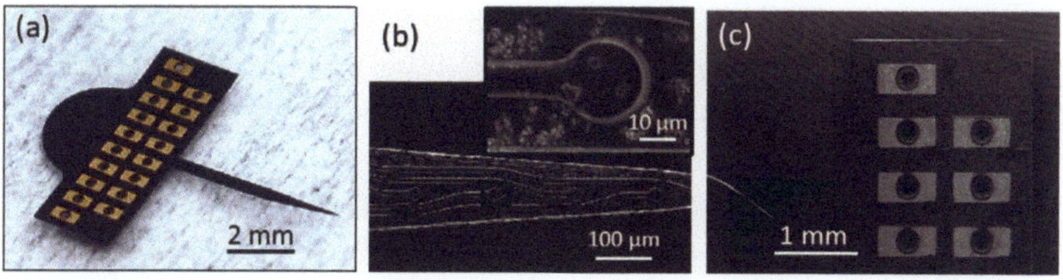

Figure 5.11 Physical characterization of the completed neural probe. (A) Optical image of a freestanding all-SiC probe after release. (B) SEM image of the shank tip showing four of the electrode sites and a magnified image of a single electrode site (inset). (C) SEM image of some of the metal contact pads with through holes. The shank is 5.1 mm long, and the length of the tapered portion is 2.4 mm. The tab is 6.64 mm wide and 2.3 mm long, excluding the semicircular top portion. The surface roughness of the electrode sites is shown in Fig. 5.10C [34].

which a commercial Omnetics connector is bonded. Two extrapads provide connections for the return and reference electrode wires. The diameter of the electrode sites is ~15 μm, and the width of the traces is ~10 μm. Fig. 5.11 shows the optical and SEM micrographs of a free-standing probe.

The probe's shank, which contains the traces and electrode sites, is shown in Fig. 5.11B. This figure shows a scanning electron micrograph of the electrode sites, which have *a*-SiC windows to allow contact with the extracellular environment. The traces and electrode sites are mesas formed from the n^+ 3C−SiC film. There are no metallic components on the shank, which is a homogeneous structure consisting entirely of SiC. The pads, which are shown in Fig. 5.11C, contain titanium and gold layers to provide ohmic connections to external electronic devices via an Omnetics connector. However, as the metallic pads are not in direct contact with brain tissue, the issues regarding delamination of metallic parts and compatibility with CNS tissue are not a concern.

3.2 Second-generation 3C−SiC on SOI

The previous sections show the progression of the SiC Group at the University of South Florida to develop an all-silicon carbide (all-SiC) based INI, as demonstrated in Bernadin et al. [33] and Beygi et al. [34] with 4H- and 3C−SiC INIs, respectively. However, to release the probes, the thickness of the bulk 4H−SiC substrate (>400 μm) must be thinned which is very time consuming and expensive. To solve this challenge, 3C−SiC devices on bulk Si and SOI were developed to allow for easy release from the handle wafer via immersion in HF solution and/or KOH etching of the silicon substrate. Unfortunately, for the first generation 3C—SiC epitaxial material used to fabricate these easy-to-release probes, the SiC material quality was marginal, resulting in higher leakage currents compared to the 4H—SiC planar MEAs developed previously. In addition, while the all-SiC monolithic INI should result in a very stable, long-term implant, it is quite expensive to fabricate and a thinner, more flexible, and lower-cost solution is needed. Work done to develop a flexible electrode consisting of a metal trace encapsulated in amorphous SiC (*a*-SiC) has been reported by Deku et al. [48]. This work demonstrated the benefit of using *a*-SiC as both insulator and support but still relies on a metal electrode with all the associated fabrication and reliability challenges. Based on all of the research reported by both our group and others, it is highly beneficial to develop an INI using the best combination of materials available, and the focus shifted to carbon electrodes sandwiched in *a*-SiC insulation. Thus, one research aim was to investigate the next generation neural interface, both in terms of using higher-quality material (3C—SiC grown on bulk silicon, for example, discussed in this section), and alternate materials (carbon thin films synthesized on *a*-SiC) to realize biocompatible interfaces as discussed in Chapter 7.

3.2.1 Device design

Two types of devices have been used to develop the all-SiC INI in our group: Device 1 is a planar MEA composed of single-ended electrodes and double-ended resistors (Fig. 5.12A). Along with these devices, there are Schottky and pn diodes for material characterization. This design can be realized with three mask layers: (1) Mesa Etch Mask, (2) *a*-SiC RIE

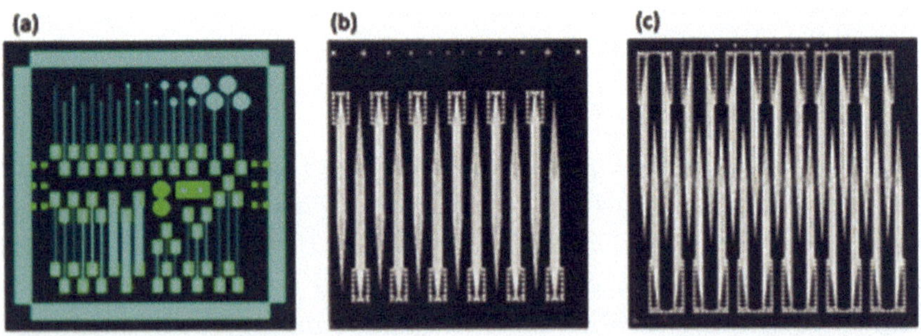

Figure 5.12 Photolithographic process masks for all-SiC INI device designs: (A) planar MEA devices for electrochemical testing and materials evaluation and implantable second generation 3C—SiC INI devices for (B) single-shank 16-electrode and (C) double-shank 32-electrode probes.

window definition mask, and (3) metal lift-off mask. Device 2 are implantable MEAs and they can be realized with 4 mask layers as follows: (1) Mesa Etch (DRIE) Mask, (2) *a*-SiC window (RIE) definition mask, (3) metal lift-off mask, and (4) probe definition (DRIE) mask.

Fig. 5.13 illustrates the fabrication process for realizing the all-SiC neural interface. The 3C–SiC epitaxial wafer was first diced into smaller pieces (die) for subsequent processing using a diamond blade in a wafer dicing tool (Dicing saw M1006, Micro Automation Inc.). Next, the die was cleaned using solvent and Radio Corporation of America (RCA) cleans to remove any organic and inorganic residues, surface oxide, and heavy metal contaminants on top of the epi wafer. After cleaning, the epiwafer was thoroughly rinsed with DI water and dried with N_2 gas to remove all water from the surface. Next, a thin layer of HMDS (hexamethyldisilazane; Microchemicals GmbH, Ulm, Germany) was spin coated onto the wafer (3000 rpm for 50 s) to enhance the adhesion between the SiC surface and photoresist. Following the adhesion promoter AZ 12xt-20PL positive photoresist (Microchemicals GmbH) was spin coated on top at 1500 rpm for 50 s that results in a thickness of ~15 μm. To minimize the edge bead influence, an 11,000 rpm spin step for 2 s was used to drive any resistance

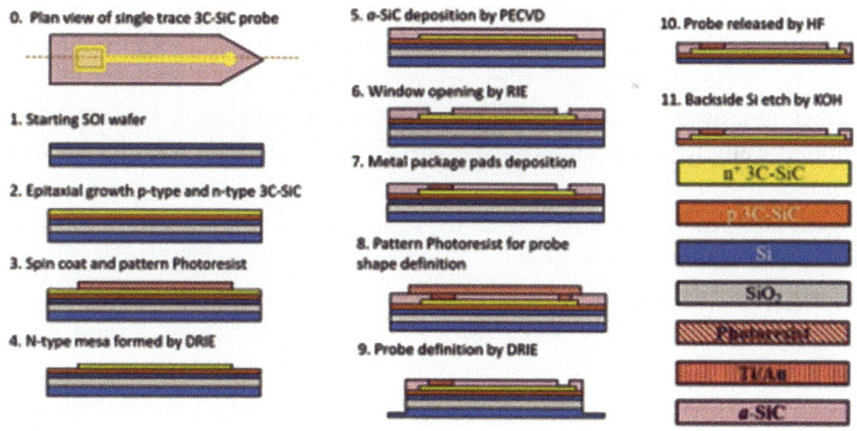

Figure 5.13 The fabrication flow of all-SiC neural probes. PPF device fabrication process steps. (1) Starting with an SOI wafer, (2) epitaxial growth p-type and n-type 3C–SiC, (3) spin-coat photoresist, (4) n-type mesa formed by DRIE etch, (5) an a-SiC film is deposited via PECVD, (6) RIE used to open windows exposing the recording tip (not shown) and bonding pad, (7) next metal is deposited on the bond pads, (8) spin-coat and pattern photoresist to define the probe shape, (9) DRIE etch through the wafer, (10) releasing probes via HF bath, and (11) the backside Si is removed by KOH bath [49,50].

that may have beaded up on the edge of the wafer/die. Following a 3 min soft-bake at 110°C, the wafer was patterned by exposure to the UV light (Quintel Mask Aligner) with an energy density of 140 mJ/cm^2. The wafer was then degassing in a dark box for 2 h, and then baked at 90°C for 1 min. Then the wafer was developed in AZ300 developer (Michrochemicals GmBH) for 2 min followed by a hard-bake at 90°C for 5 min. This completes the fabrication of the etch mask to create the semimetallic electrodes. A DRIE (Adixen AMS 100) was performed to etch the wafer for 3 min to create the n$^+$ mesa on the epi wafer surface. The etch was made ~0.5 μm deeper than needed to ensure that the n$^+$ layer was completely removed between adjacent mesas. The DRIE etch process recipe was as follows: 10 sccm O_2, and 90 sccm SF_6 under a pressure of 5.7 mTorr, the temperature on the sample holder was kept at −20°C, and the power on the sample holder was 550 W while the RF power was set to be 1800 W. The etch rate for this recipe was estimated to be ~0.9 μm/min. The etched n-type traces on the p-type substrate thus form a pn diode along the length of the mesa.

Next, a ~250 nm *a*-SiC insulation layer was deposited via PECVD (Unaxis 790). Methane (CH_4) and silane (SiH_4) served as the carbon and silicon precursors that were diluted in Ar with flow rates of 360, 12, and 700 sccm, respectively. The chamber temperature and pressure were set to 250°C and 1100 mTorr with 200 W of RF power. The high C:Si ratio helps to decrease the *a*-SiC film stress. The film stress assessment will be further discussed in Chapter 7. After mesa etch processing, the mask was stripped using Microchem 1165 and the die cleaned for the next processing step that is to open windows in the *a*-SiC layer. After cleaning AZ15nXT negative photoresist was patterned on top of *a*-SiC, and a reactive ion etch (RIE) was run for 300 s to open windows in the top *a*-SiC film for the recording sites and package pads. RIE recipe was as follows: 37 sccm tetrafluoromethane (CF_4) and 13 sccm O_2 were served as processing gases, with a power of 200 W and pressure of 50 mTorr. The RIE etch process rate was ~0.9 nm/s, and as the etch rate is much slower for 3C—SiC, an etch stop is not needed to avoid over-etching of the n$^+$ mesa region. After window definition, a metal-liftoff mask was formed using the same photolithographic procedure outlined earlier. After removal of the mask in the metal bonding pad regions, the die was again cleaned and ready for metal deposition. A Varian e-beam metal evaporator (four pockets) was used to deposit a 20 nm titanium (Ti) thick metal adhesion layer, followed by a 300 nm gold (Au) layer to create the package bonding pads for electrical and electrochemical testing. To achieve low-resistance contacts after metal liftoff a rapid thermal process (RTP) was performed on the wafer to eliminate the Schottky contact between the SiC and metal pads. The RTP was done at 650°C for 10 min at a ramping rate of 10°C/s. For free-standing probes (not yet completed at the time of this dissertation writing) an additional Ti/Au deposition is performed resulting in an Au overlayer that facilitates Au wire bonding. This completes the fabrication of the all-SiC electrodes and for planar testing this marks the end of the process.

For implantable INI devices, the final step is to release the probes from the SOI substrate. To illustrate this step the procedure developed by Beygi [34] is discussed here. Positive photoresist AZ12xt-20PL was patterned with the probe shape with a thickness of 15 μm, then the same DRIE recipe that was used for defining the n-type traces was applied to etch through the SiC layers to define the probes. The etch time was increased to 15 min to ensure that the epitaxial films were etched through and the buried oxide layer in the SOI substrate was exposed. Next, the probes were released via an HF (49%) etch to remove the sacrificial oxide layer, then cleaned with rinsing DI and dried with N_2 gas. The backside Si residue from the SOI was then removed by a diluted KOH bath.

One important discovery during the SOI-based all-SiC INI (first generation) developed in our group was the inferior quality of the epitaxial 3C−SiC films on SOI. As a consequence, a new set of epiwafers was grown in the laboratory of Dr. Francesco La Via, IMM-CNR, Catania, Sicily (IT) and were used in the work reported here. Two (2) bulk (100)Si substrates and one (1) SOI substrate were used. Probes have been fabricated on both substrates to date as part of this research and are awaiting probe definition DRIE etching. The earlier procedure will be used to release the probes on SOI, while a slightly different procedure will be used for the bulk Si substrate-supported devices. Here is the process procedure that will be used to achieve free-standing probes: After completion of the device, ending with the probe definition etch, the backside of the substrate will be thinned to ~100 μm. In this case, the probe definition etch will be run so that a ~50 μm deep etch into the bulk substrate is achieved (in Chapter 7, the same deep etch was performed for C-based INI devices and details will be provided there). Once the deep etch has been completed the wafer is flipped onto a Si handle wafer and attached using Crystal Bond. The bulk Si wafer is then "blanket etched" in DRIE until the 50 μm top-side etch is reached. At that point, the wafer is flipped (device side up) and soaked in acetone to remove the crystal bond and, thus, release, the probes. After release ~50 μm thick probes will have been harvested and will be ready for packaging and test. To completely remove the Si from the probe backside, two approaches can be used: (1) DRIE the Si using the 3C–SiC as an etch stop or (2) KOH etching that is effective in removing Si but does not etch SiC.

As the isolation between each mesa trace and substrate was provided by the p–n junction that formed between the n^+ and p-type 3C–SiC epitaxial layers, it is important to evaluate the isolation properties of the p–n diodes and the n–p–n junctions formed between traces by applying forward and reverse voltages and measuring the leakage current that flows. The current–voltage (*I–V*) curves were measured using a Keithley 2400 SourceMeter (Tektronix, Inc., Beaverton, OR). A swept voltage was applied on the p–n diode from −5 to +5 V at a rate of 0.1 V/s. The IV curves are shown in Fig. 5.14. The breakdown voltage was defined as the voltage where the current rapidly increased during the application of either a positive or negative voltage [50] (NPN case) or a negative voltage (PN diode case). The leakage current is defined as the root mean square of the current between the breakdown and zero bias potentials. Ten devices were tested, and the breakdown voltage was defined at a current flow of 1 μA. The results indicate that the breakdown voltage was ~4 V, and the average leakage current was 0.73 μA.

SEM and atomic force microscopy (AFM) were used to evaluate both the device features and material properties. In Fig. 5.15A, the cross-section view of the epitaxial wafer was used to accurately measure the thickness of each layer (n^+, p^- 3C–SiC, Si, and buried SiO_2). The top epitaxial

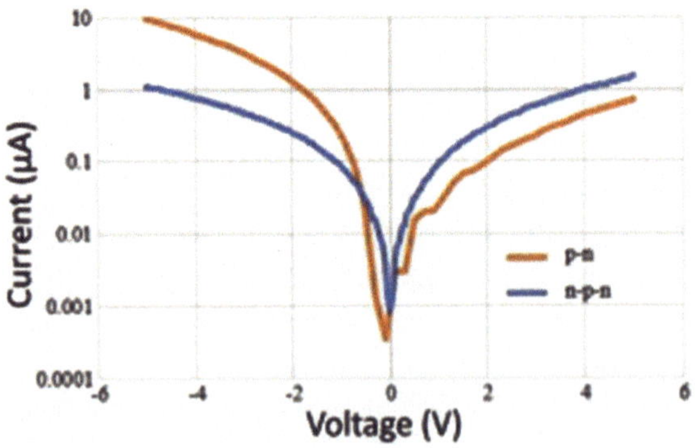

Figure 5.14 *IV* curve measurement on a typical Gen 2 p–n diode and n–p–n junction between each trace fabricated on the same wafer. By definition, the breakdown voltage was ~-4 V corresponding to a leakage current of ~0.76 μA [49].

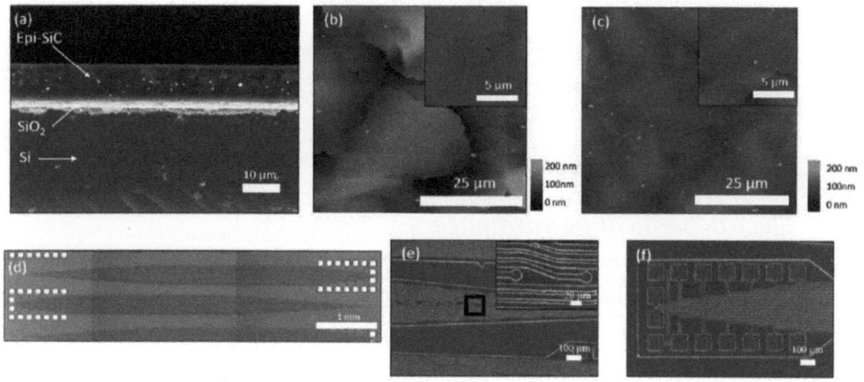

Figure 5.15 SEM and AFM analysis on Gen 2 epitaxial SiC film and a prereleased all-SiC neural probe. (A) Cross-section SEM micrograph of epitaxial 3C–SiC on SOI wafer. AFM analysis on the epitaxial 3C–SiC film, (B) edge region of the wafer, and (C) center region of the wafer. (D) Optical micrograph of to be released neural probe and (E,F) SEM micrographs of recording sites and package pads [49].

3C–SiC layer was measured to be ~10 μm thick in total comprised of 2 μm of n^+ and 8 μm of p^-. In this case, the SOI Si layer was 2 μm, and the buried SiO_2 layer was 2 μm. The roughness of the edge and center region of the die was measured by AFM (DI 3100). As shown in Fig. 5.15B and C, the mean surface roughness in the center of the die (C) was 8.86 nm while the mean surface roughness at the edge (B) was 23.7 nm. These results indicate a 90% improvement in surface roughness at the center of the wafer compared with the surface roughness of the previous batch of Gen 1 wafers (~244 nm) [34]. High surface roughness may lead to higher leakage currents in the devices fabricated from the center region.

Optical and SEM micrographs of a prereleased probe are shown in Fig. 5.15D–E. Monolithic SiC-based neural probes were fabricated from epitaxially grown 3C–SiC with an n^+ semimetallic later on a p^- base layer, forming an integral PN junction and insulated by *a*-SiC. The planar neural probes contain 16 electrodes for neural recording and stimulation. Fig. 5.15E shows the 18 metallic package pads with a length and width of 100 and 100 μm. In Fig. 5.15E, an SEM micrograph of the probe's shank (mesa traces) shows the *a*-SiC window opening on the recording site with a diameter of 15 μm that allows contact between the electrodes and neurons. The whole shank of the neural probe was made from only SiC without any metallic or polymeric components, with n^+ 3C–SiC serving as the conducting traces, and the insulation was provided by an integral p–n junction (bottom) and *a*-SiC (top). Although the package pads were made with titanium-gold layers, to provide connection to external electronic devices, they will not be implanted into the brain. Thus, SiC will be the only material in direct contact with brain tissue, thus avoiding the reliability challenges well known with metals and insulators in the brain [31,51,52].

3.2.2 Electrochemical performance

EIS and CV were utilized for electrochemical characterization on the planar 3C–SiC single-ended electrodes. A potentiostat (Reference 600, Gamry, Inc.) was used in the standard three-electrode measurement configuration: working electrode (3C–SiC), counter electrode (Pt), and reference electrode (Ag/AgCl). The charge transfer properties, charge storage capacity, and any electrochemical reactions can be obtained by CV. The potential range was chosen to be −0.6 to +0.8 V, which is the same potential water window of Pt. Therefore, a direct comparison between SiC and Pt electrodes was feasible. EIS provides both impedance and phase performance data in the frequency range of interest that is 1 kHz in this case because 1 kHz is associated with the neuron spiking frequency.

Electrochemical testing was performed on the planar test microelectrodes that were fabricated along with the neural probes from the same wafer, except that the planar test microelectrodes were not released from the substrate. All measurements were performed in N_2 aerated PBS at room temperature with a pH of 7.40 ± 0.01. During EIS measurement, the frequency range was set from 10 Hz to 1 MHz with an RMS voltage of 10 mV. Ten (10) data points were collected per decade, and three measurements were repeated and averaged. Each CV measurement cycle started with a swept potential from −0.6 to +0.8 V, and then back to −0.6V with a rate of 50 mV/s. The results were averaged from three cycles.

CV curves on four (4) SiC planar test microelectrodes with a recording area of 491 μm^2 are shown in Fig. 5.16A. The potential range (−0.6 to 0.8 V) was limited by the electrochemical window for Pt in water. The same area on top of the curve and bottom of the curve indicates the cathodic and anodic currents were charge balanced, and there was no peak along the curve that indicates that there was no oxidation or reduction reaction happening in the range of −0.6 to 0.8 V. The phase diagram in Fig. 5.16B shows a capacitive-dominant mechanism not only at higher frequencies, for instance -91.9 ± 0.29 degrees at 1 kHz, but also at lower frequencies. The average anodic and cathodic charge storage capacity (CSC_a and CSC_c) were calculated to be 56.1 and 18.2 mC/cm^2, respectively.

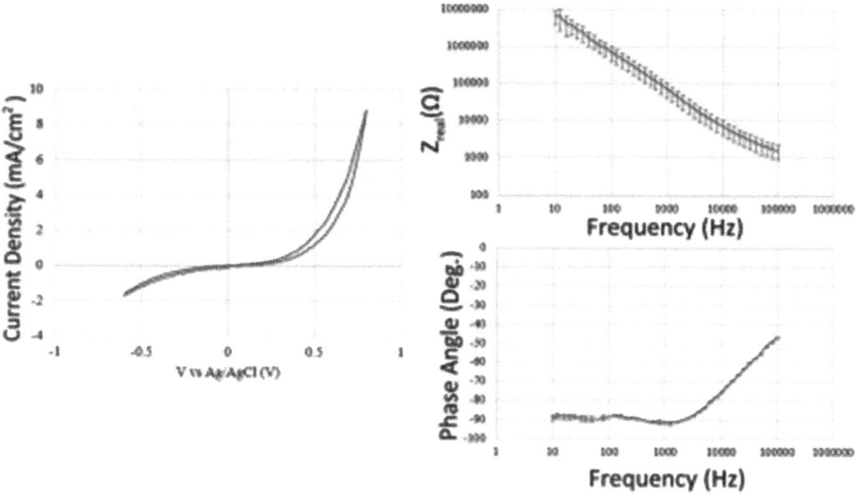

Figure 5.16 Electrochemical characterization on Gen 2 all-SiC planar test devices: (A) CV curves from −0.6 to 0.8 V with a scan rate of 50 mV/s; (B) EIS results show the impedance magnitude of 71.6 ± 29.1 kΩ and phase angle of −91.9 ± 0.29 degrees at 1 kHz [24].

The EIS results on the same microelectrodes were shown in Fig. 5.16B. It can be seen that, with increasing frequency, the impedance decreases as expected. For a recording area of 491 μm^2, the impedance at 1 kHz was 71.6 ± 29.1 kΩ with a negative phase angle of −91.9 ± 0.29 degrees. This indicates that the electrode–electrolyte interface was dominated by capacitive current, again which is expected from SiC that is a ceramic-like material.

4. Summary

For INI technology to continue to grow as a valuable therapeutic tool for individuals suffering from nervous system damage or disorders, the failure mechanisms associated with present-day neural devices must be eliminated. SiC, more specifically 3C–SiC, has demonstrated several key attributes that make it a valuable replacement for present-day INI devices. SiC has been demonstrated to be more biocompatible and hemocompatible than Si (which are used in present-day devices). The first set of devices fabricated utilized the 4H–SiC polytype followed by two generations (Gen 1 and 2) of 3C–SiC on Si and SOI. The top SiC epilayer was degenerately doped to give the material semimetallic properties, eliminating the need for metal electrode traces. SiC INI devices were fabricated by growing degenerately n-doped electrode traces on a p-doped substrate. The pn junctions between the individual traces and the substrate provided isolation between adjacent electrode traces, eliminating the need for a dielectric material between substrate and electrode traces. Conventional silicon photolithographic processing techniques were employed in the design and fabrication of the all-SiC device. The top side of the electrodes and exposed substrate were insulated with a ~250 nm conformal layer of *a*-SiC, a well-known and highly utilized biomedical grade insulator, to prevent shorting of the pn junction within the electrochemical environment.

Due to the wide bandgap nature of SiC, a turn-on voltage of ~2.3 V was observed for the 4H−SiC pn junctions (as a reference Si has a turn-on voltage of ~0.7 V). This turn-on voltage is well above the operating potential utilized within in vivo INI devices. A leakage current of ~7.5 nA_{rms} was observed between electrodes over a voltage range of −50 to 50 V (a voltage range well above the required range for chronically implanted devices). Electrochemical results show that the fabricated 4H−SiC MEAs interacted with the electrochemical environment primarily through capacitive mechanisms and have impedance comparable to that of gold electrodes. The capacitive interaction of the MEAs is preferred over a Faradaic interaction. However, electrodes that undergo Faradaic chemical reaction mechanisms (IrOx) tend to have larger CSC_C values. Therefore, 4H−SiC devices cannot deliver charge as efficiently as other conventionally used microelectrode materials but are more chemically robust. Even with that in mind, all studies and data collected thus far indicate that the monolithic SiC neural device can aid in the advancement of chronic INI use in clinical settings.

In this chapter, two generations of 3C−SiC-based all-SiC neural probes were fabricated and the electrical and electrochemical characterization results from planar MEAs were presented. The fabrication process started with the epitaxial growth of a p-type 3C−SiC layer followed by a heavily doped n-type 3C−SiC layer, all on either SOI or bulk 4 Si wafer. Each probe had 16 conducting traces and electrode sites. In addition, an *a*-SiC layer was deposited on top of the epitaxial layer by PECVD and served as the top side insulation layer. As the neural probes were fabricated via an advanced semiconductor fabrication process, the neural probes can be easily fabricated into different shapes. The probes were released from the substrate using an HF bath, and the residual Si on the backside was removed by a KOH bath at room temperature.

Table 5.2 summarizes the surface roughness and electrochemical properties of Gen 1 and Gen 2 3C−SiC devices. The highly doped top

Table 5.2 Properties comparison between Gen 1 and Gen 2 3C–SiC devices.

3C–SiC generation	Surface roughness (nm)		Impedance[a] (kΩ)	Phase angle[a] (degrees)	CSC_a (mC/cm^2)	CSC_c (mC/cm^2)
	Center	edge				
Gen 1	244.0	21.0	165 ± 14.7	-61.2 ± 3.7	15.4	15.2
Gen 2	8.8	23.7	71.6 ± 29.1	-91.9 ± 0.29	56.1	18.2

[a]Measured at 1 kHz.

n-type layer offers the neural probes excellent electrical and electrochemical properties. The surface roughness of the n-type layer was measured by AFM with the surface roughness of Gen 2 was vastly improved over Gen 1 in the wafer center region. This indicates better crystallinity and less defects in the film. The breakdown voltage of the devices was measured to be 4 V with a leakage current of 0.76 μA, which is an order of magnitude improvement over Gen 1. The electrochemical properties were characterized using planar MEA electrodes. With a surface area of 491 μm^2 the 3C−SiC all-SiC electrode (Gen 2) demonstrated an impedance of 71.6 ± 29.1 kΩ with a phase angle of -91.9 ± 0.29 degrees at 1 kHz, and CSC_a and CSC_c of 56.1, and 18.2 mC/cm^2. Compared with Gen 1, Gen 2 showed superior electrochemical properties, most likely due to the better crystal quality of the epi films. These results offer the promise that 3C−SiC all-SiC neural probes are capable to record neural signals and stimulate neurons.

In summary, while silicon is one of the most commonly used materials by today's implantable neural interface industry, it suffers from a set of complex interactions between abiotic and biotic responses and reduces the reliability for long-term implantation. Unfortunately, this limits the interest in the implantable neural interface in humans. Fortunately, previous results from our group on the biocompatibility and hemocompatibility have shown that SiC is a promising candidate for biomedical applications. Further in vivo experiments on all-SiC neural probes are needed and will be performed in the near future.

Acknowledgments

We gratefully thank J. ul-Hassain of LIU and F. La Via of CNR-IMM for providing the epitaxial wafers of 4H- and 3C−SiC, respectfully. These are the most important ingredient in the all-SiC recipe and work could not have been performed without this material. Dr. J. Pancrazio at the University of Texas, Dallas, is acknowledged for his support in characterizing and electrochemical measurements for the 4H−SiC planar devices in his laboratory. Additionally, we would like to extend our thanks to Dr. Pancrazio for hosting E. Bernardin for a summer internship to perform these measurements. We thank R. Everly of the USF NREC for his constant support in the microfab of all of our devices. We thank Ryan 'Collin' Asson of the USF SiC Group for providing the artwork shown in Fig. 5.1.

References

[1] J.J. Vidal, Toward direct brain-computer communication, in: L.J. Mullins (Ed.), Annu Rev Biophys Bioeng vol. 2, Annual Reviews, Inc., Palo Alto, CA, 1973, pp. 157−180.

[2] M.A. Lebedev, M.A.L. Nicolelis, Brain-machine interfaces: past, present and future, Trends in Neurosciences 29 (September 2006) 536–546.
[3] K.D. Wise, A.M. Sodagar, Y. Yao, M.N. Gulari, G.E. Perlin, K. Najafi, Microelectrodes, microelectronics, and implantable neural microsystems, Proceedings of the IEEE 96 (July 2008) 1184–1202.
[4] J.P. Donoghue, Connecting cortex to machines: recent advances in brain interfaces, Nature Neuroscience 5 (November 2002) 1085–1088.
[5] K.J. Miller, D. Hermes, N.P. Staff, The current state of electrocorticography-based brain-computer interfaces, Neurosurgical focus 49 (July 2020) E2.
[6] G. Buzsaki, Large-scale recording of neuronal ensembles, Nature Neuroscience 7 (May 2004) 446–451.
[7] K.H. Pettersen, G.T. Einevoll, Amplitude variability and extracellular low-pass filtering of neuronal spikes, Biophysical Journal 94 (February 1, 2008) 784–802.
[8] G.T. Einevoll, C. Kayser, N.K. Logothetis, S. Panzeri, Modelling and analysis of local field potentials for studying the function of cortical circuits, Nature Reviews Neuroscience 14 (November 2013) 770–785.
[9] M. Hämäläinen, R. Hari, R.J. Ilmoniemi, J. Knuutila, O.V. Lounasmaa, Magnetoencephalography—theory, instrumentation, and applications to noninvasive studies of the working human brain, Reviews of Modern Physics 65 (1993) 413.
[10] P.L. Nunez, R. Srinivasan, A theoretical basis for standing and traveling brain waves measured with human EEG with implications for an integrated consciousness, Clinical Neurophysiology 117 (2006) 2424–2435.
[11] S.E. Saddow (Ed.), Silicon Carbide Biotechnology: A Biocompatible Semiconductor for Advanced Biomedical Devices and Applications, second ed., Elsevier, Amsterdam, 2016 (p.p̂p. Pages).
[12] V.S. Polikov, P.A. Tresco, W.M. Reichert, Response of brain tissue to chronically implanted neural electrodes, Journal of Neuroscience Methods 148 (2005) 18.
[13] C.T. Nordhausen, P.J. Rousche, R.A. Normann, Optimizing recording capabilities of the Utah intracortical electrode array, Brain Research 637 (February 21, 1994) 27–36.
[14] S.F. Cogan, Neural stimulation and recording electrodes, Annual Review of Biomedical Engineering 10 (2008) 275–309.
[15] D.R. Kipke, Implantable neural probe systems for cortical neuroprostheses, International Conference of the IEEE Engineering in Medicine and Biology Society 7 (2004) 5344–5347.
[16] S.S. Stensaas, L.J. Stensaas, Reaction of cerebral-cortex to chronically implanted plastic needles, Acta Neuropathologica 35 (1976) 187–203.
[17] P.J. Rousche, R.A. Normann, Chronic recording capability of the Utah Intracortical Electrode Array in cat sensory cortex, Journal of Neuroscience Methods 82 (July 1, 1998) 1–15.
[18] A.M.P. Turner, N. Dowell, S.W.P. Turner, L. Kam, M. Isaacson, J.N. Turner, et al., Attachment of astroglial cells to microfabricated pillar arrays of different geometries, Journal of Biomedical Materials Research 51 (September 5, 2000) 430–441.
[19] D.H. Szarowski, M.D. Andersen, S. Retterer, A.J. Spence, M. Isaacson, H.G. Craighead, et al., Brain responses to micro-machined silicon devices, Brain Research 983 (September 5, 2003) 23–35.
[20] R. Biran, D.C. Martin, P.A. Tresco, Neuronal cell loss accompanies the brain tissue response to chronically implanted silicon microelectrode arrays, Experimental Neurology 195 (September 2005) 115–126.
[21] V.S. Polikov, M.L. Block, J.M. Fellous, J.S. Hong, W.M. Reichert, In vitro model of glial scarring around neuroelectrodes chronically implanted in the CNS, Biomaterials 27 (November 2006) 5368–5376.

[22] D.F. Williams, On the mechanisms of biocompatibility, Biomaterials 29 (July 2008) 2941–2953.
[23] K.K. Lee, J.P. He, A. Singh, S. Massia, G. Ehteshami, B. Kim, et al., Polyimide-based intracortical neural implant with improved structural stiffness, Journal of Micromechanics and Microengineering 14 (January 2004) 32–37.
[24] J.C. Barrese, J. Aceros, J.P. Donoghue, Scanning electron microscopy of chronically implanted intracortical microelectrode arrays in non-human primates, Journal of Neural Engineering 13 (2016) 26003.
[25] J.C. Barrese, N. Rao, K. Paroo, C. Triebwasser, C. Vargas-Irwin, L. Franquemont, et al., Failure mode analysis of silicon-based intracortical microelectrode arrays in non-human primates, Journal of Neural Engineering 10 (2013) 66014.
[26] B.D. Winslow, M.B. Christensen, W.K. Yang, F. Solzbacher, P.A. Tresco, A Comparison of the Tissue Response to Chronically Implanted Parylene-C-Coated and Uncoated Planar Silicon Microelectrode Arrays in Rat Cortex, Biomaterials, June 17, 2010.
[27] A. Campbell, C. Wu, Chronically implanted intracranial electrodes: tissue reaction and electrical changes, Micromachines 9 (2018) 430.
[28] B.J. Black, A. Kanneganti, A. Joshi-Imre, R. Rihani, B. Chakraborty, J. Abbott, et al., Chronic recording and electrochemical performance of Utah microelectrode arrays implanted in rat motor cortex, Journal of Neurophysiology 120 (October 1, 2018) 2083–2090.
[29] A. Prasad, Q.S. Xue, V. Sankar, T. Nishida, G. Shaw, W.J. Streit, et al., Comprehensive characterization and failure modes of tungsten microwire arrays in chronic neural implants, Journal of Neural Engineering 9 (October 2012) 056015.
[30] L.K. Massey, Permeability Properties of Plastics and Elastomers: A Guide to Packaging and Barrier Materials, 2 Ed. Norwich, NY, 2002.
[31] T.D. Kozai, K. Catt, X. Li, Z.V. Gugel, V.T. Olafsson, A.L. Vazquez, et al., Mechanical failure modes of chronically implanted planar silicon-based neural probes for laminar recording, Biomaterials 37 (January 2015) 25–39.
[32] S.E. Saddow (Ed.), Silicon Carbide Biotechnology: A Biocompatible Semiconductor for Advanced Biomedical Devices and Applications, Elsevier, Amsterdam, 2011.
[33] E.K. Bernardin, C.L. Frewin, R. Everly, J. Ul Hassan, S.E. Saddow, Demonstration of a robust all-silicon-carbide intracortical neural interface, Micromachines 9 (2018) 412.
[34] M. Beygi, J.T. Bentley, C.L. Frewin, C.A. Kuliasha, A. Takshi, E.K. Bernardin, et al., Fabrication of a monolithic implantable neural interface from cubic silicon carbide, Micromachines 10 (2019) 430.
[35] A. Henry, J. ul Hassan, J.P. Bergman, C. Hallin, E. Janzen, Thick silicon carbide homoepitaxial layers grown by CVD techniques, Chemical Vapor Deposition 12 (2006) 475–482.
[36] J. Hassan, H.T. Bae, L. Lilja, I. Farkas, I. Kim, P. Stenberg, et al., Fast growth rate epitaxy on 4 off-cut 4-inch diameter 4H-SiC wafers, Materials Science Forum 778 (2014).
[37] V. Saxena, A.J. Steckl, Building blocks for SiC devices: ohmic contacts, Schottky contacts, and p-n junctions, in: Y.S. Park (Ed.), Semiconductors and Semimetals, Elsevier, 1998, pp. 77–160.
[38] S.E. Saddow, C.L. Frewin, M. Nezafati, A. Oliveros, S. Afroz, J. Register, et al., 3C-SiC on Si: a bio- and hemo-compatible material for advanced nano-bio devices, in: Nanotechnology Materials and Devices Conference (NMDC), 2014 IEEE 9th, 2014, pp. 49–53.
[39] D. Peters, et al., Planar aluminum-implanted 1400 V 4H silicon carbide p-n diodes with low on resistance, Applied Physics Letters 71 (1997) 2996–2997.

[40] E. Bernardin, et al., Development of an all-SiC neuronal interface device, MRS Advances 1 (2016) 3679–3684.
[41] H. Mitlehner, et al., Switching behaviour of fast high voltage SiC pn-diodes, in: 10th International Symposium on Power Semiconductor Devices and ICs, 1998.
[42] P. Allongue, H. Cachet, Band-edge shift and surface-charges at illuminated n-GaAs aqueous electrolyte junctions. Surface state analysis and simulation of their occupation rate, Journal of the Electrochemical Society 132 (1985) 45–52.
[43] L.M. Peter, Semiconductor electrochemistry, in: B.J.G. S (Ed.), Photoelectrochemical Solar Fuel Production, S pringer, Cham., 2016.
[44] F. La Via, A. Severino, R. Anzalone, C. Bongiorno, G. Litrico, M. Mauceri, et al., From thin film to bulk 3C-SiC growth: understanding the mechanism of defects reduction, Materials Science in Semiconductor Processing 78 (2018) 57–68.
[45] M. Zielinski, R. Arvinte, T. Chassagne, A. Michon, M. Portail, P. Kwasnicki, et al., p-type doping of 4H-and 3C-SiC epitaxial layers with aluminum, Materials Science Forum 858 (2016) 137–142.
[46] M. Zimbone, M. Mauceri, G. Litrico, E.G. Barbagiovanni, C. Bongiorno, F.L. Via, Protrusions reduction in 3C-SiC thin film on Si, Journal of Crystal Growth 498 (2018) 248–257.
[47] R. Myers, K. Hobart, M. Twigg, S. Rao, M. Fatemi, F. Kub, et al., Structural characterization of 3C-SiC films grown on Si layers wafer bonded to polycrystalline SiC substrates, MRS Proceedings 815 (2004) J5.23.
[48] F. Deku, C.L. Frewin, A. Stiller, Y. Cohen, S. Aqeel, A. Joshi-Imre, et al., Amorphous silicon carbide platform for next generation penetrating neural interface designs, Micromachines 9 (2018) 480.
[49] C. Feng, Development of Carbon and Silicon Carbide Based Microelectrode Implantable Neural Interfaces, PhD, Electrical Engineering, University of South Florida, 2021.
[50] D.J. Spry, A.J. Trunek, P.G. Neudeck, High breakdown field P-type 3C-SiC Schottky diodes grown on step-free 4H-SiC mesas, Materials Science Forum 457–460 (2004) 1061–1064.
[51] S.M. Wellman, et al., A materials roadmap to functional neural interface design, Advanced Functional Materials 28 (2018) 1–38.
[52] T.D.Y. Kozai, e. al, Ultrasmall implantable composite microelectrodes with bioactive surfaces for chronic neural interfaces, Nature Materials 11 (2012) 1065–1073.

CHAPTER 6

The development of a fully MRI-compatible silicon carbide neural interface

Mohammad Beygi[1], William Dominguez-Viqueira[2], Gokhan Mumcu[3], Christopher L. Frewin[4], Francesco La Via[5] and Stephen E. Saddow[6]

[1]Institute of Electrical and Microengineering, École polytechnique fédérale de Lausanne, Lausanne, Switzerland; [2]Moffitt Cancer Center, Tampa, FL, United States; [3]Electrical Engineering Department, University of South Florida, Tampa, FL, United States; [4]NeuroNexus LLC, Ann Arbor, MI, United States; [5]IMM-CNR, Catania, Sicily, Italy; [6]Departments of Electrical & Medical Engineering, University of South Florida, Tampa, FL, United States

Contents

Silicon Carbide Technology for Advanced Human Healthcare Applications
ISBN 978-0-323-90609-8
https://doi.org/10.1016/B978-0-323-90609-8.00003-X

1. Introduction

As mentioned in the previous chapters, 3C–SiC is a wide bandgap semiconductor that has been proven to have a high compatibility with neural tissue [1]. SiC has a specific molecular structure with covalent bonding between silicon and carbon atoms. The bonding length is very short and this gives SiC an extremely high chemical and mechanical stability [2]. SiC also has several polytypes and one amorphous structure that gives it a wide range of physical properties. The mechanical, chemical, and electrical properties of SiC, as well as its high biocompatibility, have made SiC an attractive material for fabricating neural implants [3–8].

The utilization of neuromodulation in the treatment of neurological disorders, such as chronic pain, Parkinson's disease, tremors and dystonia, has been growing during the past decade [9]. For many of these treatments, magnetic resonance imaging (MRI) is used as a modality to map the region of interest for implants inside the body and to monitor the postoperation/treatment condition. In addition, MRI is one of the common noninvasive diagnostic tools that gives high-contrast images of soft tissue while avoiding the use of ionizing radiation. For these reasons, the ability to employ the powerful MRI technique to patients with implanted devices enables this powerful diagnostic tool, especially for pre- and postbrain implantation. Thus, the medical community is in need of neural implants that can remain in-body during MRI scans without jeopardizing patient safety. Unfortunately, "MRI safe" implants have been of limited use as the maximum static magnetic field ($\boldsymbol{B}_0$) they may be used with is limited to 1.5 T for typically [10], and recently in a few cases up to 3 T [11]. The challenge is these MRI scans generally offer insufficient resolution and are of very limited clinical use.

There are certain complications that may occur when an implant with conductive or magnetic material is placed in an MRI machine. Patient safety and complications in postimplantation monitoring are the concerns that considerably limit these materials when fabricating neural implants [12]. A neural implant can interact with the static magnetic field ($\boldsymbol{B}_0$), gradient magnetic fields ($d\boldsymbol{B}/dx$), and radiofrequency (RF) fields ($\boldsymbol{B}_1$) in an MRI machine. This interaction between the electromagnetic fields and the neural implant can damage the surrounding tissue by inducing mechanical vibrations and heat as reported in Refs. [9,10,13–16]. It can also reduce image quality by introducing image artifacts through implant interaction with $\boldsymbol{B}_0$ and $\boldsymbol{B}_1$ fields and, thus, complicates the interpretation of the images

[17–20]. One last issue is the precision with which a neurosurgeon can place a neural implant and, at 1.5 T, the resolution is on the order of cm's that is insufficient for placing probes with precision in the brain. Fig. 6.1 shows a comparison between 7 and 1.5 T MRI images illustrating the importance of MRI-compatible neural implants for human use.

To develop an implanted neural interface that possesses a higher level of safety in MRI magnetic fields in the brain, several approaches have been reported in the literature. In a recent study [17], glassy carbon (GC) microelectrodes were introduced that experimentally showed less artifacts, lower displacement, and lower interaction with RF fields. For the GC electrodes to reduce their interaction with the RF field, the conductivity of the material was kept low, in the range of 6803 S/m, in comparison with the platinum (Pt), which is 9.43×10^6 S/m. In addition, due to the negative magnetic susceptibility, χ, of GC of -1.2 ppm, it is believed that the artifacts caused by the magnetic susceptibility difference are minimized [17]. In another work, to reduce the magnetic coupling between the penetrating electrodes and RF fields, the electrodes were coated with high dielectric materials [9], thus the RF energy was substantially reduced inside the dielectric material. Reported approaches to develop a more MRI-compatible neural implant are mainly based on low electrical conductivity materials, materials with magnetic susceptibility compatible with tissue, and the shielding of electrodes with high dielectric materials or conductive coils [22–28]. Although many of the reported works have shown an improvement in MRI compatibility, neural implants that possess

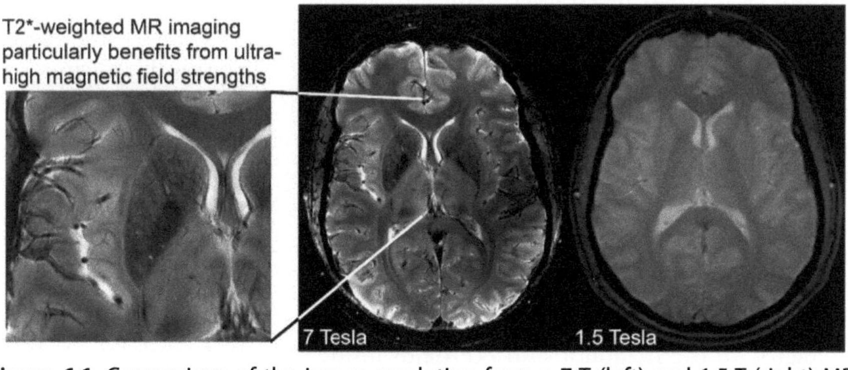

Figure 6.1 Comparison of the image resolution from a 7 T (left) and 1.5 T (right) MRI brain scan. This illustrates the need for higher $\boldsymbol{B_0}$ MRI imaging due to the significantly higher contrast and resolution available to the neurosurgeon during probe placement in the brain [21].

mechanical and chemical robustness, high compatibility with tissue, and MRI safety are still absent.

In our previous work [29], we developed a monolithic planar neural probe from cubic silicon carbide (3C−SiC). The *all*-SiC neural probe was monolithically fabricated from 3C−SiC (reported in Chapter 5), except on the contact pads that contained titanium/gold (Ti/Au) to facilitate wire bonding to the package that resides outside of the brain. This fabrication method can potentially reduce the chance of delamination of probe films inside the tissue environment. It also eliminates any metallic parts that come into contact with tissue thus increasing the compatibility with the tissue and decreasing the electric conductivity of the shank part of the probe. In addition, due to the high thermal conductivity of 3C−SiC (3.6−3.7 W/cm-K for SiC compared to Si (1.49 W/cm-K), which is close pure copper ~ 3.8 W/cm-K), and its tissue-compatible magnetic susceptibility (−12.87 ppm for SiC vs −9.05 ppm for human tissue), SiC has an intrinsic MRI compatibility advantage over conventional probe materials. When one considers the ability to form relatively high-resistivity conductive traces, in comparison with metals, neural probes fabricated monolithically from 3C−SiC may reduce the magnetic perturbation caused by magnetic susceptibility differences and decrease the heat generated by MRI-induced currents on the neural probe conductive traces.

In this chapter, the magnetic compatibility of 3C−SiC, in comparison with Pt and Si, is studied. The focus of the current work is mainly on the artifacts caused by the magnetic susceptibility difference and the induced heat under MRI excitation. Multiple finite element method (FEM) simulations developed in ANSYS Multiphysics, and a Fourier based method for artifact measurement in MATLAB, as well as MRI experiments at 7 T with fabricated devices inside polyacrylic acid (PAA) tissue phantoms, are utilized to study the MRI compatibility of 3C−SiC neural implants. Before we discuss the experiments and the results, we review the concept of MRI safety and the related theories in the next section.

2. MRI safety

An implant's metallic parts, in a patient with an implanted device, can interact with the magnetic and RF fields inside the MRI machine resulting in implant heating and/or induced torque. The resulting implant heating and displacement may damage the surrounding tissue and consequently cause serious injury to the patient. To avoid these disastrous situations several standard procedures and tests have been defined to examine implant safety during MRI operation [30–32]. In this section, implant interaction with gradient magnetic fields, RF fields, and static magnetic fields are studied, and the nature of each interaction is elaborated.

2.1 MRI RF fields and induced heat

MRI images from the body are created based upon the interaction between a static magnetic field ($\boldsymbol{B_0}$), a low-frequency time domain magnetic field gradient ($\mathrm{d}\boldsymbol{B}/\mathrm{dx}$), and a high-frequency electromagnetic field ($\boldsymbol{B_1}$). MRI RF coils consist of either a transmitter or receiver, or both transmitter and receiver. The $\boldsymbol{B_1}$ is applied perpendicular to the static field $\boldsymbol{B_0}$ at the Larmor frequency of interest [33].

The induced electric field ($\boldsymbol{E_i}$) can be calculated using the incident electric field ($\boldsymbol{E_0}$) radiated by the RF coils. Then, using a reaction integral on the conductive parts of the implant, the induced current can be calculated. The incident electric field ($\boldsymbol{E}_0$) and $\boldsymbol{E_i}$ are determined by Eqs. (6.1) and (6.2), respectively [34]:

$$\boldsymbol{E}_0 = -j\omega \boldsymbol{A}(r) + \frac{\nabla(\nabla.\boldsymbol{A}(r))}{j\omega\varepsilon\mu} \tag{6.1}$$

$$\boldsymbol{E}_i = -\boldsymbol{E}_0.\hat{z} \tag{6.2}$$

where $\boldsymbol{A}$ is the magnetic vector potential, and ε and μ are the medium permittivity and magnetic permeability, respectively. Then, the deposited power, which is expressed by the specific absorption rate, specific absorption rate (SAR) (W/kg) [35], is calculated via Eq. (6.3):

$$SAR = \frac{\sigma \boldsymbol{E}^2}{\rho} \tag{6.3}$$

where σ is the electric conductivity and ρ is the mass density.

The heat transferred from the surface of the conductor to the surrounding tissue is obtained by the heat transfer equation for a nonperfused material with an internal heat source [30], as indicated by Eq. (6.4):

$$\rho c_p \frac{d\boldsymbol{T}}{dt} = \nabla.(k\nabla \boldsymbol{T}) + SAR\rho \tag{6.4}$$

where ρ is the density of material, c_p is the specific heat, $\boldsymbol{T} = \boldsymbol{T}(r, z, t)$ is the temperature function (°C), and k is the thermal conductivity (W/m-K) with K temperature in Kelvin.

2.2 Gradient magnetic field and induced heat

The use of a gradient magnetic field creates a spatial variation in the static magnetic field profile by adding a field gradient to $\boldsymbol{B_0}$. The intensity of the gradient magnetic field is given by d$\boldsymbol{B}$/dx in T/m. Early MRI systems could generate gradient magnetic fields with a maximum strength d$\boldsymbol{B}$/dt = 100 mT/m [33]. The gradient coils are usually specified by their switching rate in T/s.

The time-varying magnetic field with the switching frequency of f can be modeled using a sine function as shown in Eq. (6.5):

$$\boldsymbol{B} = |B|\sin(2\pi ft) \tag{6.5}$$

where $\boldsymbol{B}$ is the magnetic field vector that is time dependent and has a direction in space and $|\boldsymbol{B}|$ is the amplitude, or intensity, of the magnetic field. Considering that d$\boldsymbol{B}$/dt is the switching rate, we can find the intensity of the magnetic field in the initial time using Eq. (6.6):

$$|\boldsymbol{B}| = \frac{d\boldsymbol{B}}{dt}\,\frac{1}{2\pi f} \tag{6.6}$$

As this magnetic field is time varying, it can induce an electric field in the conductive parts of the neural probe according to the Maxwell–Faraday equation, shown in Eq. (6.7):

$$\oint \mathbf{E}.dl = -\frac{\partial}{\partial t}\iint_s \mathbf{B}.ds \tag{6.7}$$

The result of this induced electric field is an Eddy current that flows in the conductive parts of the probe. This current results in joule heating, also referred to as Ohmic heating, where $P \propto I^2R$, *Watts*. This explains the basic mechanism behind MRI-induced heating in neural implants.

2.3 Static magnetic field

In addition to induced joule heating in implants, the static field $\boldsymbol{B}_0$ can induce a torque on the implanted neural probe. The induced current generated by the gradient fields can produce a magnetic moment on the implant, and this magnetic moment, in the presence of the static magnetic field, can generate a torque via the Lorenz Force Law, $\boldsymbol{F} = q[\boldsymbol{v} \times \boldsymbol{B}]$. The induced torque causes a high-frequency mechanical vibration in neural probes [10].

The magnetic moment for a volume with a nonuniform charge distribution is defined by the differential magnetic moment as shown in Eq. (6.8):

$$\boldsymbol{\mu} = r \times \boldsymbol{J} \tag{6.8}$$

where $\boldsymbol{\mu}$ is the magnetic moment, r is the position vector, and $\boldsymbol{J}$ is the electric current density. The magnetic torque is defined by the cross product of the magnetic moment and the static magnetic field:

$$\tau = \boldsymbol{\mu} \times \boldsymbol{B} \tag{6.9}$$

As mentioned before, since the current inducing this torque in the presence of the static magnetic field ($\boldsymbol{B}_0$) is a time-varying current, induced by the gradient magnetic field, it causes a vibration on the implant with a frequency similar to the switching frequency of the gradient coils.

3. Magnetic perturbation and MRI imaging artifacts

In temporal and spatial mapping of the brain, and during intracortical electrode implantation, MR imaging is essential. However, due to the magnetic susceptibility (χ) difference between the electrodes and the tissue, the static magnetic field ($\boldsymbol{B}_0$) around the electrodes may be distorted and artifacts observed. This can simply compromise the anatomical information that is obtained by the MRI scans and degrades the quality of the images taken [17,36]. Another condition that may lead to unwanted artifacts is the high conductivity of the metallic parts used in the implants. Thus highly conductive materials can distort the $\boldsymbol{B}_1$ field around the implant resulting in image artifacts. The focus of this section, however, relates to artifacts caused by the magnetic susceptibility difference, $\Delta\chi$.

Magnetic susceptibility is a magnetic property of all materials, denoted by χ, that shows the degree of magnetization in materials when they are exposed to $\boldsymbol{B}_0$. χ can be positive or negative depending on whether the magnetization vector aligns in the direction of $\boldsymbol{B}_0$ or opposite to it, respectively. If the magnetization vector is the same direction as $\boldsymbol{B}_0$, then the material is called paramagnetic, and if the magnetization vector is opposite to the $\boldsymbol{B}_0$, it is called diamagnetic [37]. Magnetic susceptibility of human tissue and some of the materials commonly used for neural implant fabrication are listed in Table 6.1.

Magnetic perturbation surrounding an arbitrarily shaped electrode placed inside a tissue-like material can be calculated using a Fourier-based

Table 6.1 Magnetic susceptibility of neural implant materials and human tissue [36].

Material	Magnetic susceptibility, χ_v (ppm)
Human tissue	−9.05
Silicon carbide	−12.87
Silicon	−4.2
Gold	−34
Platinum	279

method explained elsewhere [36,38]. In these mathematical models, the magnetic perturbation caused by a magnetic susceptibility difference is defined as an offset in the magnetic field from the main static magnetic field ($\boldsymbol{B_0}$) that the set-up is exposed to, and it is denoted by $\Delta\boldsymbol{B_z}(\boldsymbol{r})$. The z subscript in the $\Delta\boldsymbol{B_z}(\boldsymbol{r})$ term is due to the direction of $\boldsymbol{B_0}$ that is assumed to be in z direction. To find the value of $\Delta\boldsymbol{B_z}(\boldsymbol{r})$, first the magnetization needs to be calculated in space:

$$\boldsymbol{M}_z(\boldsymbol{r}) = \boldsymbol{\chi}(\boldsymbol{r})\frac{\boldsymbol{B}_0}{\mu_0(1+\boldsymbol{\chi}(\boldsymbol{r}))} \tag{6.10}$$

where $\boldsymbol{\chi}(\boldsymbol{r})$ is the magnetic susceptibility in space, $\boldsymbol{M}_z(\boldsymbol{r})$ is the magnetization in space in the z direction, and μ_0 is the magnetic permeability of free space. Then, the 3D Fourier transform of $\boldsymbol{M}_z(\boldsymbol{r})$ is used to transform to *k*-space, as shown in Eq. (6.11):

$$\boldsymbol{M}_z(\boldsymbol{k}) = \mathscr{F}_{3D}\{\boldsymbol{M}_z(\boldsymbol{r})\} \tag{6.11}$$

Considering that β is the angle between the direction of the $\mathbf{B_0}$ and the $\boldsymbol{k}$ vector defining a point in *k*-space, the magnetic perturbation in *k*-space, $\Delta\boldsymbol{B_z}(\boldsymbol{k})$, is calculated via Eq. (6.12):

$$\Delta\boldsymbol{B_z}(\boldsymbol{k}) = -\frac{\mu_0\boldsymbol{M}_z(\boldsymbol{k})}{3}\left(3cos^2\beta - 1\right) \tag{6.12}$$

In Eq. (6.12), $cos\ \beta$ is calculated using Eq. (6.13):

$$cos\beta = \frac{-k_x sin\theta + k_y cos\theta sin\psi + k_z cos\theta cos\psi}{\sqrt{k_x^2 + k_y^2 + k_z^2}} \tag{6.13}$$

In Eq. (6.13), θ indicates a rotation about the y axis and ψ about the x axis. Finally, $\Delta\boldsymbol{B_z}(\boldsymbol{r})$ is calculated in *r*-space after finding the inverse Fourier transform of the $\Delta\boldsymbol{B_z}(\boldsymbol{k})$ as shown in Eq. (6.14):

$$\Delta B_z(r) = \mathscr{F}_{3D}^{-1}\{\Delta B_z(k)\} \tag{6.14}$$

Using the earlier equations, the magnetic perturbation caused by the susceptibility difference between the probe and brain can be mathematically modeled and calculated using MATLAB for any arbitrary shaped electrode placed inside a tissue-like material.

4. Simulations and experiments

To evaluate the MRI compatibility of 3C−SiC neural implants, we took advantage of several FEM simulations, a Fourier-based method to estimate the image artifacts caused by magnetic susceptibility differences, and finally multiple MRI experiments at 7T to measure the artifacts of the samples and the temperature rise caused by electromagnetic coupling [39]. Throughout this work, the MRI compatibility simulations and measurements were limited to artifacts under MRI excitation caused by susceptibility differences, and the induced heat and SAR caused by electromagnetic coupling between the conductive parts of the samples and $\boldsymbol{B_1}$. The other possible scenarios, such as displacement and vibration under MRI, will be addressed in future studies. In addition, artifacts surrounding the *all*-SiC probe [29] are also shown.

4.1 Sample preparation

Various samples were fabricated for this study to compare artifacts and induced heating under 7 T MRI excitation. This includes 3C−SiC and Si samples with various doping types and concentrations, and platinum (Pt) metal on various substrates. The samples were fabricated using two different designs depending on whether they were used for image artifact or induced heat assessments. The samples used for artifact measurements were a rectangular-shaped base electrode (15 mm × 4 mm) representing stimulating and recording electrodes used in neural probes. Other sets of samples were fabricated on various substrates with similar dimensions as the base electrode, but this time with three parallel single-ended electrodes of various lengths (8, 6, and 4 mm) on the base substrate. This design was chosen to study the effect of electrode length on both the artifacts and the resulting induced heat. It also helped us to determine how the electromagnetic coupling between the electrodes can influence the SAR distribution surrounding each electrode. In addition, since the electrodes were not large enough to produce enough of a measurable heat rise under 7T MRI excitation, a pair of extended stainless-steel wires (40 mm long) was attached to the electrodes to increase induced current in the electrodes to better measure the induced heating. These measurements were used to verify the FEM simulations results. The SAR and the heat measurements using the FEM simulations proved to provide a better picture of the electromagnetic interactions between the electrodes and $\boldsymbol{B}_1$ under MRI in this study as the temperature resolution of the fiber-optic probes used proved to be insufficient to measure accurately volumetric heating in the tissue phantom.

Several samples were fabricated from different materials and a combination of these materials. By using a combination of different materials during the experiments we were able to recognize, first, the effect of each material during MRI scanning and, second, the effect of multiple stacks of materials in generating artifacts. The samples fabricated for the MRI experiments are shown in Fig. 6.2. These samples are as follows:

(1) ~2 μ m Heavily doped n-type (n^+) 3C–SiC epi-film on ~8 μ m low doped p-type (p) 3C–SiC epi-film (n^+/p) on a silicon on insulator (SOI) substrate.

(2) ~2 μ m Heavily doped p-type (p^+) 3C–SiC epi-film on ~8 μ m low doped n-type (n) 3C–SiC epi-film (p^+/n) on a similar SOI substrate.

(3) ~2 μ m Heavily doped n-type (n^+) 3C–SiC epi-film on ~8 μ m low doped p-type (p) 3C–SiC epi-film (n^+/p) on a p-type Si substrate.

(4) Sample (1) after etching away the oxide film in HF diluted in water (50:1) and etching away the remaining Si from the sample using KOH resulting in a free-standing n^+/p 3C–SiC base electrode.

(5) Sample (2) after etching away the oxide film in HFdiluted in water (50:1) and etching away the remaining Si from the sample using KOH resulting in a free-standing p^+/n 3C–SiC base electrode.

(6), (7), (8) ~ 1 μ m Pt film deposited on a polyimide (PI) film, n-type Si substrate, and p-type Si substrate, respectively.

(9), (10), (11) PI film, n-type Si substrate, and p-type Si substrate, respectively.

(12) ~100 nm Pt deposited on an n-type Si substrate and microfabricated into three parallel electrodes with pads and recording sites. Two 40 mm PFA-coated stainless steel (coated diameter of 330 μm) were also soldered on the pads.

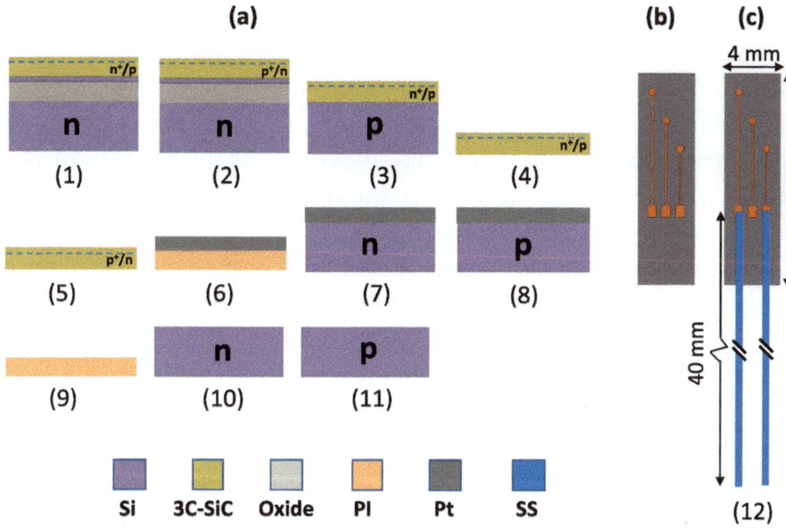

Figure 6.2 Samples fabricated for the MRI experiments. (A) Cross-section of the samples fabricated for the experiments to measure artifacts. Each number is related to the number of sample given in Section 4.2.1. Si stands for silicon, 3C–SiC for cubic silicon carbide, PI for polyimide, Pt for platinum, and SS for stainless steel. (B) Top view of the sample with triple electrodes (8, 6, and 4 mm) used for SAR measurements. (C) Sample used for heat measurement under MRI with two 40 mm extended PFA-coated stainless-steel wires (coated diameter of 330 μm).

Fabrication details are provided in our published work [29]. To summarize, 3C–SiC epitaxial layers (n^+ and p) were grown on three 100 mm diameter substrates, two of which were SOI ((100) Si-oriented) wafers, and the other wafer was a p-type Si (100) wafer. Then, n- and p-type 3C–SiC films were grown on the substrates using a hot-wall reactor (LPE Epitaxial Technology Center, Catania, Italy). Hydrogen (H_2) and ethylene (C_2H_4) were used as the carrier and carbon (C) precursor gases, respectively. Trichlorosilane ($SiHCl_3$) was used as the Si precursor gas.

Aluminum (Al) and nitrogen (N_2) were added to the growth process as the p and n dopants, respectively. The doping density of the n^+ and p^+ layers was $\sim 10^{19}$ dopants/cm^3. Finally, portions of the three wafers were diced into 15 mm × 4 mm die and used as the previously described base electrodes. Extra fabrication steps were necessary to release the n^+/p and p^+/n 3C–SiC films from the SOI wafers. First, samples (1) and (2) were soaked in HF (49%) until the epitaxial films were released from the substrate. However, a thin (~27 μm) thick layer of Si remained on the backside of the films. To etch this thin layer of Si from the backside of the samples, they were soaked in hot

KOH. Fig. 6.3 shows cross-section SEM micrographs of the 3C–SiC samples before and after the oxide and silicon etches.

Platinum was deposited on three dies: PI, n-type Si, and p-type Si. Various substrates were selected to verify the substrate's influence on MRI artifacts surrounding the Pt electrodes. Nevertheless, in the case of neural probes, Pt was deposited on another substrate. This substrate is typically either Si or a polymer film such as PI [17].

An ~1 μ m thick Pt film was deposited via Ebeam evaporation on two (2) p-type and n-type Si substrates. Using a 4-probe configuration, the resistivity of the p-type and n-type Si substrates was measured. The resistivity of the p-type substrate was ~9 Ω-cm and the value for the n-type substrate was ~0.5 Ω-cm. Before Pt deposition, a very thin (20 nm) layer of titanium (Ti) was deposited in the same sputtering chamber that acts as an adhesion layer for Pt [40]. The base electrodes were ready for MRI testing after this step in the process. Another set of samples was fabricated with three parallel Pt electrodes on the substrate. Using a lift-off photolithography process, the Pt was patterned into the three electrodes as illustrated in Fig. 6.2B. The details of the lift-off process are explained in our previous work [29]. Another Pt sample was prepared with two (2) 40 mm extended

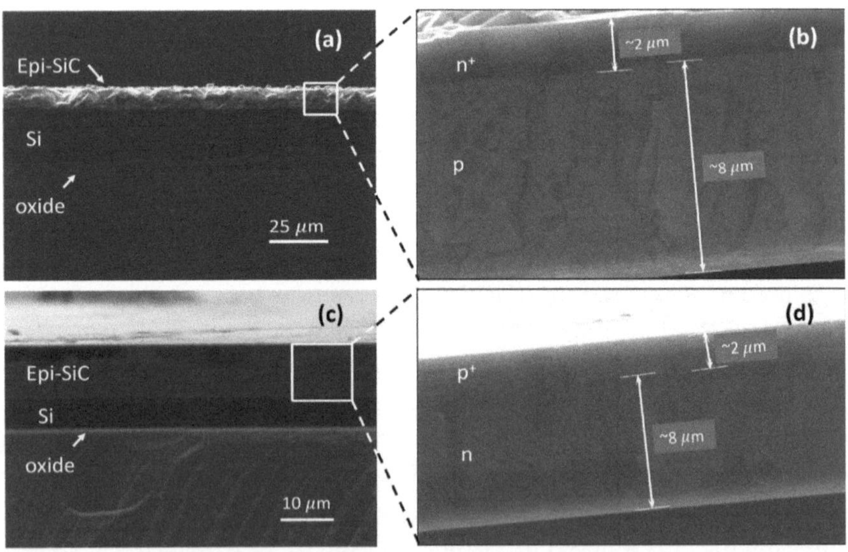

Figure 6.3 Cross-section SEM micrographs of the 3C–SiC samples. (A) Cross-section view of the n^+/p 3C–SiC on SOI substrate. (B) Free-standing n^+/p sample after etching oxide in HF and Si in KOH solution. (C) Cross-section view of the p^+/n 3C–SiC on SOI substrate. (D) Free-standing p^+/n sample.

stainless-steel wires to increase electromagnetic coupling and, therefore, induced heat (Fig. 6.2C).

4.2 Birdcage coil implementation for 7 T small animal MRI

A transmitter/receiver resonator coil that can allow for imaging at ~300 MHz was developed for the MRI experiments. As the birdcage coil is a common resonator coil used for volume imaging [41], this design was chosen for the current work. The length of the birdcage was 150 mm so that it enclosed a full wavelength of the RF signals at ~300 MHz inside a dielectric material (PAA phantom with dielectric constant $\varepsilon_r = \sim 52$). With this length, the maximum electromagnetic coupling happens between the conductive parts inside the coil and the RF signals. To have a homogeneous RF field inside the coil and an acceptable SNR at this length, the effective length of the rungs should be shorter. The effective length can be shortened by splitting the rungs and placing capacitors between them. This realizes a hybrid, or band-pass, coil configuration. As a rule of thumb, the length of the rungs may not exceed $\lambda/20$ to have an acceptable SNR [35]. Another important factor in designing a coil is the number of capacitors that are required to build a coil. An optimized design was a hybrid coil with rungs split into two by capacitors. The diameter of the designed coil was 70 mm, and it consisted of 12 rungs. The number of rungs and the diameter were optimum values to achieve high SNR values and field homogeneity inside the coil.

Power was fed into the coil through a quadrature configuration on the top end ring. In a quadrature configuration, two ports are physically 90 degrees apart and have a 90 degrees phase difference. Through this configuration, a circularly polarized RF field was generated. Impedance matching was performed using a balanced matching circuit with a variable capacitor. Tuning each channel was also obtained by two variable capacitors placed at 180 and 270 degrees around the top end ring. The details of the implemented coil are presented in Table 6.2.

To select values for the capacitors, an online application (BirdcageBuilder [42]) was initially used that estimated the capacitors values. As these values were not accurate, a more accurate model was defined using ANSYS HFSS (19.2, Ansys, Inc. Canonsburg, PA) and Advanced Design System (ADS, 2019, Keysight Technologies, Santa Rosa, CA). First electromagnetic simulations were performed in HFSS and a 36-port S-parameter matrix was imported into ADS. The capacitors and the matching circuits were added to the design with the ideal capacitor values and the actual values calculated using BirdcageBuilder.

Table 6.2 Birdcage coil resonator specifications for a 7 T small animal bore MRI system.

Coil type	12-Leg band-pass birdcage coil
Leg capacitors	1.5 pF
End-ring capacitors	17.5 pF
Tuning cap	18.5 pF (two trimmers installed on the ports)
ESR resistance	0.05–0.07 Ω
Matching components	20 pF capacitor and 123.5 nH inductor
Frequency	~300 MHz
Dimensions	Coil-diameter = 70 mm, length = 150 mm, leg-width = 6.35 mm (0.25-in copper tape), port-width = 2 mm

A considerable offset was observed in the power reflection and isolation (S_{11}, S_{22}, and S_{21}) and the resonance frequency comparing to the values expected. Then, using an optimization method in ADS, the values for the capacitors were extracted.

However, because we used ideal capacitors, we expected a large offset between the simulation results and experiments. To compensate for these mismatches, the ideal capacitors were replaced with realistic capacitor models (Modelithics, Inc, Tampa, FL). Then, the coil was built with the dimensions and capacitor values presented in Table 6.2. Fig. 6.4 shows both the resonator coil model and the implemented coil.

4.3 Modeling and simulation

As discussed earlier, in this study different computer simulations were used to predict and compare both the artifacts surrounding various samples and also to calculate the SAR (W/kg) and, consequently, any induced heat surrounding the samples. In this section, details of the Fourier-based simulations used to predict the magnetic perturbation caused by the magnetic susceptibility difference ($\Delta\chi$) between the sample and the tissue phantom (PAA) to model image artifacts and the FEM simulations to calculate the SAR and the induced heating are elaborated.

4.3.1 Magnetic perturbation simulations

A Fourier-based method was used and formulated in MATLAB (R2017b, MathWorks, Natick, MA) to predict image artifacts caused by $\Delta\chi$. The MATLAB codes were written based on the method reported in

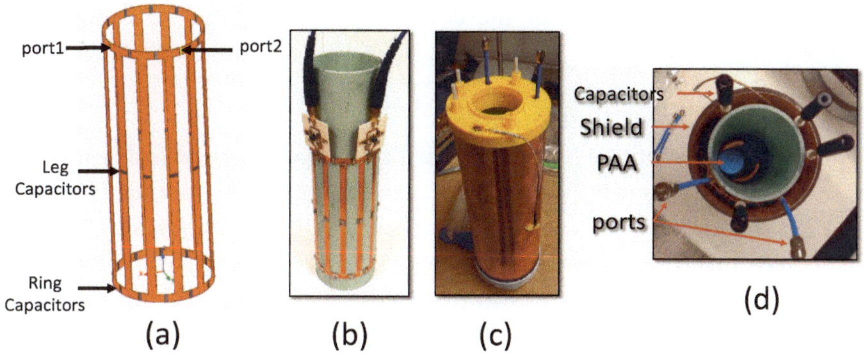

Figure 6.4 The 300 MHz birdcage coil resonator designed and built for MRI experiments. (A) The model used in HFSS for s-parameter calculation. Locations of the ports, the end-ring capacitors, and the rung capacitors are indicated with *arrows*. (B) The implemented resonator without the RF shield. Here, the two matching circuits, implemented using surface mount nonmagnetic capacitors and inductors, are shown. (C) Fabricated coil with two power ports, two variable capacitors for matching, and two for tuning. (D) The top view of the coil without the upper cap. The PAA tubes were used as loads to tune and match the coil using a network analyzer, pre-MRI experiment.

Refs. [36,38]. For simulation purposes, the following were used: Pt film on Si substrate, 3C—SiC free-standing sample, and Si substrates (both n-type and p-type). The background material in which the samples were placed was a PAA tissue phantom [39]. The magnetic susceptibility of these materials is provided in Table 2.1. These were the main materials whose artifacts were observed via experiments under 7 T MRI excitation. Using these simulations, $\boldsymbol{B}_0$ perturbation caused by each material of interest was predicted. The magnetic interaction between a stack of layers was not captured in these simulations, but rather they were experimentally measured. By combining the simulation and experimental results, one can better understand the artifacts patterns occurring during the MRI experiments. The experiments also helped verify and validate the numerical models, a very important point as direct measurement of minute temperature rise in the tissue phantom was not possible due to resolution limits of available temperature probes.

In these simulations, $\boldsymbol{B}_0$ was set to 7 T, the field of view (FOV) was 256 × 256 × 256 pixels, length and width of the samples were 150 and 40 mm, respectively, and the voxel size was 1 × 1 × 1 mm. More details about the implementation of the codes and variables can be found elsewhere [43].

4.3.2 Finite element simulations

One essential benefit of simulations is to control all aspects of a physical phenomenon that is often not possible during actual experiments. Here, the goal of these simulations was to compare the SAR distribution surrounding the various materials under 7 T MRI excitation. However, as the length of the samples is short in comparison with the wavelength of the RF fields inside the tissue phantom, the electromagnetic coupling consequently was reduced, which, as a result, decreases the induced heating effect. The induced heat is thus expected to be very low and not measurable during actual experiments. Although low in intensity, the heat may increase dramatically if the length of the samples becomes comparable to the wavelength of the RF signals inside the MRI. This can also be modeled using FEM simulations after validation of the numerical models.

ANSYS HFSS (19.2, Ansys, Inc., Canonsburg, PA) was used to perform FEM electromagnetic simulations. Via these simulations, the electromagnetic coupling between the $\boldsymbol{B}_0$ field and the Pt and 3C–SiC samples was modeled. For simulation purposes, a high-pass birdcage resonator with 16 legs was used in the simulations that were tuned at ~300 MHz in HFSS. The Pt and 3C–SiC samples (Fig. 6.2B and C) were placed inside a tube using a 3D-printed polylactic acid (PLA) holder. The tube was filled with the PAA tissue phantom. This was also modeled in ANSYS HFSS as illustrated in Fig. 6.5. The electromagnetic simulation conversion accuracy was set to $\Delta S < 0.01$, which may guarantee an acceptable accuracy in the calculation of Maxwell's equations. After mesh generation, each part of the model was individually inspected to ensure a good quality mesh. The simulations were run on the advanced computing resources at the University of South Florida that provided 5 × 64 GB of RAM and 24 CPU cores (2x Intel Xeon CPU E5-2650 v4 @ 2.20 GHz). The electromagnetic simulations were done in ~3 h.

Another FEM electromagnetic simulation without the sample was done to validate the simulation results using the experiments under a 7 T horizontal magnet (Agilent-Technologies) and Bruker electronics (BioSpec AV3HD). The results of the electromagnetic simulations were then connected to thermal simulations in ANSYS Workbench and ANSYS Mechanical to measure the temperature rise inside the tube and compare it with the experimental results to validate the simulations.

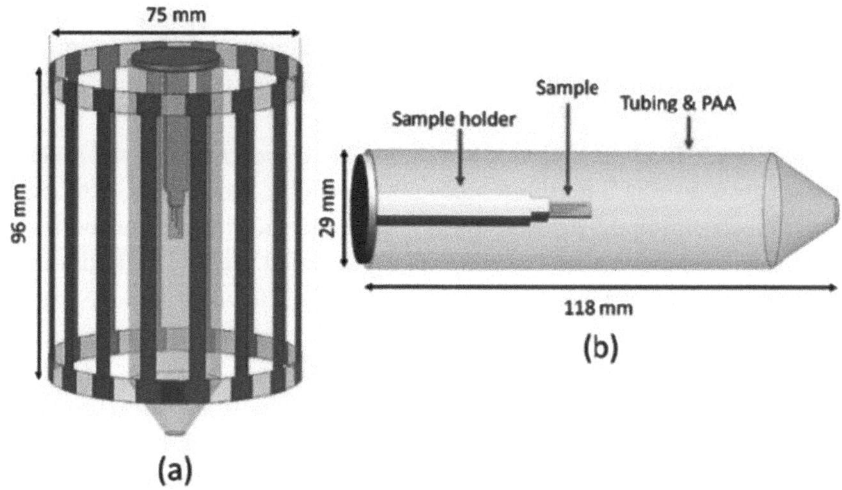

Figure 6.5 Illustration of the models used in ANSYS HFSS for electromagnetic and thermal simulation. (A) High-pass birdcage designed for the simulations. This birdcage resonator has 16 rungs and is tuned to ~300 MHz. (B) Sample tube that is filled with the PAA tissue phantom and a 3D-printed PLA holder that holds the sample inside the tubing.

5. MRI experiments

The MRI experiments were performed in a 7 T horizontal magnet (Agilent-Technologies) with Bruker electronics (BioSpec AV3HD) and a 35-mm M2M birdcage coil (M2M imaging corp.) at the Moffit Cancer Center. Two different sets of experiments were conducted to measure both image artifacts and induced heating under MRI excitation. The experiments were performed using the samples fabricated as described in the previous sections that were inserted into a saline gel (i.e., PAA) used as a human tissue phantom. In the following sections, the recipe to make the phantom, and the two sets of MRI experiments are explained.

5.1 Saline gel phantom preparation

As mentioned earlier, a saline gel was used as the tissue phantom that simulates the electrical, thermal, and magnetic properties of human brain tissue. To accurately achieve the properties of human tissue, the synthesis was exactly and carefully followed according to the relevant standards [30]. The phantom was made by mixing PAA (Sigma—Aldrich, St. Louis, MO, USA) and pure NaCl (reagent grade, purity >99%) dissolved in distilled water. The ratio of NaCl and water was set to 1.32 g/L, while the value for PAA and water was 10 g/L. The electrical conductivity of the phantom can be adjusted by changing the ratio of NaCl to water, and by changing the ratio of PAA to water the dielectric constant of the phantom may be changed. The electrical conductivity and dielectric constant of the mixture were measured using a network analyzer (Keysight, Santa Rosa, CA, USA) and a dielectric probe. The setup used to measure the electrical properties of the phantom is shown in Fig. 6.6. The measured electrical conductivity of the phantom at 25°C and a frequency of 300 MHz was $\sigma \approx 0.5$ S/m and its relative dielectric constant was $\varepsilon_r \approx 70$. According to the applicable standards [30], this recipe should result in a diffusivity of 1.3×10^{-7} m^2/s and a heat capacity of 4150 J/kg-C, which are the thermal properties of the human tissue. 500 mL of this phantom was made, carefully stirred, and refrigerated in a sealed container for future use. Each time before use, the phantom was carefully stirred to remove any lumps inside the mixture.

5.2 MRI experiments to measure image artifacts

Multiple samples were fabricated to measure image artifacts under 7 T MRI scans as mentioned in Section 3.1. The apparatus used for image artifact measurement is shown in Fig. 6.7. The setup consisted of a plastic tube that was filled with the PAA saline gel. A 3D-printed PLA holder was used to place the sample inside the plastic tube. The holder was glued to the screw cap of the tube. The sample was also glued to the holder. The cap was carefully tightened, checked for the absence of air bubbles, and the tube was

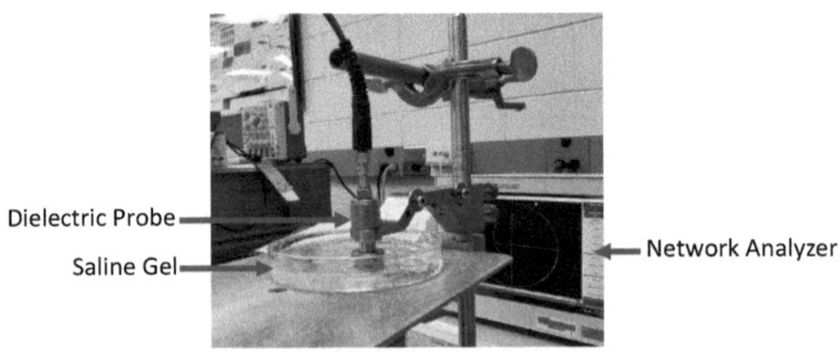

Figure 6.6 The setup used to measure the electrical conductivity and dielectric constant of the tissue phantom. The saline gel phantom was made by mixing polyacrylic acid (PAA) and pure NaCl (reagent grade, purity >99%) dissolved in distilled water. The ratio of NaCl and water was set to 1.32 g/L and the ratio for PAA and water was 10 g/L. The measured electrical conductivity of the phantom at 25°C and 300 MHz was $\sigma \approx 0.5$ S/m and its relative dielectric constant $\varepsilon_r \approx 70$.

FOV of the sequence was 35 mm × 35 mm and with 256 × 256 pixels.

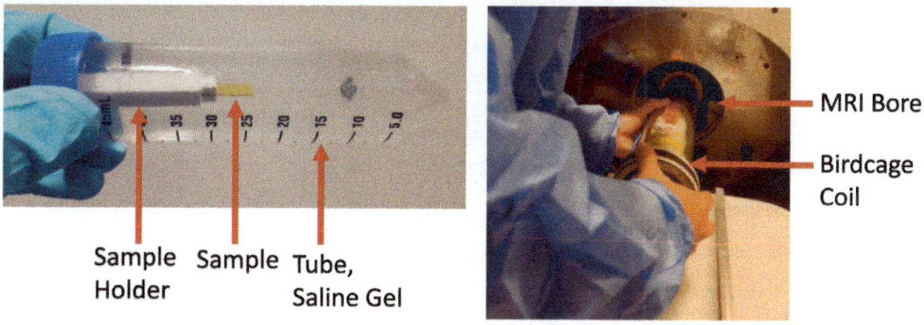

(a) (b)

Figure 6.7 Apparatus used to measure image artifacts under MRI excitation. (A) Plastic tube filled with saline gel phantom and the sample with 3D-printed polylactic acid (PLA) holder used to hold the sample in place. The holder was glued to the screw cap and the sample to the PLA holder. (B) Coil insertion into the MRI bore used for all MRI experiments.

placed inside the MRI bore for the experiments. The samples were tested individually in each MRI scan.

The following MRI sequence was used for image artifact measurement. A similar sequence was used for all the samples tested for image artifacts, while the location of the tubes was carefully inspected to ensure consistent placement in the coil during measurement. T2 axial and coronal images of the devices were obtained with a rapid acquisition with relaxation enhancement (RARE) sequence with TR/TE 2220/32 ms, nine slices, with the slice thickness of 0.3 mm. The FOV of the sequence was 35 mm × 35 mm and with 256 × 256 pixels.

5.3 MRI experiments to measure induced heat

Another set of MRI experiments was designed to measure the induced heat surrounding the test samples. As mentioned earlier, for these experiments samples with three electrodes were used. However, the induced heat was very low, and measuring it was very difficult. For this reason, two extended SS wires were soldered to the electrodes to increase the physical length of the electrodes and, thus, the RF field electromagnetic coupling to the electrodes inside the MRI tool.

Overall, accurate measurement of induced heating is very laborious as there are multiple factors that might influence heat generation and distribution inside the MRI [9,30]. For this reason, FEM simulation is an alternative strategy that offers higher precision observation of the relevant physical phenomena and, if validated by a simple experimental setup, very complex problems can be analyzed using this method. Therefore, in the current work, we took advantage of accurate electromagnetic and thermal numerical simulations to predict the SAR (W/kg) distribution surrounding the electrodes. In addition, two MRI experiments were conducted to validate these simulations and to predict the expected maximum temperature rise in the sample with the highest electrical conductivity (i.e., Pt). The thermal and electrical properties of the materials used for these simulations and experiments are presented in Table 6.3.

The setup that was used to measure the induced heating was very similar to the one used for image artifact measurement, except the holder was designed to encompass two fiber-optic temperature sensors (SA Instruments, Inc., Stony Brook, NY, USA). One of the fiber-optic sensors was in the vicinity of the longest of the three electrodes on the sample to measure the temperature rise surrounding the tip region and the other sensor was placed further away from the sample, closer to the inner wall of the plastic tube, to measure the temperature rise inside the PAA saline gel phantom. The setup used to measure the temperature inside the plastic tube is shown in Fig. 6.8.

The following MRI sequence was used for these experiments. Each scan was 15 min long to give enough time for heat accumulation. The T2 axial and coronal images of the devices were obtained with a RARE (Rapid Acquisition with Relaxation Enhancement) sequence with TR/TE 425/12 ms, 11 slices, with a slice thickness of 0.5 mm. The FOV of the sequence was 30 mm × 30 mm and with 256 × 256 pixels.

5.4 RF coil simulation and experimental results

In this section, S-parameter values for the birdcage coil, the simulated and experimental results indicating image artifacts for the various samples, and

Table 6.3 Properties of materials used to calculate MRI-induced heating.

Material	Electric conductivity ($\times 10^6$ S/m)	Thermal conductivity (W/m-K)
Human tissue	0.5×10^{-6}	0.4
Doped SiC ($\sim 10^{19}$ dopants/cm^3)	~ 0.17	360
Doped Si ($\sim 10^{18}$ dopants/cm^3)	~ 0.1	148
Platinum	9.3	71

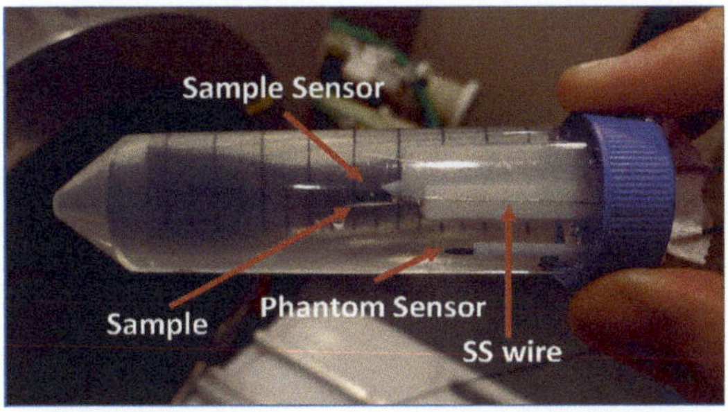

Figure 6.8 Photograph of the sample and holder used to measure the temperature rise surrounding a Pt sample with three electrodes and two extended stainless-steel (SS) wires soldered to the electrodes. Two fiberoptic temperature sensors were used for temperature measurement. One placed in the vicinity of the long electrode on the sample to measure the temperature rise at the tip and the other further away from the sample, closer to the inner wall of the plastic tube, to measure the temperature rise inside the PAA—saline gel phantom.

the simulated and experimental results showing the induced heat and SAR for the various samples tested and simulated are presented. Although the birdcage coil built in this work was not ultimately utilized in the experiments due to insufficient SNR, the experimental results are presented as they show the impact of the PAA phantom placed in the coil. Furthermore, the simulated and experimental results specifying the difference between MRI compatibility of the materials used are compared.

5.4.1 Birdcage coil

As discussed earlier in this chapter, the birdcage coil designed was a 16-rung hybrid birdcage tuned at ~300 MHz for use in the 7 T MRI machine for small laboratory animals. Before the coil was tested in the MRI machine, the S-parameter characteristics for both loaded and unloaded conditions were measured. Two plastic phantom tubes, similar to the ones used for the MRI experiments, were filled with the saline gel and used as loads to tune and match the resonator coil, as shown in Fig. 6.4D. First, the frequency response of the coil was simulated in HFSS and ADS. Using this method, power reflection and isolation between ports were simulated and the S-parameter plotted as shown in Fig. 6.9. These plots show nine resonance frequencies, one of which is the resonance of the end-rings. The other eight resonances belong to loops that the rungs are built from. The last resonance frequency is the end-ring resonance and the one before this resonance frequency is the actual resonance frequency that was set to 300 MHz.

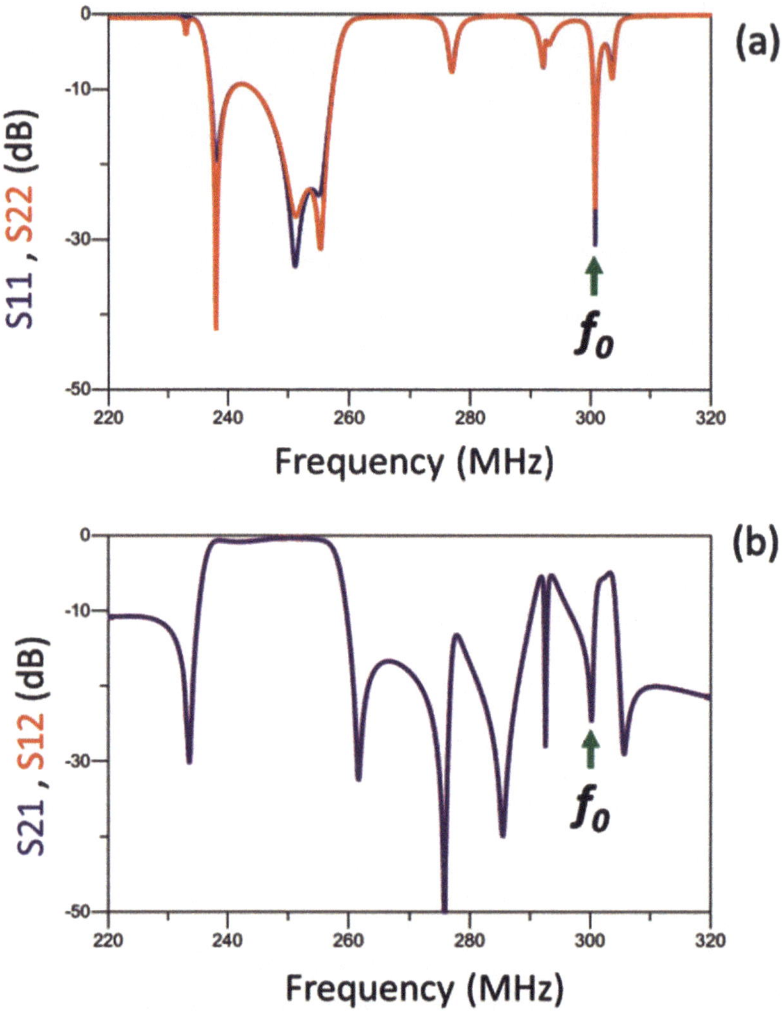

Figure 6.9 Simulated S-parameters using HFSS and ADS showing the power reflection (S_{11} and S_{22}) and isolation (S_{21}, S_{12}) between two ports on the RF coil. In these plots, f_O shows the main resonance frequency of the hybrid birdcage coil. (A) Reflected power of the two ports indicating that the ports are nearly symmetric. (B) Transmitted power between the ports. At f_O, the reflected power (S_{11}) is below −25 dB, which is suitable for the birdcage resonator.

Therefore, this particular resonance frequency needs to have a very low power reflection (i.e., $S_{11} \leq 20$ dB) and also very low transmitted power between two ports to be able to isolate the ports at the frequency of interest.

After tuning and matching the resonance frequency of interest in software, and after the optimum capacitor values were calculated, the coil was built. To test for reflected power and port isolation, a network analyzer was used. The test was done with and without saline gel loads to fine-tune the loaded and unloaded coil, respectively. S-parameters for reflected power for the two ports (S_{11}, S_{22}) are shown in Fig. 6.10.

As shown in Fig. 6.10, the load can distort resonance coil tuning and matching at the frequency of interest. The resonance frequency was not exactly 300 MHz, as prior tests had shown a ~1.5 MHz offset when the coil was placed inside the MRI bore. This frequency offset could be due to the coupling of the coil with the MRI magnets. The offset was observed even when a copper shield was used around the coil. Thus, the coil was retuned and rematched before use in the MRI machine.

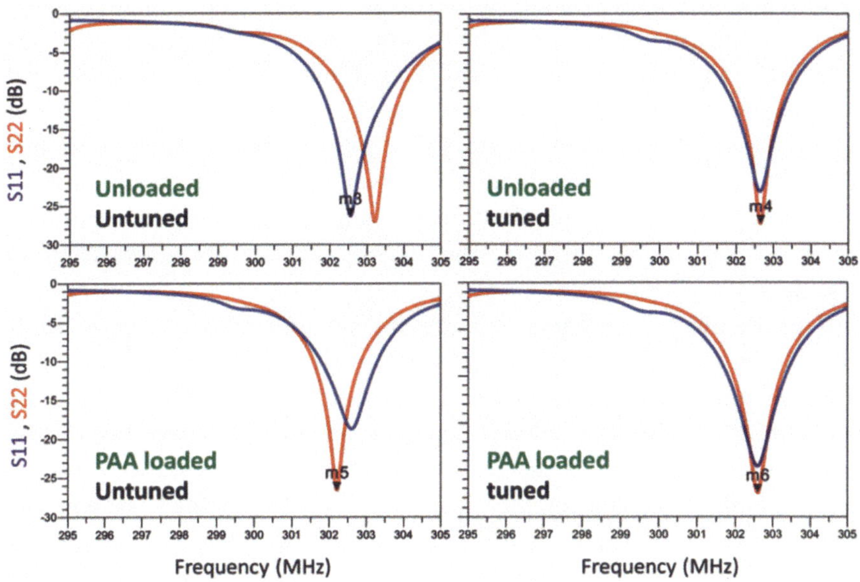

Figure 6.10 Measured S-parameters indicating reflected power at the resonance frequency of interest. The resonance was not accurately set at 300 MHz, due to frequency offset caused by magnetic coupling inside the MRI bore. Two saline gel (PAA) tubes were used as loads to tune and match the coil before use in the MRI tool. (A) Reflected power values for the two ports in the unloaded coil before tuning. (B) Reflected power in the unloaded coil after tuning and matching with a 50-Ω impedance load. (C) Tuned and matched coil after loading with saline gel (PAA). (D) Tuned and matched loaded coil.

6. MRI compatibility simulations and experiments

6.1 Image artifacts

Image artifacts reduce image quality during MRI analysis and may be caused by interactions between the sample and the $\boldsymbol{B}_0$ and $\boldsymbol{B}_1$ fields. The samples prepared previously were placed inside the 7 T MRI machine and the coronal and sagittal images from the samples were obtained. The image artifacts can extend a noticeable distance in all the directions surrounding the sample. They can be either dark or bright depending if $\Delta\chi$, which is the difference between the tissue phantom magnetic susceptibility and the sample magnetic susceptibility, is less than zero or greater than zero. Also, another phenomenon may play a role in determining the severity and contrast of image artifacts, such as the interaction between the sample conductive parts and $\boldsymbol{B}_1$ field. This may lead to $\boldsymbol{B}_1$ distortion surrounding the sample.

Fortunately, the influence of these two phenomena can be distinguished via numerical simulations. The simulations, then, can be compared to the MRI experimental data for a better understanding of the interactions involved. The Fourier-based simulation results that estimate $\boldsymbol{B}_0$ field perturbation due to $\Delta\chi$ are shown in Fig. 6.11. The results indicate a shift in the $\boldsymbol{B}_0$ field. As expected, regarding the χ for SiC in comparison with Pt and Si, the 3C−SiC sample displayed a lower amount of $\boldsymbol{B}_0$ field distortion surrounding the sample while Pt displayed the highest. The minimum $\Delta\ \boldsymbol{B}_0$ was $\sim\ -0.3\ \mu T$ in 3C−SiC, and the maximum $\Delta\ \boldsymbol{B}_0$ was $\sim 100\ \mu T$ in the Pt sample.

The Results of the MRI experiments are presented in Fig. 6.12. As observed in this figure, all the materials, except 3C−SiC, showed an extended image artifact surrounding the samples. The 3C−SiC samples were almost invisible in the MRI images as seen in the figure. For the rest of the materials studied image artifacts covered the whole device and distorted the shape of the sample. However, for the silicon substrates, the severity of the image artifacts was also related to the doping type and also concentration. This can be seen for the higher resistivity p-type Si substrate, which did not show any extended image artifacts caused by magnetic field distortion. This will be elaborated further in the discussion section.

6.2 Induced heat and SAR

To estimate induced sample heating we must take advantage of FEM simulations due to the low resolution of the available temperature probes.

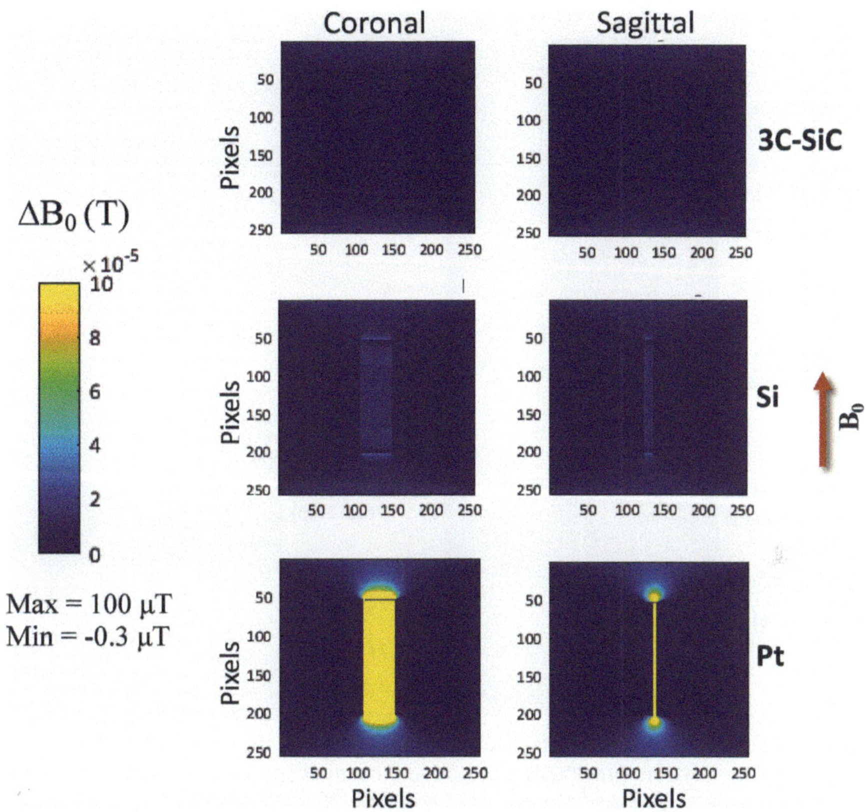

Figure 6.11 The results of the Fourier-based simulations to calculate the image artifacts caused by magnetic susceptibility difference ($\Delta\chi$) between the saline gel phantom and the material used for the experiments. Two coronal and sagittal views of each sample are presented. The red *arrow* shows the direction of the static magnetic field (B_0). The minimum and maximum magnetic field shift caused by $\Delta\chi$ in the materials used for these simulations were ~ -0.3 and $\sim 100\ \mu T$, respectively. The lowest simulated B_0 field distortion was observed in 3C–SiC material and the highest in Pt. This is due to the negligible $\Delta\chi$ between the saline gel phantom and the 3C–SiC material.

This is because the samples are small in size, resulting in a minute temperature rise. However, as the size of the samples becomes larger and larger (relatively large in comparison to the wavelength inside the dielectric material), so does the SAR and induced heating. Therefore, these results can be used as a reference that compares the SAR and induced heating in the materials of interest despite their small dimension.

To validate the simulations, the temperature inside the saline gel phantom (no samples present) was measured using fiberoptic temperature

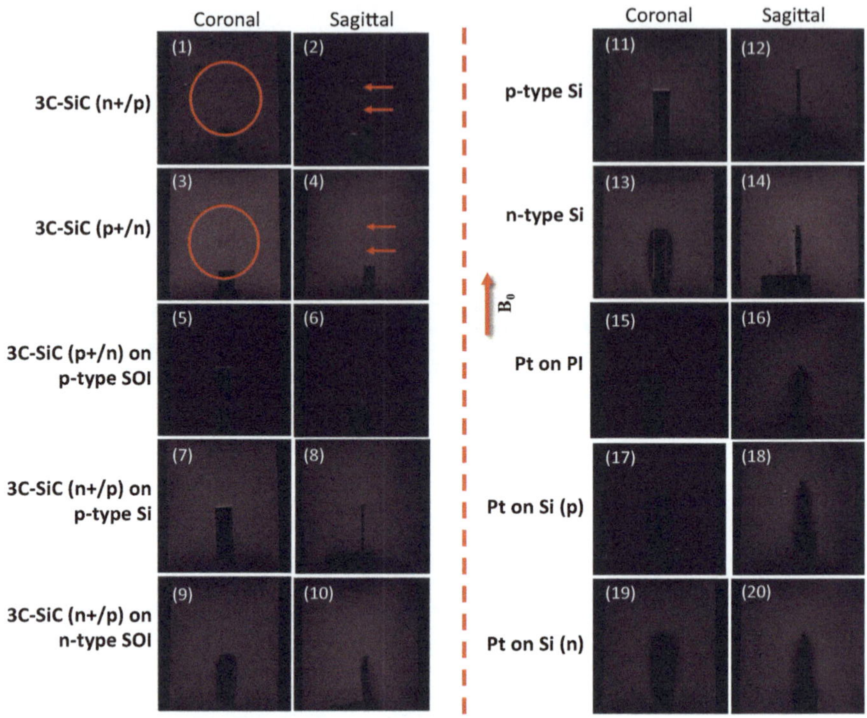

Figure 6.12 7 T MRI experimental scan images indicating the intensity of the image artifacts in the samples previously developed. The direction of the $\boldsymbol{B_0}$ filed is shown with the *arrow* in this figure. (1) Coronal view of the 3C—SiC sample (n^+/p). This was a free-standing sample released after HF and KOH etching; therefore, there was no Si substrate on this sample. As seen, this thin sample (~10 μm) was almost invisible in the scans. This is also true for the sagittal view of the similar sample (2). Similarly, the 3C—SiC sample (n^+/p) did not display any footprint in the scans (3,4). The image artifacts were minimum for all 3C—SiC samples grown on p-type Si substrates (5—8). However, all of these samples were visible in the MRI scans when the Si substrate remained on the sample. On the other hand, 3C—SiC samples grown on n-type Si created image artifacts when the Si substrate remained on the sample (9,10). Opposite to the p-type Si substrate (11,12) that did not show any image artifacts, the n-type Si substrate generated a comparatively high image artifact (13,14). All the Pt samples showed severe image artifacts, regardless of the substrate that they had deposited on (15—20).

probes. Then, these results were compared with the simulation results for this setup. While the value of the measured $\boldsymbol{B}_0$ at the isocenter of the coil with the saline gel load was ~29 μT, this value in the simulations was ~20 μT. This can be due to a different coil used for the simulations and the experiments and also the quality of the simulation mesh. The measured and estimated results for the temperature rise for an MRI scan duration of 15 min is presented in Fig. 6.12.

The initial temperature of the phantom was 27.4°C and, after 15 min of MRI exposure, the temperature in the middle of the tube, where the sample was attached in the other experiments, increased to 29.1°C. By way of comparison, the estimated value from the FEM simulation was 29.08°C, as shown in Fig. 6.13B.

The next set of simulations was performed to estimate the SAR distribution around each electrode for the three electrode samples. The results

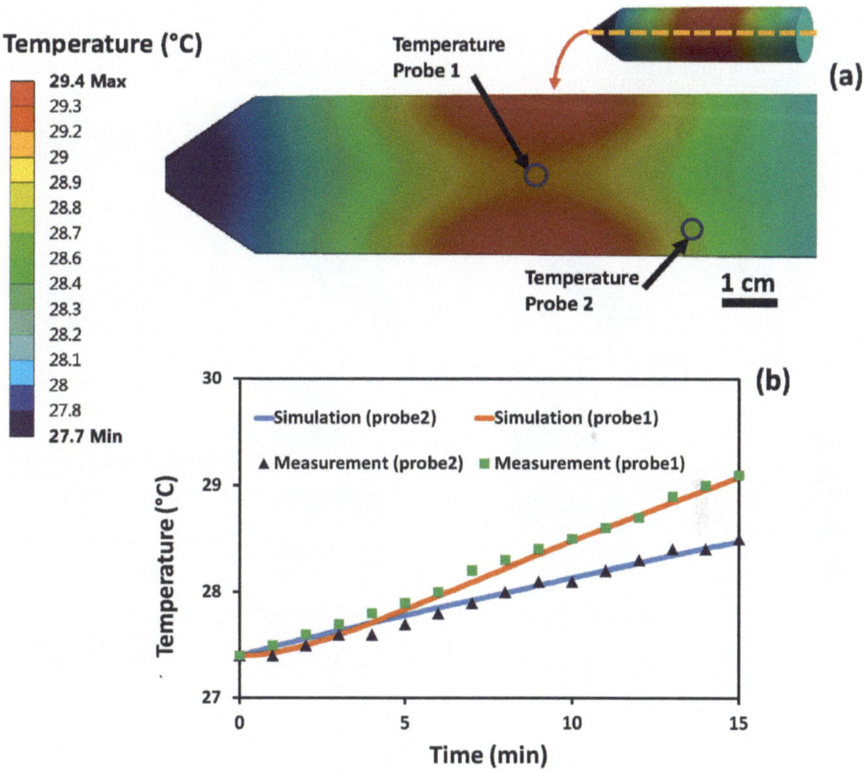

Figure 6.13 Measured and simulated gel phantom temperature rise without any samples present. (A) Cross-section view of the simulated tube temperature profile after 15 min of exposure to ~300 MHz RF field excitation. (B) Measured and simulated temperature profiles at probe 1 (probe tip) and probe 2 (tissue phantom) locations. Initial temperature 27.4°C, and after 15 min exposure to MRI scan, it increased to 29.1°C at probe 1 and to 28.5°C at probe 2. Estimated FEM simulated value at probe 1 location 29.08°C and at probe 2 location 28.47°C, which is in very good agreement with experimental results.

for the FEM simulations indicating the SAR_{1mg} distribution in two Pt and 3C–SiC samples are shown in Fig. 6.14.

As expected, and shown in Fig. 6.14, the highest SAR_{1mg} values occurred at the sample extremities where the electric current flows out of the electrodes. However, the hot spot area in the 3C–SiC sample showed less intensity compared to the Pt sample. While the estimated SAR_{1mg} was very low in both cases, if the size of the electrodes were scaled up, the SAR_{1mg} values would also increase. The SAR_{1mg} value for 3C–SiC showed ~30% reduction compared to the Pt sample. This value would be reduced further if the thermal conductivity of materials is taken into account.

One of the MRI experiments performed to measure the induced heating was on the Pt sample with the extended SS wires. The main

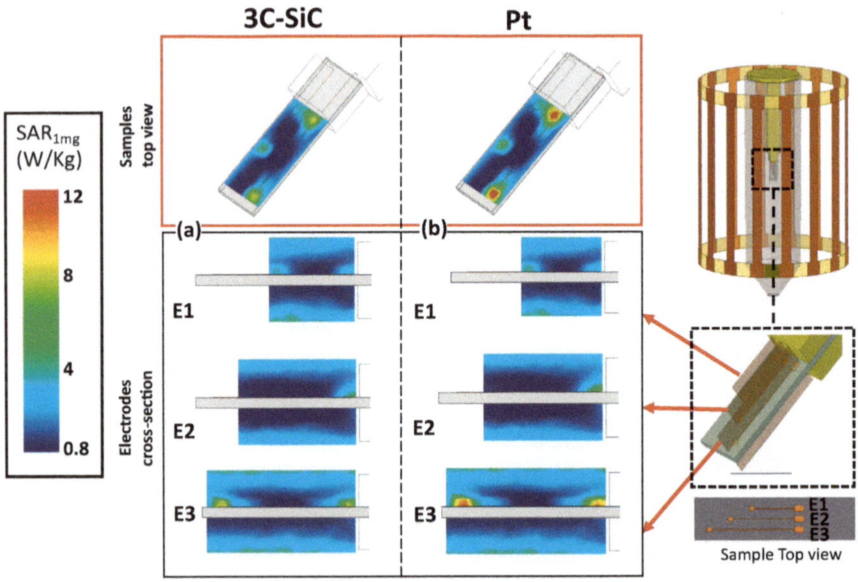

Figure 6.14 Estimated SAR1mg around the three Pt and 3C–SiC electrode samples. E1 stands for the shortest electrode, E2 for the middle electrode, and E3 for the longest electrode. (A) Estimate SAR1mg results for 3C–SiC via FEM electromagnetic simulations in ANSYS HFSS. Both the top view and cross-section view for each electrode is illustrated. The maximum estimated SAR for the 3C–SiC sample appeared at the tip of the longest electrode (SAR_{1mg} ~8 W/kg) while the averaged $\boldsymbol{B}_1$ at the coil isocenter was ~20 μT. (B) Estimated SAR_{1mg} distribution of the Pt sample. Maximum SAR_{1mg} was estimated to be ~12 W/kg and occurred at the tip of the longest electrode. These results indicate a ~30% reduction in the maximum SAR_{1mg} for 3C–SiC compared to Pt.

purpose of this measurement was to measure the temperature rise in the sample and connect the measured temperature rise to the estimated simulated SAR values. The Pt sample was chosen for this measurement as high electrical conductivity Pt was expected to induce more heating than 3C−SiC. The Pt induced enough heat so that the fiberoptic probes were able to measure the temperature rise accurately. In addition, another set of FEM electromagnetic simulations was conducted on the same Pt sample to connect the measured data to the simulation. Similar simulations were performed on the 3C−SiC sample with extended SS wires to compare the results with the Pt sample. The results are illustrated in Fig. 3.15. As expected, the difference in the maximum temperature rise for the Pt and 3C−SiC samples was negligible (Fig. 6.15A and B). The negligible difference in the temperature rise occurred because the highest amount of electromagnetic coupling happened in the SS wires, as they were longer than the electrodes (and identical SS wires were soldered to both samples).

The temperature measurement at the tip of the E3 electrode on the Pt sample is shown in Fig. 6.15C. This plot shows the normalized temperature rise, that is, the difference between the temperature measured with probe 1 in Fig. 6.13A and the temperature measured with probe 2. In addition, the temperature measurement results for the saline gel, when no sample was present, are also shown in this plot. A higher slope for the wired-Pt sample indicates a faster increase in temperature during the time of MRI exposure.

6.3 3C−SiC neural probe under 7 T MRI

For this experiment, the free-standing functional 3C−SiC probe was glued to the PLA holder and placed inside the plastic tube along with the saline gel phantom. The same MRI sequence used for measuring the image artifacts was used in this case. The setup and the sagittal and coronal images of the probe are shown in Fig. 6.16. The image artifacts before and after etching backside Si layer are also shown in this figure. The images indicating artifacts after backside Si etch were taken from the samples used for the comparison of the image artifacts in Section 6.1.

7. Summary

In this chapter, the magnetic resonance compatibility of single-crystalline cubic silicon carbide (3C−SiC) probes was evaluated. It was hypothesized that a brain implant fabricated monolithically from 3C−SiC material may remarkably improve the MRI compatibility of these implants. Most

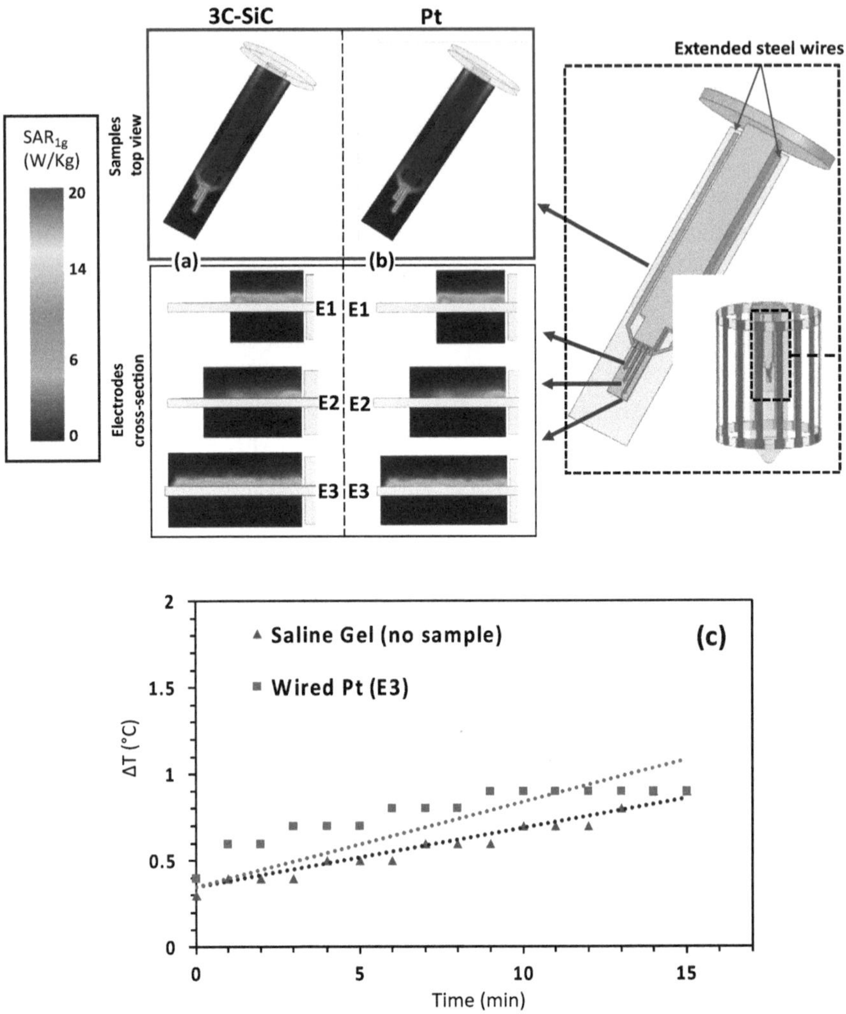

Figure 6.15 Temperature measurement and FEM electromagnetic simulation results for the samples with extended SS wires. (A) SAR_{1g} for the 3C–SiC sample with extended SS wires. (B) SAR_{1g} for the Pt sample with extended SS wires. The maximum SAR_{1g} values for the two samples were approximately identical as the highest amount of electromagnetic coupling happened in the SS wires, as they were longer than the electrodes. (C) Measured temperature at the tip of the E3 electrode on the Pt sample. Plot shows the normalized temperature rise, that is, the difference between the temperature measured with probe 1 and probe 2. Temperature measurements for the saline gel, when no sample was present, are also shown.

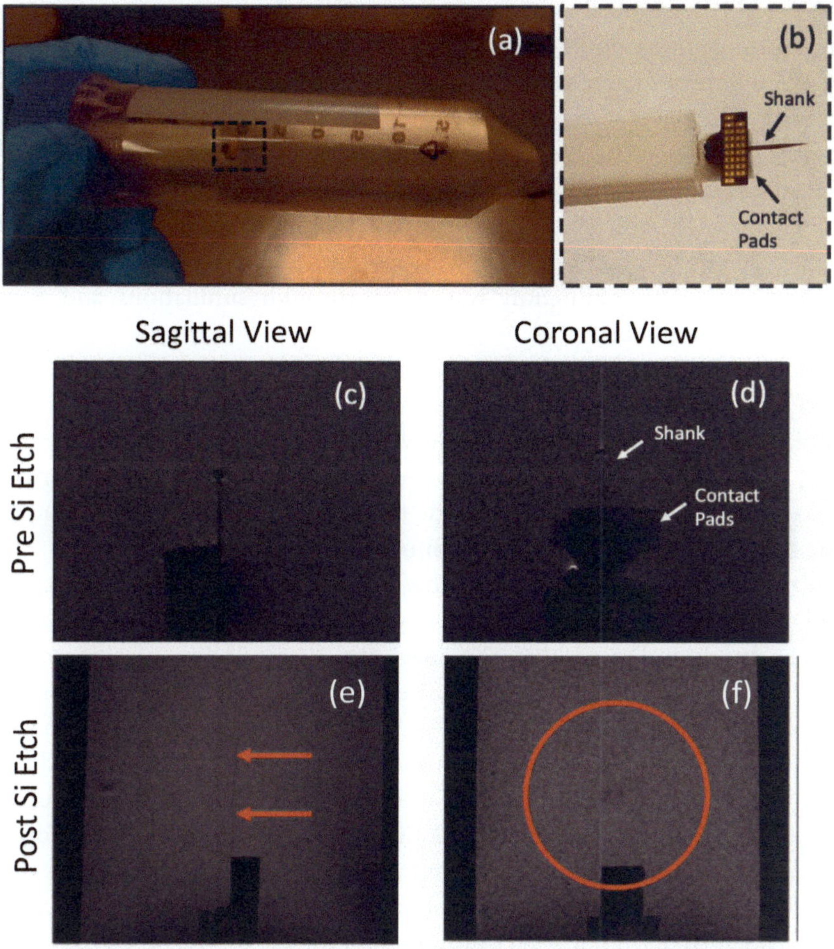

Figure 6.16 MRI scans of the fabricated 3C−SiC probe under 7 T MRI scanning. The same MRI sequence used for image artifact analysis was used in this experiment. (A) Photograph of experimental setup consisting of PLA holder, plastic tube, saline gel phantom, and the neural probe. (B) A close-up image of the 3C−SiC neural probe glued on the PLA holder. (C) Sagittal view of the neural probe under 7 T MRI. The tip of the probe showed a circular image artifact. (D) Coronal view of the neural probe. The shank generated less image artifacts than the pads, due to the metallic pads that would be outside of the brain during probe use and is not an issue. (E) Sagittal view of the 3C−SiC sample after etching the backside Si in a KOH bath. (F) Coronal view of the same sample after etching the backside Si.

importantly, the 3C−SiC implants may allow for an increase in the standard $\boldsymbol{B}_0$ intensity that would permit the use of implants in 7 T MRI tools. Therefore, to evaluate the MRI compatibility of 3C−SiC neural implants, a 7 T MRI machine for small laboratory animals was used in this work. Silicon, of various doping types and concentrations, and platinum were used as reference materials to compare the MRI compatibility of 3C—SiC material. The MRI compatibility criteria in this work were limited to the severity of image artifacts surrounding the samples and induced heating and SAR distribution under MRI scans. Various samples were fabricated from 3C—SiC, Si, Pt, and PI. Si and PI were mainly used as the substrate to deposit Pt on, while Si and SOI were used to grow thin epitaxial films of 3C—SiC on. The evaluation was done through simulations and tissue phantom experiments.

As seen in Fig. 6.13, the simulated results indicated a meaningful difference in the SAR distribution between the Pt and 3C—SiC samples. The simulations predicted a ~30% lower maximum SAR for 3C—SiC compared to Pt. Although both samples experienced very low amounts of SAR, in the case of a longer electrode this difference was more evident and thus this was used to validate the simulation.

One of the observations during this work was the difference in magnetic field perturbation in p-type and n-type silicon. The experiments in the current work indicated that the magnetic susceptibility of silicon, and consequently the extent to which it caused magnetic field perturbation and image artifacts under MRI, is highly dependent on their doping type. As observed in the experimental results shown in Fig. 6.11, p-type Si induced fewer image artifacts while n-type Si displayed severe image artifacts under MRI. The magnetic susceptibility of Si, and its dependence on the doping type and concentration, was reported in other works [44—46]. However, this dependence on the doping concentration and type was not observed in epitaxially grown thin 3C—SiC films used in these experiments. One reason for this can be due to the very thin nature of the film that causes fewer image artifacts as reported elsewhere [36]. The reason why it was possible for the 3C—SiC samples to be fabricated very thin (~10 μm) was because of the monolithic fabrication method that is only possible in 3C—SiC because of its high mechanical strength, flexibility, and chemical stability.

Another important point observed during the MRI experiments was the image artifacts measured for the fabricated all-3C—SiC neural probe. The probe showed very little footprint inside the 7 T MRI scans. However, the tip of the probe had visible dark image artifacts that might be caused by the sharp point of the tip. The effect of the shape and sharp points in creating image artifacts has been studied elsewhere [36] where it is believed that sharp points can increase image artifacts under MRI. However, one of the reasons that the probe showed some visibility during MRI imaging was believed to be due to the very thin (~27 μm) Si substrate film that remained on the probe backside. Once the Si was etched away, the 3C–SiC neural probe was virtually transparent at 7 T, which is a highly significant result.

Acknowledgments

The assistance of Richard Everly and Chenyin Feng with microfabrication process in the University of South Florida Nanotechnology Research and Education Center (NREC) is appreciated.

References

[1] S.E. Saddow, C.L. Frewin, M. Reyes, J. Register, M. Nezafati, S. Thomas, 3C-SiC on Si: a biocompatible material for advanced bioelectronic devices, ECS Transactions 61 (7) (2014) 101–111.

[2] S. E. Saddow, Silicon Carbide Biotechnology: A Biocompatible Semiconductor for Advanced Biomedical Devices and Applications. Elsevier, © 2012.

[3] C.L. Frewin, C. Locke, L. Mariusso, E.J. Weeber, S.E. Saddow, Silicon carbide neural implants: in vivo neural tissue reaction, IEEE/EMBS Conference on Neural Engineering (2013) 661–664.

[4] G.L. Knaack, D.G. McHail, B. German, B. Koo, N. Peixoto, S.F. Cogan, T.C. Dumas, J.J. Pancrazio, In vivo characterization of amorphous silicon carbide as a biomaterial for chronic neural interfaces, Frontiers in Neuroscience 10 (2016) 301.

[5] Knaack, G.L., Hamid C., S.F. Cogan, and J.J. Pancrazio. "Amorphous silicon carbide for neural interface applications." In S. E. Saddow, Silicon Carbide Biotechnology: A Biocompatible Semiconductor for Advanced Biomedical Devices and Applications. Elsevier, © 2016.

[6] X. Lei, S. Kane, S. Cogan, H. Lorach, G. Ludwig, P. Huie, M. Keith, T. Kamins, J. Harris, D. Palanker, SiC protective coating for photovoltaic retinal prosthesis, Journal of Neural Engineering 13 (4) (2016) 046016.

[7] F. Deku, C.L. Frewin, A. Stiller, Y. Cohen, S. Aqeel, A. Joshi-Imre, B. Black, T.J. Gardner, J.J. Pancrazio, S.F. Cogan, Amorphous silicon carbide platform for next generation penetrating neural interface designs, Micromachines 9 (10) (2018) 480.

[8] H.-P. Phan, Y. Zhong, T.-K. Nguyen, Y. Park, T. Dinh, E. Song, R. Kumar Vadivelu, et al., Long-lived, transferred crystalline silicon carbide nanomembranes for implantable flexible electronics, ACS Nano 13 (10) (2019) 11572–11581.

[9] L. Golestanirad, L.M. Angelone, J. Kirsch, S. Downs, B. Keil, G. Bonmassar, L. Lawrence, Wald. Reducing RF-induced heating near implanted leads through high-dielectric capacitive bleeding of current (CBLOC), IEEE Transactions on Microwave Theory and Techniques 67 (3) (2019) 1265–1273.

[10] J.A. Nyenhuis, S.M. Park, R. Kamondetdacha, A. Amjad, F.G. Shellock, A.R. Rezai, MRI and implanted medical devices: basic interactions with an emphasis on heating, IEEE Transactions on Device Materials and Reliability 5 (3) (2005) 467–479.

[11] Medtronic PERCEPT PC Neurostimulator. Available online: https://www.medtronic.com/us-en/healthcare-professionals/products/neurological/deep-brain-stimulation-systems/percept-pc.html (accessed on 20 December 2020).

[12] J.B. Erhardt, E. Fuhrer, O.G. Gruschke, J. Leupold, M.C. Wapler, J. Hennig, T. Stieglitz, J.G. Korvink, Should patients with brain implants undergo MRI? Journal of Neural Engineering 15 (4) (2018) 041002.
[13] L. Golestanirad, L.M. Angelone, M.I. Iacono, H. Katnani, L.L. Wald, G. Bonmassar, Local SAR near deep brain stimulation (DBS) electrodes at 64 and 127 MHz: a simulation study of the effect of extracranial loops, Magnetic Resonance in Medicine 78 (4) (2017) 1558−1565.
[14] F.G. Shellock, Radiofrequency energy-induced heating during MR procedures: a review, Journal of Magnetic Resonance Imaging 12 (1) (2000) 30−36.
[15] L. Golestanirad, M. Ida Iacono, B. Keil, L.M. Angelone, G. Bonmassar, M.D. Fox, H. Todd, et al., Construction and modeling of a reconfigurable MRI coil for lowering SAR in patients with deep brain stimulation implants, Neuroimage 147 (2017) 577−588.
[16] L.P. Panych, B. Madore, The physics of MRI safety, Journal of Magnetic Resonnce Imaging 47 (1) (2018) 28−43.
[17] S. Nimbalkar, E. Fuhrer, S. Pedro, T. Nguyen, M. Sereno, S. Kassegne, K. Jan, Glassy carbon microelectrodes minimize induced voltages, mechanical vibrations, and artifacts in magnetic resonance imaging, Microsystems Nanoengineering 5 (no. 1) (2019) 1−11.
[18] S. Louis, On the AJR Viewbox MRI : A Hairy Situation," Image (Rochester, N.Y.), No. February, 2004, pp. 532−535.
[19] G. Schramm, "Review Article Metal Artifact Correction Strategies in MRI- - Based Attenuation Correction in PET/MRI," No. July, 2019.
[20] H. Scherberger, I. Fineman, S. Musallam, D.J. Dubowitz, K.A. Bernheim, B. Pesaran, B.D. Corneil, B. Gilliken, R.A. Andersen, Magnetic resonance image-guided implantation of chronic recording electrodes in the macaque intraparietal sulcus, Journal of Neuroscience Methods 130 (1) (2003) 1−8.
[21] M.E. Ladd, P. Bachert, M. Meyerspeer, E. Moser, A.M. Nagel, D.G. Norris, S. Schmitter, Oliver Speck, S. Straub, M. Zaiss, Pros and cons of ultra-high-field MRI/MRS for human application, Progress in Nuclear Magnetic Resonance Spectroscopy 109 (2018) 1−50.
[22] G. Bonmassar, K. Fujimoto, A.J. Golby, PTFOS: flexible and absorbable intracranial electrodes for magnetic resonance imaging, PLoS One 7 (9) (2012).
[23] P.A. Bottomley, A. Kumar, W.A. Edelstein, J.M. Allen, P.V. Karmarkar, Designing passive MRI-safe implantable conducting leads with electrodes, Medical Physics 37 (7) (2010) 3828−3843.
[24] D. Li, X. Ji, J. Zheng, C. Pan, J. Chen, W. Kainz, A novel design of implantable esophageal stent to reduce the MRI RF-induced heating, IEEE Transactions on Electromagnetic Compatibility 59 (3) (2017) 805−812.
[25] C.J. Yeung, R.C. Susil, E. Atalar, RF safety of wires in interventional MRI: using a safety index, Magnetic Resonance in Medicine 47 (1) (2002) 187−193.
[26] H.S. Ho, Safety of metallic implants in magnetic resonance imaging, Journal of Magnetic Resonance in Imaging 14 (4) (2001) 472−477.
[27] S.A. Mohsin, J. Nyenhuis, R. Masood, Interaction of medical implants with the MRI electromagnetic fields, Progress in Electromagnetic Research 13 (2010) 195−202.
[28] S. Zhao, X. Liu, Z. Xu, H. Ren, B. Deng, M. Tang, L. Lu, et al., Graphene encapsulated copper microwires as highly MRI compatible neural electrodes, Nano Letters 16 (12) (2016) 7731−7738.
[29] M. Beygi, J.T. Bentley, C.L. Frewin, C.A. Kuliasha, A. Takshi, E.K. Bernardin, Francesco La via, and Stephen E. Saddow. "Fabrication of a monolithic implantable neural interface from cubic silicon carbide, Micromachines 10 (7) (2019) 430.

[30] ASTM F2182-11a, Standard Test Method for Measurement of Radio Frequency Induced Heating on or Near Passive Implants during Magnetic Resonance Imaging, ASTM International, West Conshohocken, PA, 2011. www.astm.org.
[31] ASTM F2052-06e1, Standard Test Method for Measurement of Magnetically Induced Displacement Force on Medical Devices in the Magnetic Resonance Environment, ASTM International, West Conshohocken, PA, 2006. www.astm.org.
[32] ASTM F2119-07(2013), Standard Test Method for Evaluation of MR Image Artifacts from Passive Implants, ASTM International, West Conshohocken, PA, 2013. www.astm.org.
[33] J.P. Hornak, The Basics of MRI, vol. 68, 2008. *URL*, http//www.cis.rit.edu/htbooks/mri/index.html.
[34] C.A. Balanis, Antenna Theory: Analysis and Design, John wiley & sons, 2016.
[35] J.T. Vaughan, J.R. Griffiths, RF Coils for MRI, John Wiley & Sons, 2012.
[36] F.M. Martinez-Santiesteban, S.D. Swanson, D.C. Noll, D.J. Anderson, Magnetic field perturbation of neural recording and stimulating microelectrodes, Physics in Medicine and Biology 52 (8) (2007) 2073–2088.
[37] J.H. Duyn, J. Schenck, Contributions to magnetic susceptibility of brain tissue, NMR in Biomedicine 30 (4) (2017) 1–37.
[38] J.P. Marques, R. Bowtell, Application of a fourier-based method for rapid calculation of field inhomogeneity due to spatial variation of magnetic susceptibility, Concepts in Magnetic Resonance Part B Magnetic Resonance Engineering 25 (1) (2005) 65–78.
[39] M. Beygi, W. Dominguez-Viqueira, C. Feng, G. Mumcu, C.L. Frewin, F. La Via, S.E. Saddow, Silicon carbide and MRI: towards developing a MRI safe neural interface, Micromachines 12 (2) (2021) 126.
[40] T. Maeder, L. Sagalowicz, P. Muralt, Stabilized platinum electrodes for ferroelectric film deposition using Ti, Ta and Zr adhesion layers, Japanese Journal of Applied Physics 37 (4R) (1998) 2007.
[41] F.D. Doty, E. George, J. Kulkarni, K. Pamarthy, P. John, Staab, Radio frequency coil technology for small-animal MRI, NMR in Biomedicine: An International Journal Devoted to the Development and Application of Magnetic Resonance In Vivo 20 (3) (2007) 304–325.
[42] C.-L. Chin, et al., BirdcageBuilder: design of specified-geometry birdcage coils with desired current pattern and resonant frequency, Concepts in Magnetic Resonance: An Educational Journal 15 (2) (2002) 156–163.
[43] J.G. Bouwman, C.J.G. Bakker, Alias subtraction more efficient than conventional zero-padding in the Fourier-based calculation of the susceptibility induced perturbation of the magnetic field in MR, Magnetic Resonance in Medcine 68 (2) (2012) 621–630.
[44] M.P. Sarachik, D.R. He, W. Li, M. Levy, J.S. Brooks, Magnetic properties of boron-doped silicon, Physical Review B 31 (3) (1985) 1469–1477.
[45] H.G. Schlager, H.V. Löhneysen, Susceptibility of local magnetic moments in phosphorus-doped silicon near the metal-insulator transition, Europhysics Letters 40 (6) (1997) 661–666.
[46] W. Sasaki, J. Kinoshita, Piezoresistance and magnetic susceptibility in heavily doped n-type silicon, Journal of the Physical Society of Japan 25 (6) (1968) 1622–1629.

CHAPTER 7

Ultrathin neural interfaces constructed from carbon and amorphous silicon carbide

Chenyin Feng[1,2], Christopher L. Frewin[3], Md Rubayat-E Tanjil[2], Richard Everly[5], Jay Bieber[5], Ashok Kumar[2], Michael Cai Wang[2] and Stephen E. Saddow[4]

[1]Department of Electrical Engineering, University of South Florida, Tampa, FL, United States; [2]Department of Mechanical Engineering, University of South Florida, Tampa, FL, United States; [3]NeuroNexus LLC, Ann Arbor, MI, United States; [4]Departments of Electrical & Medical Engineering, University of South Florida, Tampa, FL, United States; [5]Nanotechnology Research & Education Center, University of South Florida, Tampa, FL, United States

Contents

1. Introduction

Neural interfaces have continued to gain significant interest over the last few decades [1], especially microelectrode implantable neural probes (mINP), which may be attributed to advances in microfabrication processes from the semiconductor industry [2]. A fully neural-compatible material is necessary to obtain a reliable and long-term implantable device. However, conventional devices are typically made with silicon and noble metals, as well as polymeric materials [3,4]. To date, none of these devices have

Silicon Carbide Technology for Advanced Human Healthcare Applications
ISBN 978-0-323-90609-8
https://doi.org/10.1016/B978-0-323-90609-8.00011-9

proved to be suitable for long-term implanted use in humans due to in vivo issues that relate to a set of complex abiotic and biotic processes [5,6]. For instance, the environment into which the devices are implanted has a high oxidative species concentration that may cause significant reliability challenges such as device corrosion, film cracking and delamination just to name a few [7—9]. Thus, the development and investigation of new materials for mINP applications are urgently needed.

In this chapter, amorphous silicon carbide (*a*-SiC) was chosen as the primary material for a novel, flexible mINP as both the base and top side conformal insulator [10—13]. Carbon, derived from pyrolyzed photoresist film (PPF), was used as the conductor and sandwiched between the insulating *a*-SiC layers. The previous research of our group has demonstrated that *a*-SiC has excellent biocompatibility, hemocompatibility, and mechanical properties [10,13]. Moreover, the relative dielectric constant of *a*-SiC can be controlled in the range of 2.7—10 by optimizing the stoichiometry of the film, which means it can reduce the capacitive coupling between each trace during neural stimulation [14,15]. Besides that, as an insulator, *a*-SiC has demonstrated excellent insulation properties. It showed a low leakage current (<20 nA) at $\pm$ 50 V under both dry and wet phosphate-buffered saline (PBS) conditions when testing an interdigitated electrode (IDE) device [7]. Compared with other commonly used insulating materials in mINPs, *a*-SiC demonstrates superior chemical inertness that can prevent ionic diffusion and device failure due to implantation in harsh environments [16—18].

For long-term human use, mINP electrode materials must possess reliable electrical performance without stimulating the human immune system response that damages tissue in addition to reducing implant reliability. Typically, platinum (Pt) and gold (Au) along with an adhesion layer of titanium (Ti), are used as the recording electrode materials for mINP applications. However, during chronic neural stimulation/recording, the electrodes are in contact with the harsh environment of the brain. This means that metal electrodes may be degraded due to corrosion and dissolution. Moreover, metal electrodes can also cause an inflammatory reaction in the tissue. Thus, the proper choice of compatible conductive materials for mINP electrodes is crucial. As one of the most versatile materials in the periodic table, carbon has a variety of allotropes attributed to their sp, sp^2, and sp^3 hybridization [19]. It has been used in nearly all device fields, which include implantable neural interfaces. To date, numerous papers have reported about carbon-based mINPs that include graphene [20], carbon nanotubes (CNTs) [21], glassy carbon (GC) [22], and PPF [23,24].

In 2004, Novoselov and Geim first exfoliated graphene from highly oriented pyrolytic graphite using scotch tape. Since then, more than 2 million publications have been reported on this carbon allotrope [25]. Graphene contains a single layer of carbon atoms that forms into a hexagonal structure that is only sp^2 hybridized [26–28]. Thanks to the unique structure of graphene, it displays extraordinary mechanical and electrical properties, and it has been utilized in many fields. In addition, it is a promising candidate for brain–machine-interface applications because of the high area-volume ratio and two-dimensional nature. Park et al. [29] have demonstrated a graphene-based electrode array neural interface. The device can offer optogenetic activation of cortical areas and imaging the vasculature by fluorescence microscopy in meantime. Usmani et al. [30] have successfully fabricated a 3D CNT foam (CNF) that could help spinal cord cell growth and reconnection. The ex vivo results indicated that the spinal organotypic slices cultured on CNF had significant outgrowth [31].

However, there are many debates on the biocompatibility and neurotoxicity of CNT and graphene-related nanomaterials [32,33]. In addition, the fabrication processes of CNT and graphene devices are complex, relatively high cost, and hard to be mass produce. Comparing two of the most promising carbon materials for mINP applications, GC and PPF, PPF has demonstrated a smooth surface and excellent electrochemical performance [22,24,34]. Therefore, PPF was chosen as the material for both the C conductive traces and electrodes for the mINP developed in this work. It can be directly synthesized from pyrolyzing standard photoresist, a patternable polymeric material commonly used in semiconductor processes. The thickness and the uniformity of the photoresist can be easily and accurately controlled by adjusting the spin speed during the photoresist spin-coating step, and it can be easily fabricated into the desired pattern. Previous research from our group has demonstrated the biocompatibility of PPF and graphene [24]. Thus, it is worthwhile to develop a carbon-based mINP using PPF as the conductive traces and electrodes along with *a*-SiC as the insulation material. Compared with conventional silicon and noble metals-based mINPs, this work does not require metal evaporation/sputtering and lift-off processes of small features, which can simplify the fabrication process and increase cost-efficiency.

In this chapter, both 16 and 32 channel PPF-based planar mINP devices will be presented. In addition, a set of planar single-ended electrodes with various recording areas were fabricated for electrochemical testing to demonstrate the properties of PPF for this challenging application. The mINP contains two layers of *a*-SiC: the bottom support and top conformal insulator along with a PPF interlayer serving as conducting the traces and electrodes. Each electrode has a window with a diameter of 25 μm that contacts the neural environment. For the single-ended electrodes, there were five different electrode areas which were 502, 125, 7.8, 1.9, and 0.49 kμm^2, respectively. In addition, there is a 50 μm thick silicon layer that served as a physical support layer for the base *a*-SiC film.

2. Fabrication process and methods

The PPF/*a*-SiC mINP can be fabricated via standard semiconductor micromachining processes. As shown in Fig. 7.1, it started with *a*-SiC deposition by plasma enhanced chemical vapor deposition (PECVD). 12 sccm SiH_4 and 360 sccm CH_4 served as silicon and carbon precursors along with 700 sccm Ar served as the carrier gas. The chamber was preheated to 250°C at a pressure of 1100 mTorr with an RF power of 200 W. Then, the positive photoresist (AZ12xt) was spin-coated on the *a*-SiC coated wafer at 500 rpm for 20 s, 3000 rpm for 50 s, and 11,000 rpm for 2 s. The first spin stage was to distribute the photoresist on the wafer uniformly, the second stage set the thickness of the photoresist, in this case ~7 μm as measured by a stylus profilometer, and the last stage was used to eliminate the edge bead. The coated substrate was then soft-baked at 120°C for 3 min, followed by UV exposure at an intensity of ~120 mJ/cm^2. Next, a 1-min postexposure bake at 95°C was performed. Pyrolyzation was performed by annealing the photoresist in a tube furnace at atmospheric pressure and at different temperatures from 500 to 900°C under an Ar and H_2 environment of 100 sccm and 5 sccm, respectively. The thermal ramp rate was 10°C/min, followed by a thermal soak at the desired temperature for 1 hour. After annealing the sample was cooled down to room temperature under the same of Ar and H_2 flow. The top conformal *a*-SiC insulator layer was then deposited on the PPF layers using the identical PECVD conditions as the base layer. Contact and electrode windows were opened in the top insulator through reactive ion etching (RIE) employing the following parameters: 37 sccm CF4 and 13 sccm O_2, RF power 200 W, and a base pressure of 50 mTorr for 5 minutes time. The etch rate was 0.9 nm/s thus a timed etch was used, and complete removal of the *a*-SiC layer as confirmed after this step was completed using a stylus profilometer. In future work, an etch

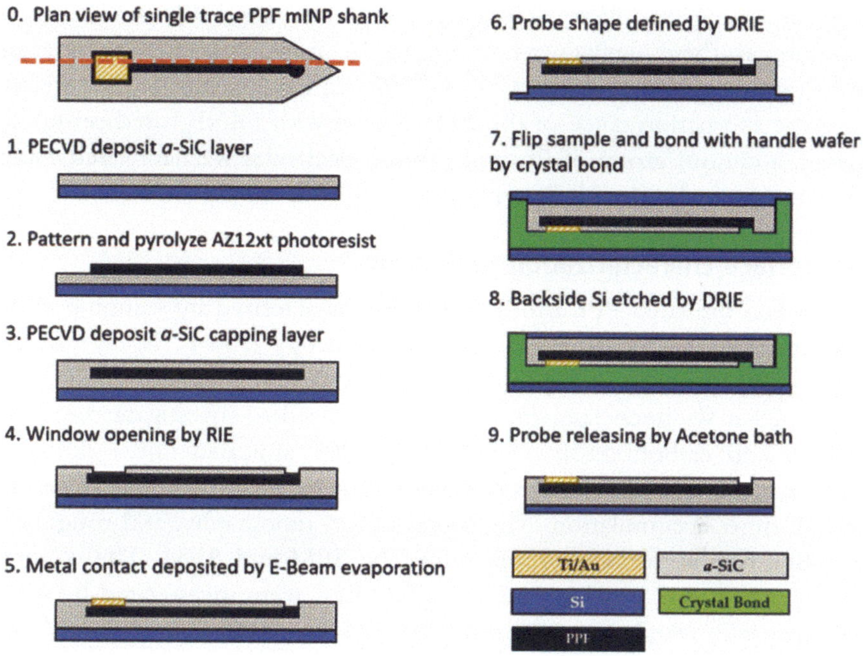

Figure 7.1 Sketch of a single trace PPF mINP shank for process illustration purposes. (**0**) Top view of completed device; dashed line shows cross-section cut for (**1**–**9**). (**1**) Starting with an oxide-coated Si wafer, an *a*-SiC film is deposited via PECVD. (**2**) Positive photoresist is spun, patterned, and thermally annealed to pyrolyze the photoresist into PPF carbon traces. (**3**) Wafer is coated with another layer of *a*-SiC. (**4**) RIE is used to open windows exposing the recording tip and bonding pad. (**5**) Metal is deposited on the bond-pads using a lift-off process and (**6**) probe is defined by DRIE (mINP only, singled ended electrode process completed at step (**5**)). (**7**) Die is flipped and bonded to Si handle wafer using crystal bond. (**8**) Backside Si is thinned to ~50 μm by DRIE. (**9**) Probes are released from Si handle wafer via crystal bond dissolution in acetone [7].

stop will be employed to ensure window opening is consistent from batch to batch and across a full wafer. Bond pads were formed on the contact mesas via E-beam evaporation starting with 50 nm of Ti as an adhesion layer followed by 300 nm of Au to facilitate device packaging. The die was then bonded to a Si handle wafer device side down using crystal bond (Ted Pella, Inc.) and the silicon substrate thinned using deep reactive ion etching (DRIE) to achieve a 50 μm Si supporting layer. The final process step was to harvest the probes from the Si handle wafer via dissolution of the crystal bond adhesion layer in acetone. The influence of the electrode geometric area on PPF performance was investigated through single-ended electrodes fabricated using variable recording areas. In this case, we did not thin the Si substrate as these devices were not to be implanted. Electrode areas investigated are 0.49, 1.9 7.8, 125, and 502 kμm^2, respectively. To directly compare the performance of the PPF devices with mINP based on noble metals, a control group of Pt single-ended electrodes was fabricated using the same procedure, with Pt replacing the PPF layer [7].

2.1 Surface characterization of PPF mINP

The *a*-SiC insulated PPF mINP has been characterized by scanning electron microscopy (SEM), atomic force microscopy (AFM), X-ray photoelectron spectroscopy (XPS), and Raman spectroscopy. JASCO NRS-4500 with a 20-mW green laser (532 nm) was utilized to investigate the crystallinity and carbonization degree of the PPF annealed under different temperatures, and each data point was collected with 5 seconds exposure and 15 times accumulation. The morphology, topography, and roughness of *a*-SiC film and PPF were examined by SEM and AFM. The oxygen concentration and stoichiometry of *a*-SiC film were investigated by XPS depth profile, which was performed via Ar ion milling [7].

2.2 Evaluation of PECVD-deposited *a*-SiC film stress

Film stress is one of the most important criteria that will influence the shape of the released probes and their reliability during high-temperature annealing. A Dektak D150 profilometer was used in this work to analyze the film stress by measuring the curvature before and after deposition, as well as the influence of high-temperature annealing. The film stress was calculated using Stony's equation:

$$\sigma = \frac{1}{6}\left(\frac{1}{R_{\text{post}}} - \frac{1}{R_{\text{pre}}}\right)\frac{E}{1-\nu}\frac{t_S^2}{t_f}$$

where E is Young's modulus and ν, Poisson's ratio that the intrinsic properties of the substrate, which is Si in this work. R_{pre} and R_{post} represent the curvature before and after the deposition processes, while the t_s and t_f are the thickness of the substrate and film, respectively.

2.3 Electrical and electrochemical characterization of PPF mINP

Electrical and electrochemical testing were conducted on the double-ended resistors and single-ended electrodes on the planar microelectrode array. The PPF electrode resistivity was calculated via current-voltage analysis. The insulating properties of the *a*-SiC insulation were characterized by applying a swept voltage range of −50 V to +50 V using IDE devices under both dry and wet (PBS) environments. Each IDE device consists of two comb electrodes traces of 50 μm width, 1 mm length, separated by 100 μm (i.e., pitch), and contains 22 digits. The leakage current was measured between the traces using a Keithley IV plotter (model no. 2400). Electrochemical impedance spectroscopy (EIS) and cyclic voltammetry (CV) testing were performed using a potentiostat (Reference 600, Gamry, Inc.) with a standard three-electrode set up, where the PPF served as the working electrode, Pt as the counter electrode, and Ag/AgCl as the reference electrode. All electrochemical testing was performed in 30 min N_2 aerated PBS with a room temperature pH value of 7.4.

3. Results and discussion

The annealing temperature range for PPF synthesis was chosen from 500°C, to 900°C in 100°C steps. Shown in Fig. 7.2A is a cross-section SEM image of a PPF electrode annealed at 900°C. The thickness of each layer can be clearly observed, and the PPF trace has a thickness of 387 nm while the pre-PPF synthesis photoresist has a thickness of 7 μm. Thus, the thickness shrinkage rate was 92%, which indicates a significant size decrease of the mINP in the vertical direction, which is a positive feature of this electrode. Fortunately, there was virtually no change in the lateral dimension after pyrolyzing. This was due to performing the pyrolyzation in several stages. First, the resist was hard-baked at 150°C, after which the solvent phenols inside of the photoresist were evaporated completely. After the temperature rises above 300°C, C=O bonds start to break resulting in C−C bonds and, ultimately, C=C bonds are formed. As the *a*-SiC/PPF interfacial C atoms were bonded with dangling bonds at the *a*-SiC surface before pyrolyzation, this inhibits PPF lateral shrinkage as observed. Thus, the photoresist film is expected to shrink in the vertical dimension while the lateral dimension should not experience appreciable change during pyrolyzation. When combined with the top and bottom *a*-SiC insulation layers, the total thickness of the PPF mINP was below 1 μm; However, in this work, a 50 μm backside Si layer from the handle wafer was left in-place from the backside Si removal step to serve as a support layer.

A photograph of a free-standing functional PPF mINP with 16 channels is shown in Fig. 7.2B. The device was 5 mm in length, 500 μm in width, and 1 μm in thickness supported by a 50 μm Si layer on the backside of the

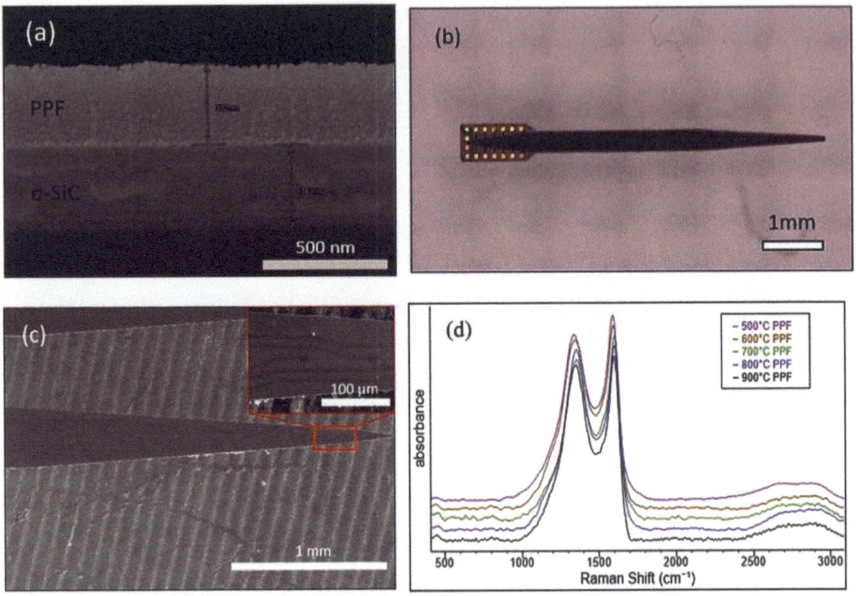

Figure 7.2 Fabricated PPF on a-SiC probe characterization data: (A) SEM cross-section micrograph after PPF annealing at 900°C. Photoresist thickness 7.4 μm before annealing and of 387 nm after annealing indicating a ~92% vertical shrinkage. (B) Composite optical image of single shank *a*-SiC/PPF mINP. (C) SEM plan view micrograph showing electrode and recording tip detail. (D) Raman spectra of PPF films versus annealing temperature show a 10 cm^{-1} red shift with increasing annealing temperature indicating improved PPF film structure.

device. Fig. 7.2C shows a planar SEM image of a double-shank PPF mINP with 16 channels per shank. Each recording site is 314 μm^2 with a trace width of 10 μm. The influence of annealing temperature on PPF crystallinity was investigated by Raman spectroscopy, and the results are shown in Fig. 7.2D. As a carbon-based material, the bands located at ~1360 cm^{-1} and ~1580 cm^{-1}, the so-called "D" and "G" bands, have been investigated extensively. The presence of the D and G bands verifies carbon sp^2 hybridization during high-temperature annealing, and the I_D/I_G ratio can be used to observe the structural order and crystallinity of the PPF film. Unfortunately, Raman spectra of pristine photoresist were not measured due to the high fluorescence of the films which overlapped with the D and G peaks. As shown in the figure, with increasing annealing temperature the I_D/I_G ratio increased, which indicates better crystallinity of the PPF film annealed at higher temperatures. Moreover, the D and G bands become more distinguishable, and there is a 10 cm^{-1} (red shift with increasing annealing temperature further indicating a better PPF film crystallinity and structure.

3.1 *a*-SiC film characterization

The surface roughness of the base *a*-SiC layer was examined by tapping mode AFM, and results are shown in Fig. 7.3. Fig. 7.3A was measured at the center region of the wafer, while Fig. 7.3B was measured at the edge region. The results indicate that the PECVD deposit *a*-SiC film (250 nm) was pretty smooth with a surface roughness of 0.763 ± 0.17 nm at the center region and 0.919 ± 0.11 nm at the edge region.

To study the film, chemical composition XPS measurements were conducted. The XPS depth profile, as well as high-resolution C 1s and Si 2p spectra, is shown in Fig. 7.4A–C. Ar ion milling was utilized to obtain a depth profile with a beam energy of 3.5 kV, raster size of 25 mm^2, and an X-ray power of 350W. Fig. 7.4A indicates that the oxygen content was mainly on the film surface with very low oxygen concentration in the *a*-SiC film bulk. For *a*-SiC films, a low oxygen content is critical to ensure that carbon-doped oxide layers were not formed, which are water-soluble Si–O–C bonds instead of robust Si–C bonds. In addition, Si–O–C bonds may cause device failure during chronic implantation [35]. As shown in Fig. 7.4A, within approximately 15 nm of the film surface the oxygen content dramatically dropped to the detection limit, which indicated that the oxygen atoms were mainly located on the surface that may be attributed to a small amount of surface oxidation. The C 1s and Si 2p high-resolution spectra further indicate that *a*-SiC was indeed deposited. XPS survey data

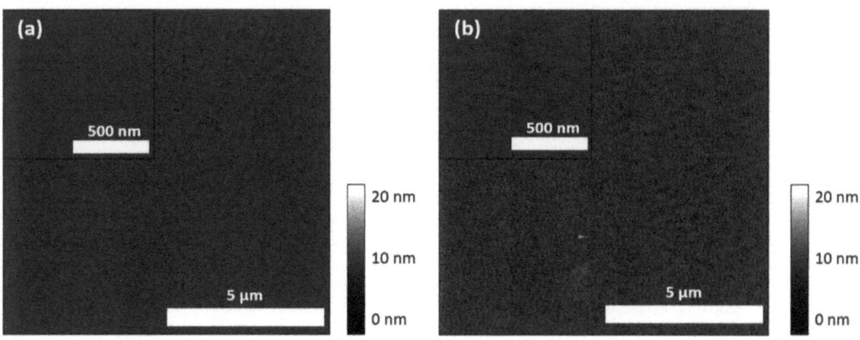

Figure 7.3 AFM analysis on PECVD deposited base layer *a*-SiC film with a roughness of (A) 0.763 ± 0.17 nm and (B) 0.919 ± 0.11 nm for the wafer center and edge regions, respectfully. Film thickness ~250 nm.

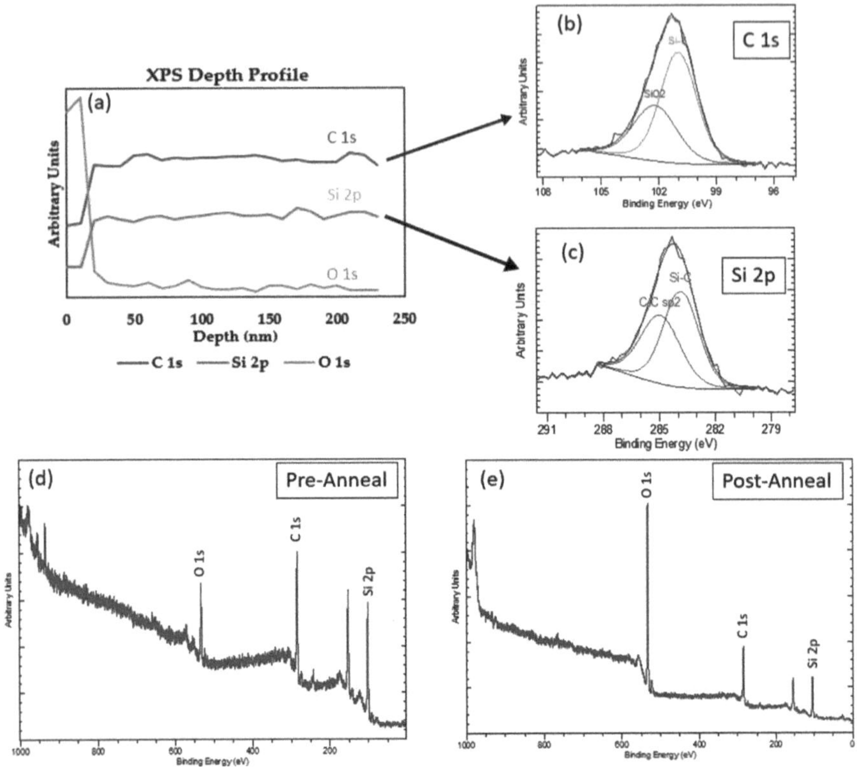

Figure 7.4 XPS analysis on 300 nm thick *a*-SiC film deposited on a Si wafer. (A) XPS depth profile by Ar sputtering. The concentration of oxygen is below the detection limit at ~15 nm depth indicating no oxygen in the a-SiC bulk. (B) and (C) are high resolution spectras of C 1s and Si 2p. XPS survey on a-SiC (D) before annealing and (E) after annealing. Note that binding energy of Si 2p and C 1s indicates Si—C bonding achieved.

on *a*-SiC before and after annealing are shown in Fig. 7.4 E—F, and Table 7.1 indicates C:Si ratios of 0.9 and 1.1 before and after annealing at 900°C, respectively. In addition, there was a significant increase in oxygen

Table 7.1 XPS *a*-SiC film atomic concentration pre- and postanneal.

Species	Preanneal	Postanneal
Carbon	43.10	34.46
Silicon	48.37	29.97
Oxygen	8.53	35.57
C:Si ratio	0.9	1.1

content after annealing, most likely due to trace oxygen present in the annealing system during high-temperature annealing. Thus, the same sample was then dipped in an hydrofluoric acid (HF) (49%) bath for 30 s, and put back to the XPS chamber immediately to measure the change in surface chemistry. The surface XPS survey is shown in Fig. 7.5A, the result shows a significant drop in oxygen and silicon content compared with Fig. 7.4E. This indicates that there was a thin layer of SiO_2 formed during annealing. As was done on the deposited *a*-SiC film, ~10 nm of *a*-SiC was removed by Ar^+ milling within an area of 5 × 5 mm^2, and another XPS measurement was performed (Fig. 7.5B). After Ar^+ milling of 10 nm, the silicon content increased while oxygen was slightly reduced. This illustrates that the bulk film was still *a*-SiC, but the stoichiometry changed due to the 900°C annealing compared with as-deposited *a*-SiC. This was expected because thermal annealing is known to release the film stress, which implies that it alters the physical structure in the film such as the C:Si ratio.

The *a*-SiC film stress is very important for neural probe applications. High film stress in the *a*-SiC layers may cause the film to crack and delaminate during high-temperature annealing PPF formation. In addition, after releasing the probes from the substrate, high film stress will cause the probe to bend and curl, which renders them very difficult to implant in tissue. In this work, the results were shown in Fig. 7.6, the as-deposited *a*-SiC film has a compressive film stress of 250 MPa, and the film stress converts to 200 Mpa tensile stress after annealing under 900°C for 1 hour. After another 250 nm *a*-SiC film deposition (to mimic the top-side insulating cap layer), the film stress changed to 50 MPa of compressive stress. A final annealing of 900°C for 10 min was applied with a ramping rate of

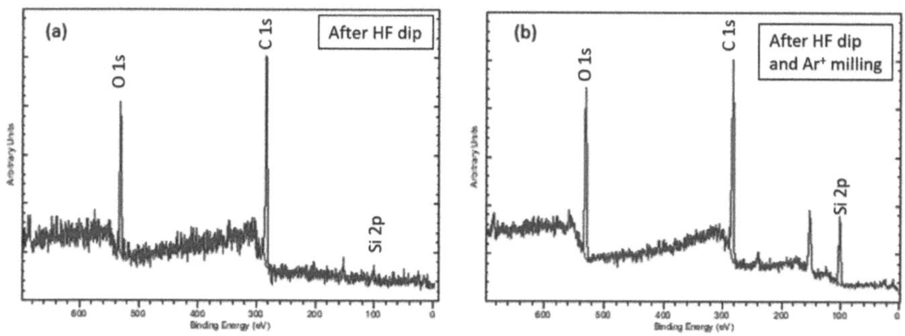

Figure 7.5 XPS analysis of *a*-SiC film after annealing studied in Fig. 7.4E. (A) HF dipped *a*-SiC surface and (B) HF dipped with Ar^+ milled surface (5 × 5 mm^2) and a depth of 10 nm.

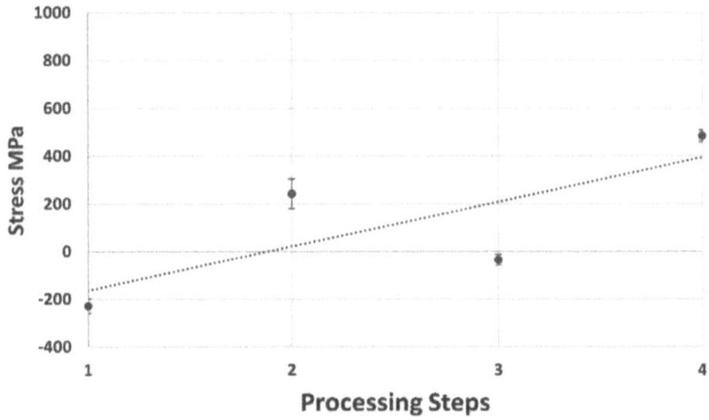

Figure 7.6 Plot of *a*-SiC film stress versus process steps as estimated by wafer curvature analysis. Stress measured after each process step: Step 1 base film *a*-SiC deposition, Step 2 after annealing under 900°C for 1 hour, Step 3 after cap film *a*-SiC deposition, Step 4 after RTP annealing at 900°C. *Dotted line* least squares fit to aid the eye.

10°C/s to reduce any film stress mismatch between the base and cap layers. The resulting stress was measured to be tensile with a value of 480 MPa. These results indicate that thermal annealing reduces the film stress and converts it from tensile to compressive strain. Although the final device displayed 480 MPa of tensile stress, it is low enough to obtain a straight probe shank that has a 50 μm backside Si as a support layer (shown in Fig. 7.2B).

3.2 PPF film characterization

Two double-ended resistors were used to characterize the electrical properties of the PPF electrodes. Each PPF resistor had a length of 3 mm, a width of 50 μm, and the thickness varied depending on the annealing temperature. Table 7.2 shows a comparison of PPF resistivity and thickness versus annealing temperature. The results show that the resistivity decreases with increasing annealing temperature, as expected based on the Raman data presented earlier. The PPF thickness was measured using a stylus profilometer, the resistance determined by IV measurement (Keithley 2400 SMU), and the resistivity calculated by the following equation:

Table 7.2 Measured PPF resistivity versus annealing temperature.

Annealing temperature (°C)	500	600	700	800	900
PPF thickness (nm)	~599	~498	~459	~424	~387
Resistivity (mΩ·cm)	24	11	8	4	3

$$\rho = R \times \frac{A}{L}$$

where ρ is the resistivity in Ω-cm, R the resistance in Ω, A the cross-section area of the resistor, and L is the length of the resistor.

3.3 PPF mINP device characterization

The next material property to characterize is the insulation properties of the *a*-SiC cap and base layer. Fig. 7.7 is the IV curve of the IDE device under both dry and wet (PBS) conditions. The *a*-SiC insulation leakage current at ±50 V were less than 7 and 19 nA dry and wet (PBS), respectfully. These results indicate the excellent insulating properties of the as-deposited *a*-SiC films.

Electrochemical tests were performed on the PPF single-ended electrodes versus electrode area. We will focus this discussion on the 900°C annealed PPF electrodes for electrochemical characterization, as they displayed the best crystallinity, the lowest resistivity, and (we will see) the lowest impedance at 1 kHz. The potentiostat from Gamry (Reference 600) was utilized to investigate the electrochemical properties of both PPF and Pt reference electrodes versus recording area. As shown in Fig. 7.8A, five different recording areas (502, 125, 7.8, 1.9, and 0.49 kμm^2) were investigated. The impedance of the PPF electrode with a recording area of 0.49

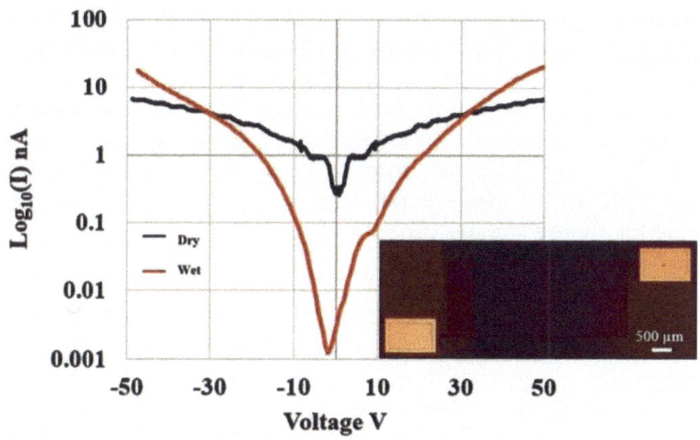

Figure 7.7 Electrical field breakdown data used to evaluate *a*-SiC insulation properties via IV measurement of leakage current from a PPF IDE device. Two dies were tested under dry/wet conditions, and the average leakage current at ±50 V was 7 nA (dry) and 19 nA (wet). Photograph of IDE device (inset) showing contact pads and 100 μm spacing between PPF mesas.

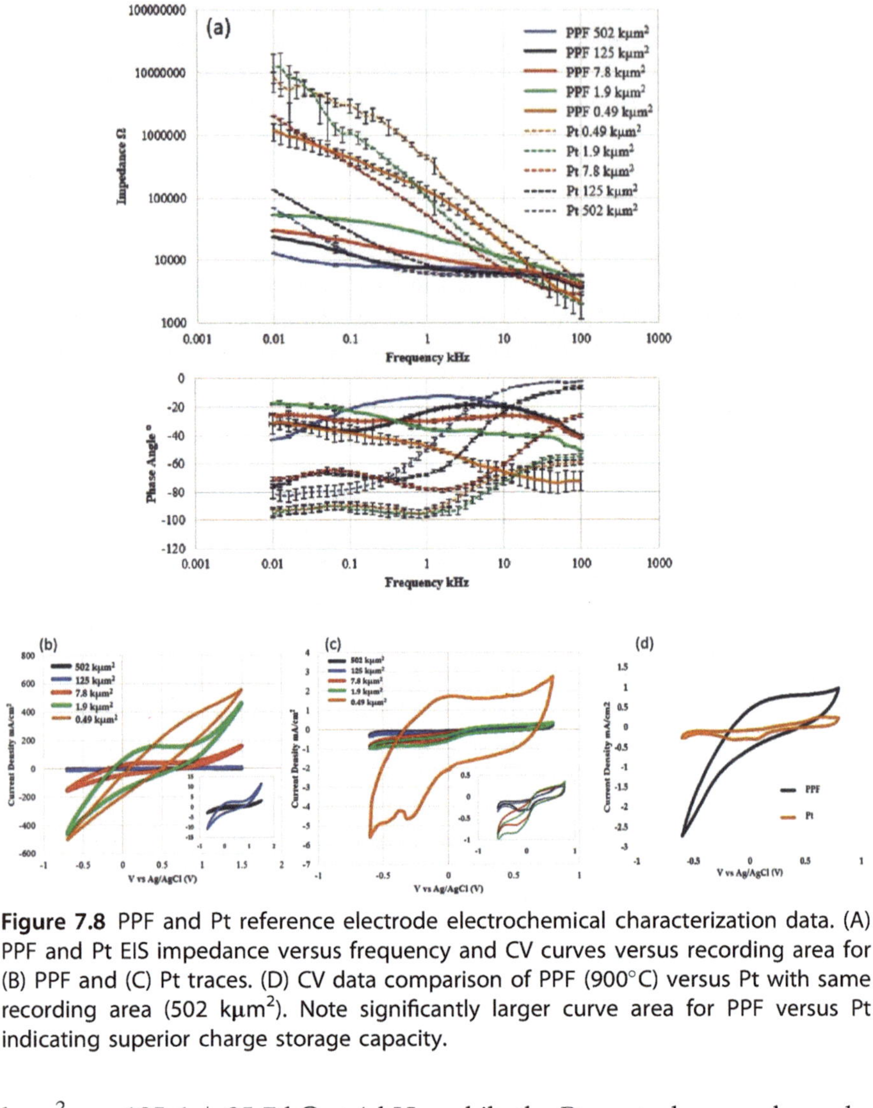

Figure 7.8 PPF and Pt reference electrode electrochemical characterization data. (A) PPF and Pt EIS impedance versus frequency and CV curves versus recording area for (B) PPF and (C) Pt traces. (D) CV data comparison of PPF (900°C) versus Pt with same recording area (502 kμm^2). Note significantly larger curve area for PPF versus Pt indicating superior charge storage capacity.

kμm^2 was 125.6 ± 25.7 kΩ at 1 kHz, while the Pt control group showed a nearly three-times higher impedance of 437.8 ± 35.9 kΩ with the same recording area. Therefore, the PPF electrode demonstrated a 71% lower impedance than the Pt reference electrode. In addition, as expected, the impedance decreased with increasing electrode area. The impedance of the PPF electrode with 1.9 kμm^2 recording area was 24.8 ± 0.4 kΩ, comparing with the Pt reference electrode (103.8 ± 2.2 kΩ) with the same recording area. Although the phase angle of the PPF electrode at 1 kHz was

-35.9 ± 0.6 degrees, this is consistent with other carbon-based materials [ref]. This result indicates that PPF has both faradaic and capacitive charge transfer mechanisms at the electrode—electrolyte interface, which means the surface of the PPF carbon electrodes were oxidized and reduced to transfer electron flow from the electrode to ion flow in the electrolyte. This differs from the Pt control group that has a phase angle of 94.5 ± 2.8 degrees, which indicates a capacitive charge transfer mechanism.

The CV curves of the PPF and the Pt control group are presented in Fig. 7.8B—D; however, the smallest electrodes showed significant measurement noise; thus, we will focus on the other electrodes hereafter. By comparing Fig. 7.8B and C, it is clear that the PPF electrodes showed a much larger electrochemical window of −0.7 V to +1.5 V compared with the Pt electrode of −0.6 V to +0.8 V. Charge storage capacity (CSC), which is one of the most crucial characteristics for mINPs, was calculated from the CV curve and illustrates the total charge available for injection during stimulation. Table 7.3 has summarized the PPF and Pt electrode EIS data at 1 kHz as well as the anodic CSCa and cathodic CSC_c from the CV data. The 1.9 kμm^2 PPF electrodes showed excellent CSC_a and CSC_C of 8.9 C/cm^2 and 5.3 C/cm^2, respectfully, with a scanning range of −0.7V to +1.5V. We believe that the larger CSC_a and smaller CSC_c values were caused by the anodic oxidation of carbon on the PPF electrodes. In addition, a comparison of the CV curves of our PPF electrode and Pt control group under the same electrochemical window (−0.6 V to +0.8 V) is shown in Fig. 7.8D. The results indicate that PPF showed a CSC_a and CSC_c of 11.88 mC/cm^2 and 16.08 mC/cm^2, respectively, while Pt showed

Table 7.3 The impedances were measured on 900°C PPF versus Pt at 1 kHz.

Electrode	Area (kμm^2)	Impedance at 1 kHz (kΩ)	CSC_a (mC/cm^2)	CSC_c (mC/cm^2)
PPF	0.49	125.6 ± 25.7	5600	3000
Pt	0.49	437.8 ± 35.9	53.2	33.2
PPF	1.9	24.8 ± 0.4	8900	5260
Pt	1.9	103.8 ± 2.2	4.7	7.4
PPF	7.8	11.4 ± 0.04	2870	1600
Pt	7.8	51.8 ± 1.1	4.9	6.4
PPF	125	7.4 ± 0.04	193	107
Pt	125	8.4 ± 0.2	4.1	5.6
PPF	502	7.7 ± 0.01	50	27
Pt	502	6.3 ± 0.1	3.9	5.2

a CSC_a and CSC_c of 3.9 mC/cm^2 and 5.2 mC/cm^2, respectively. This result indicates that the PPF electrodes have ~4 times higher CSC than Pt electrodes of the same recording area—a very significant result. The large CSC of the PPF electrodes is likely attributed to electron transfer mechanisms through faradaic chemical reactions [7].

In Table 7.4, we have compared the electrochemical impedance and CSC of commonly used electrode materials for mINP. In this work, the PPF electrode demonstrated a low impedance at 1 kHz and the largest CSC among the other materials, which further indicate that PPF is a promising candidate for next-generation mINP devices. The final device that was packaged with a commercial 16-pin style package from NeuroNexus is shown in Fig. 7.9. This device is ready for in vitro and in vivo testing, which will be reported at a later date [7].

Table 7.4 Electrochemical properties of PPF and common mINP electrode materials.

Material	Recording area (kμm^2)	Impedance @1 kHz (kΩ)	Charge storage capacity[a] (mC/cm^2)
PPF/*a*-SiC	1.9	24.8	14,160
Pt	1.9	103.8	12
PEDOT/CNT	2.83	15.0	6
Carbon-nanotube fiber	1.450	14.1	372
Graphene fiber	0.749	37.9	798
IrO_x	0.177	132.9	29
TiN	2.83	54.8	5

[a]Charge storage capacity (CSC) value sum of anodic and cathodic phases.

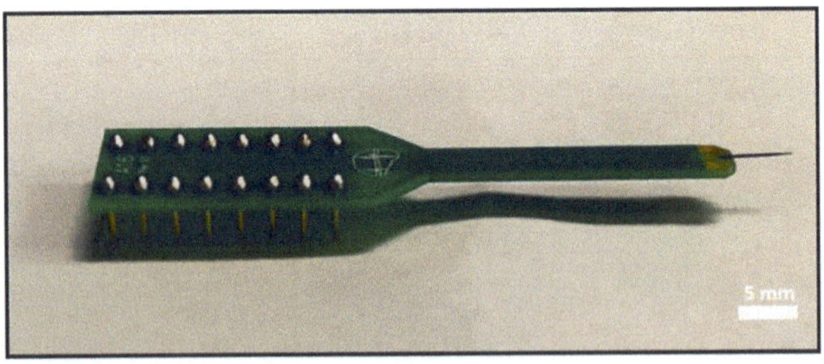

Figure 7.9 Final packaged 16-channel PPF mINP on a commercial probe header (NeuroNexus). Next step is to package more devices for an $n = 10$ to conduct in vivo recording that will be reported at a later date.

4. Summary

In this chapter, we have presented a novel PPF based mINP. Compared with commonly used silicon and noble metals-based mINPs that continue to suffer from long-term reliability issues, the presented PPF mINP may solve these challenges as the preliminary results presented here indicate. The PPF probe was fabricated by pyrolyzing photoresist on an *a*-SiC layer deposited on a Si wafer and then conformally insulated using an *a*-SiC capping layer. The patterned C conducting traces and electrodes eliminates the need for noble metal evaporation/sputter and lift-off on small features, thus simplifying the fabrication process. The *a*-SiC film showed very low oxygen incorporation via XPS and the films withstood thermal annealing up to 900°C. The PPF neural probes have 16/32 conducting traces (single and double shank implants) and recording sites that were patterned on the *a*-SiC layer via standard microfabrication processes and are awaiting packaging for continued testing and implantation into an animal model [7].

The electrochemical properties were investigated on both PPF and Pt planar single-ended electrodes with different recording areas that were fabricated via the same fabrication process as the mINP, except there were no probe release and backside Si etch steps. The surface characterization was conducted via SEM and AFM indicating that the *a*-SiC and PPF films were smooth and pin-hole free. In addition, the PPF film was analyzed by Raman spectroscopy that indicated carbon sp^2 hybridization at 900°C, which is an indication of high crystallinity and C—C bonding. The electrochemical impedance of the PPF electrodes ($24.8 \pm 0.4\ \Omega$) showed a 71% lower value than the Pt control group ($103.8 \pm 2.2\ \Omega$) at 1 kHz for an electrode area of 1.9 kμm^2. The PPF electrodes also demonstrated a four times greater CSC than the Pt control group with the same recording area and bias scanning range. Furthermore, the PPF electrodes showed a wider electrochemical window (−0.7 to 1.5 V) than Pt (−0.6 to 0.8 V). These results illustrate the feasibility of neural recording and stimulation with the fabricated PPF mINP and that it is worth further development for next-generation neural interfaces.

Acknowledgments

The authors wish to thank: J. Bieber of Nanotechnology Research and Education Center (NREC) at USF for XPS analyzing of *a*-SiC film; R. Everly of the NREC for help with the PECVD deposition of *a*-SiC; M.R. Tanjil and M.C. Wang of the Mechanical Engineering Dept. at USF for assistance with electrochemical testing; Y. Emirov of NREC for help with the AFM data analysis. Research performed by C.L. Frewin was partially supported by grant no. 1R43NS120753-01 from the NIH National Institute of Neurological Disorders and Stroke (NINDS).

References

[1] C.L. Gooch, E. Pracht, A.R. Borenstein, The burden of neurological disease in the United States: a summary report and call to action, Annals of Neurology 81 (4) (2017) 479–484, https://doi.org/10.1002/ana.24897.

[2] Introduction to Microfabrication, second ed., Wiley. https://www.wiley.com/en-us/Introduction+to+Microfabrication%2C+2nd+Edition-p-9781119991892. (Accessed 04 May, 2021).

[3] J. Bong, et al., Radiolucent implantable electrocardiographic monitoring device based on graphene, Carbon New York 152 (2019) 946–953, https://doi.org/10.1016/j.carbon.2019.06.069.

[4] N. Goshi, et al., Glassy carbon MEMS for novel origami-styled 3D integrated intracortical and epicortical neural probes, Journal of Micromechanics Microengineering 28 (6) (2018) 065009, https://doi.org/10.1088/1361-6439/aab061.

[5] J.C. Barrese, et al., Failure mode analysis of silicon-based intracortical microelectrode arrays in non-human primates, Journal of Neural Engineering 10 (6) (2013) 066014, https://doi.org/10.1088/1741-2560/10/6/066014.

[6] E.K. Bernardin, Demonstration of Monolithic-Silicon Carbide (SiC) Neural Devices, 2018, https://doi.org/10.1093/imamci/dnt037.

[7] C. Feng, et al., A flexible a-SiC-based neural interface utilizing pyrolyzed-photoresist film (C) active sites, Micromachines 12 (7) (2021) 821, https://doi.org/10.3390/MI12070821.

[8] J.C. Barrese, J. Aceros, J.P. Donoghue, Scanning electron microscopy of chronically implanted intracortical microelectrode arrays in non-human primates, Journal of Neural Engineering 13 (2) (2016), https://doi.org/10.1088/1741-2560/13/2/026003.

[9] H. Chen, L. Wang, Y. Lu, X. Du, Bioinspired microcone-array-based living biointerfaces: enhancing the anti-inflammatory effect and neuronal network formation, Microsystems and Nanoengineering 6 (1) (2020) 1–8, https://doi.org/10.1038/s41378-020-0172-0.

[10] F. Deku, et al., Amorphous silicon carbide platform for next generation penetrating neural interface designs, Micromachines 9 (10) (2018), https://doi.org/10.3390/mi9100480.

[11] S.E. Saddow, et al., 3C-SiC on Si: a bio- and hemo-compatible material for advanced nano-bio devices, in: 2014 IEEE 9th Nanotechnol. Mater. Devices Conf. NMDC 2014, 2014, pp. 49–53, https://doi.org/10.1109/NMDC.2014.6997419.

[12] G.L. Knaack, H. Charkhkar, S.F. Cogan, J.J. Pancrazio, Chapter 8: Amorphous Silicon Carbide for Neural Interface Applications, second ed., Elsevier Inc., 2016.

[13] C. Feng, et al., Silicon carbide biotechnology: carbon-based neural interfaces, in: TMS 2021 150th Annual Meeting & Exhibition Supplemental Proceedings, 2021, 2021, pp. 777–790.

[14] D. Brassard, M.A. El Khakani, Dielectric properties of amorphous hydrogenated silicon carbide thin films grown by plasma-enhanced chemical vapor deposition, Journal of Applied Physics 93 (7) (2003) 4066–4071, https://doi.org/10.1063/1.1555676.

[15] X. Li, T.K.S. Wong, Rusli, D. Yang, Structural and electronic properties of low dielectric constant carbon rich amorphous silicon carbide, Diamond and Related Materials 12 (3–7) (2003) 963–967, https://doi.org/10.1016/S0925-9635(02)00220-0.

[16] S.F. Cogan, D.J. Edell, A.A. Guzelian, Y.P. Liu, R. Edell, Plasma-enhanced chemical vapor deposited silicon carbide as an implantable dielectric coating, Journal of Biomedical Materials Research Part A 67 (3) (2003) 856–867, https://doi.org/10.1002/jbm.a.10152.

[17] M. Beygi, et al., Fabrication of a monolithic implantable neural interface from cubic silicon carbide, Micromachines 10 (7) (2019) 430, https://doi.org/10.3390/mi10070430.

[18] M. Beygi, et al., Silicon carbide and MRI: towards developing a MRI Safe neural interface, Micromachines 12 (2) (2021) 126, https://doi.org/10.3390/mi12020126.

[19] R. Rauti, M. Musto, S. Bosi, M. Prato, L. Ballerini, Properties and behavior of carbon nanomaterials when interfacing neuronal cells: How far have we come? Carbon 143 (2019) 430–446, https://doi.org/10.1016/j.carbon.2018.11.026.

[20] A.G. Richardson, et al., Transparent and flexible low noise graphene electrodes for simultaneous electrophysiology and neuroimaging, Nature Communication 5 (1) (2014) 1–10, https://doi.org/10.1038/ncomms6259.

[21] M. David-Pur, L. Bareket-Keren, G. Beit-Yaakov, D. Raz-Prag, Y. Hanein, All-carbon-nanotube flexible multi-electrode array for neuronal recording and stimulation, Biomedical Microdevices 16 (1) (2014) 43–53, https://doi.org/10.1007/s10544-013-9804-6.

[22] C. Fairman, G. Liu, D.B. Hibbert, J.J. Gooding, Comparing the electrochemical performance of pyrolysed photoresist film electrodes to glassy carbon electrodes for sensing applications, in: ICONN 2010 -Proceedings of the 2010 International Conference on Nanoscience and Nanotechnology, 2010, pp. 308–311, https://doi.org/10.1109/ICONN.2010.6045208.

[23] J.A. Lee, S. Hwang, J. Kwak, S. Il Park, S.S. Lee, K.C. Lee, An electrochemical impedance biosensor with aptamer-modified pyrolyzed carbon electrode for label-free protein detection, Sensors Actuators, B Chemical 129 (1) (2008) 372–379, https://doi.org/10.1016/j.snb.2007.08.034.

[24] A. Oliveros, C. Coletti, S.E. Saddow, Carbon based materials on SiC for advanced biomedical applications, Silicon Carbide Biotechnology (2012) 431–458, https://doi.org/10.1016/B978-0-12-385906-8.00012-X.

[25] K.S. Novoselov, et al., Electric field effect in atomically thin carbon films, Science 306 (5696) (2004) 666–669, https://doi.org/10.1126/science.1102896.

[26] D. Convertino, et al., Graphene promotes axon elongation through local stall of nerve growth factor signaling endosomes, Nano Letters 20 (5) (2020) 3633–3641, https://doi.org/10.1021/acs.nanolett.0c00571.

[27] H.C. Tian, et al., Graphene oxide doped conducting polymer nanocomposite film for electrode-tissue interface, Biomaterials 35 (7) (2014) 2120–2129, https://doi.org/10.1016/j.biomaterials.2013.11.058.

[28] S. Iijima, Helical microtubules of graphitic carbon, Nature 354 (6348) (1991) 56–58, https://doi.org/10.1038/354056a0.

[29] D.-W. Park, et al., Graphene-based carbon-layered electrode array technology for neural imaging and optogenetic applications, Nature Communications 5 (1) (2014) 5258, https://doi.org/10.1038/ncomms6258.

[30] S. Usmani, et al., 3D meshes of carbon nanotubes guide functional reconnection of segregated spinal explants, Science Advances 2 (7) (2016), https://doi.org/10.1126/sciadv.1600087.

[31] K. Pulskamp, S. Diabaté, H.F. Krug, Carbon nanotubes show no sign of acute toxicity but induce intracellular reactive oxygen species in dependence on contaminants, Toxicology Letters 168 (1) (2007) 58–74, https://doi.org/10.1016/j.toxlet.2006.11.001.

[32] Z. Guo, et al., Elucidating the mechanism of the surface functionalization dependent neurotoxicity of graphene family nanomaterials, Nanoscale 12 (36) (2020) 18600–18605, https://doi.org/10.1039/d0nr04179c.
[33] S.F. Hansen, A. Lennquist, Carbon nanotubes added to the SIN list as a nanomaterial of very high concern, Nature Nanotechnology 15 (1) (2020) 3–4, https://doi.org/10.1038/s41565-019-0613-9.
[34] M. Vomero, et al., Highly stable glassy carbon interfaces for long-term neural stimulation and low-noise recording of brain activity, Science Reports 7 (2017), https://doi.org/10.1038/srep40332.
[35] S. Gallis, V. Nikas, A.E. Kaloyeros, Silicon Oxycarbide thin films and Nanostructures: synthesis, properties and applications, in: Modern Technologies For Creating The Thin-Film Systems and Coatings, 2017, https://doi.org/10.5772/66992.

CHAPTER 8

A silicon carbide electrochemical sensor for glucose detection

Kavyashree Puttananjegowda, Arash Takshi and Sylvia Thomas
Department of Electrical Engineering, University of South Florida, Tampa, FL, United States

Contents

1. Introduction

The research arena of bioelectronics, at the intriguing convergence of hardware, science, and biotechnology, has garnered significant interest over the most recent years, primarily due to the capability of using biomedical devices for diagnostics and medical care. Bioelectronic gadgets include electronic components such as electrodes, semiconductors, and piezoelectric devices, which are interfaced with biological inferred systems such as enzymes, tissues, microorganisms, catalysts, antibodies, nucleic acids, proteins, biomarkers, and natural analytes. In fact, the developing interest of established researchers in bioelectronics is concerned with imagining and acknowledging progressive devices and frameworks, which focus on usability, cost, and versatility with living creatures [1,2].

Silicon Carbide Technology for Advanced Human Healthcare Applications
ISBN 978-0-323-90609-8
https://doi.org/10.1016/B978-0-323-90609-8.00010-7

Bioelectronics research and cutting-edge advances for biomedical applications continue to increase as advances in both our understanding of biological systems and materials that can interface with these systems grows. The revelation and enhancement of materials with improved biological, electrical, and mechanical properties, as suggested by the specific biomedical applications to which they are presented, is one of the main drivers in the field. The prominent features of silicon carbide (SiC), namely its excellent properties as discussed in Chapter 1 of this book, have resulted in an expanding number of potential biomedical devices in this specific scenario, as stated in the literature [3,4].

This chapter provides a thorough overview of silicon carbide materials and their uses in biosensor applications. A cursory review of the fundamental material properties is presented here to pave the way for using SiC for bio and electrochemical detection. As presented in Chapter 1, the silicon and carbon atoms that make up the SiC crystal lattice are grouped into SiC tetrahedrons, which form a Si—C bilayer structure. SiC's peculiarity lies in its ability to display a wide range of crystal formations, totaling more than 250 unique polymorphs. SiC polytypes that outcome upon crystallization in twofold constructions made of indistinguishable layers that are either cubic (C), hexagonal (H), or rhombohedral (R)-like stacked SiC bilayers. The majority of feasible polytypes are not stable. For technological applications, three main polytypes, one cubic (3C—SiC) and two hexagonal (4H—SiC, and 6H—SiC), have been developed mostly for electronic device applications [5—9].

Silicon carbide is generally viewed as the most appropriate material for high operating frequency and high power-efficient electronic devices with better performance compared to silicon-based circuits and devices [10—14]. Hence, for higher speed and gain devices, SiC is considered as one of the best materials, particularly for high-temperature applications. More importantly, the recent focus on the biocompatibility of SiC showed better cell propagation and adhesion to SiC when interfaced with various biological tissues and cells [15]. Specifically, in comparison to other crystalline semiconductors, SiC displays a better hemocompatibility and chemical inertness, which is suitable for long-term stability under normal biological conditions. Hence SiC is suitable for in vivo applications for wearable and implantable devices [16—19]. Additionally, SiC has excellent mechanical properties such as a high elastic modulus and hardness with a low friction coefficient helping to prevent damage of biological tissues and cells when inserted into the body [20,21]. SiC is a wide bandgap material with very high n-type and p-type charge carrier mobility and high thermal conductivity; hence, it has better electrical properties compared to silicon [22,23]. SiC has good optical properties in terms of ultraviolet wavelength absorption, better transparency to visible light, high refractive index. In addition, the photoluminescence of SiC nanoparticles makes it an attractive material for optical biosensor-based applications [24]. SiC materials can be functionalized very easily in terms of better immobilization of enzymes for a stable interface that is particularly attractive for biosensor applications [25].

There are numerous extraordinary properties that make SiC an especially reasonable material for biosensors and their applications. In the literature, a large number of devices and systems dependent on SiC have been reported, including orthopedic implants, cardiovascular stents, drug delivery systems, biosensors, biomembranes, and tissue scaffolds [26,27]. Among them, biosensors are capable of detecting biological signals from tissues, enzymes, and cells that help to develop fast, reliable, highly sensitive point-of-care detection and diagnostics for implantable, portable, and wearable sensors for healthcare and biomedical applications. Biosensors are analytical devices that are often integrated with biologically driven systems and have a transducer that can be electrochemical, mechanical, optical, thermometric, piezoelectric, or magnetic. The biosensing community is paying special attention to SiC technology in an attempt to overcome the real and anticipated limitations of present-day approaches for the clinical diagnosis of numerous diseases and the detection of biomolecules. In addition, most SiC-based biosensors are used for electrochemical detection through cyclic voltammetry, chronoamperometry, impedance spectroscopy, or electrical detection where SiC is used as a functionalized electrode in the sensor [28,29].

The latest advancements in the field of bioelectronics show that SiC material is one of the most promising alternatives to organic semiconductors (OSs). OSs are mainly pi-bonded molecules or conducting polymers that include polypyrrole, polyaniline, poly(3,4-ethylenedioxythiophene):poly(styrene sulfonic acid) (PEDOT:PSS), and poly(3-hexylthiophene), resulting in expanded interest for numerous biomedical applications [30–35]. The advantages of some of these compounds are technological in nature, the most notable of which is the ease with which their multifunctional properties can be tailored by chemical design, incorporating functional groups while manipulating physical conditions to meet specific low-cost processing requirements. Organic thin films are made using low-cost solution-based processing techniques like spin coating and inkjet printing, as well as room-temperature thermal evaporation [36]. Furthermore, several of these organic compounds are particularly promising for new biosensors due to their conformability, biocompatibility, and unique conducting properties. Indeed, the porous nature of OS for biomedical applications is one of the most intriguing features. Direct exposure of OS to biological media highlights one of their key advantages, which is the potential to change their conductive characteristics as a result of ionic species exchange with the liquid environments to which they are exposed [37]. As a direct corollary conducting polymers have been used for various applications, including enzymatic and nucleotide biosensors [38,39], microelectrode arrays [40], organic thin-film transistors [41], and memory devices [42].

Electrochemistry plays such an important role in SiC biosensors detection that this chapter will focus on electrochemical devices that rely on SiC biosensors. The major goal is to examine these applications within the context of a large number of models described in the literature, with the conducting polymer serving primarily as a reference material. We will now briefly discuss the biomedical applications of SiC, such as biosensors and tissue engineering, providing a complete overview of the most recent work on SiC-based biosensors. A special focus on electrochemically controlled SiC-based devices, where redox processes are used to detect analyte molecules, will be provided.

This chapter focuses on the fabrication and morphological and electrochemical characterization of SiC nanostructures (particles, fibers, laminates, thin films) used to develop electrochemical glucose biosensors. Glucose oxidase (GO_x) enzymes coimbedded in a conductive polymer (CP) with silicon carbide nanostructures that exhibit high sensitivity, quick response time, and an enhanced limit of detection (LOD) and durability. SiC nanoparticles (SiCNPs), spin-coated-thin-films (SCTFs), and SiC-NP electrospun-nanofibrous-membranes (ENFMs) have been implemented as glucose-sensing electrodes, and a comparative analysis of SiCNPs with both ENFMs and SCTFs is presented. Prior research has shown that conducting polymers could be utilized as a mediator for the detection of glucose. This is presumably due to direct electron transfer between glucose oxidase and the conducting polymer support, which is an oxygen-independent detection mechanism. This chapter presents the feasibility of using electrodes containing embedded SiC nanostructures as an emerging approach to fabricating highly sensitive glucose biosensors.

2. SiC for biomedical applications

Silicon carbide is a semiconducting material that is physically stable and chemically inert to acids, alkalis, and salts that makes an ideal candidate for liquid environments. Coupled with its proven excellent biocompatibility and hemocompatibility, along with better sensitivity and longevity compared to peer materials it is well suited for in vivo implantable biosensing applications [43,44].

SiC is a durable and dynamic material used in biosensors that could be one of the most recent breakthroughs in point-of-care detection and diagnostics. Because of its excellent mechanical, chemical, and electrical capabilities, numerous biosensor architectures in which SiC plays an important role have been reported to date. Biosensors that use SiC as a functional material in biorecognition interactions are primarily electrical in nature. SiC nanocomposites and nanostructures are commonly used as a functionalizing electrode material in combination with nanoparticles of Pt, NiO, Au, Pd, and TiO_2 in this case [45—51].

2.1 SiC electrode for neurotransmitters

Neuronal impulses can be transmitted by microelectrodes implanted in the brain. The use of a composite fiber (SiC—C) electrode for neural activity monitoring and biochemical detection of electroactive neurotransmitters was investigated, as illustrated in Fig. 8.1. A method for producing electrode tips from SiC—C composite fibers was also developed using electrolytic etching. Various tip geometries and morphologies were studied using scanning electron microscope (SEM). Electrochemical analysis and modeling were performed using cyclic voltammetry (CV) and electrochemical impedance spectroscopy (EIS). The current generated was due to the charging and discharging of the capacitive double layer [55], with no appreciable redox reaction, as evidenced by almost square voltammograms. The electrodes have a capacitive interaction with the electrolyte solution around them, which is ideal for safe charge transfer. The SiC—C composite electrodes were utilized to biochemically detect neurotransmitters including dopamine hydrochloride and vitamin C, and oxidation currents were shown to vary linearly with concentration. In vivo action potential recordings from an anesthetized rat's brain were made with a high signal-to-noise ratio.

Fig. 8.2 shows a SiC/carbon-fiber-sensing electrode for diagnosing neural activity and biological detecting of neurotransmitters such as

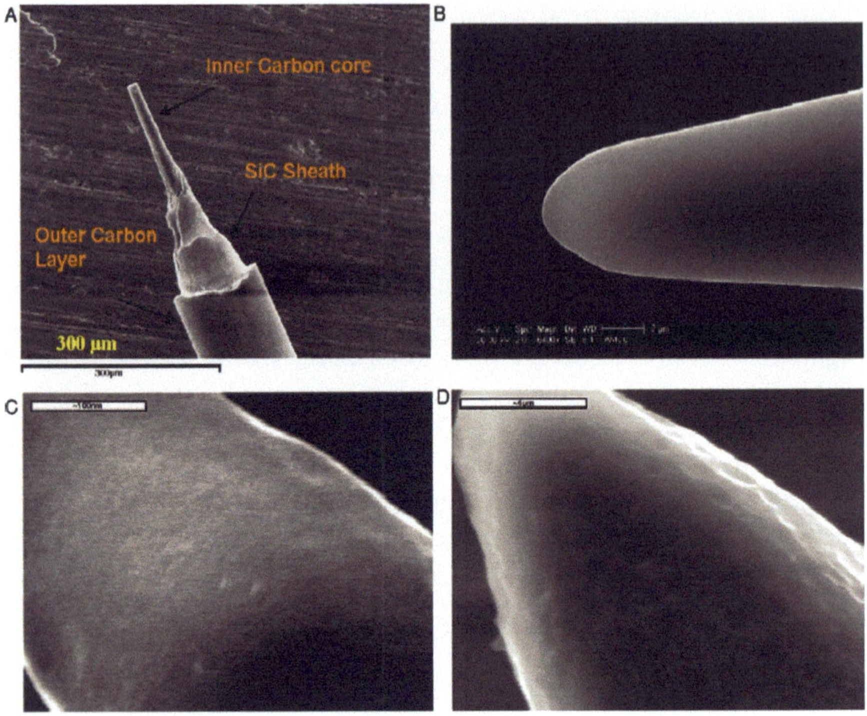

Figure 8.1 SEM pictures of (A) silicon carbide carbon composite fiber's etched section, (B) carbon recording tip, (C) low voltage etch, and (D) high voltage etch. *(From Ref. [55], with permission of Elsevier.)*

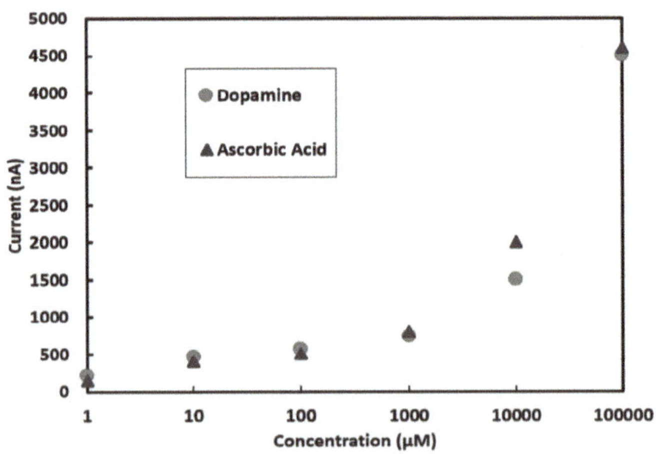

Figure 8.2 Electrochemical biosensor current response from SiC–C electrodes versus molar concentration of dopamine and ascorbic acid. *(Adapted from Ref. [55] and reprinted with permission.)*

vitamin-C and dopamine [55]. For the electrochemical measurements of the device EIS and CV analysis was used, while for the detection of both neurotransmitters, they used the analogous redox activity of labile hydroxyl groups on their molecules, with a detection limit of less than 10 mM. In vivo recording of action potentials from rat brain with a very high signal-to-noise (S/N) ratio was also reported [55]. The capacity of the SiC-based electrodes to transmit electrical charge with the charging/discharging of the electrical double layer demonstrated a reversible electrochemical behavior. One of the remarkable findings of their research was that electrodes had a capacitive contact, which is extremely beneficial to electrodes' chemical and electrochemical stability [52–55].

2.2 SiC electrode for antenna-based glucose sensor

In the development of an implanted biosensor, SiC was also utilized as a thin film biocompatible substrate material. Fig. 8.3A shows a 10 GHz SiC microstrip patch antenna system that uses radiofrequency (RF) for long-term, real-time, and continuous glucose monitoring [56,57]. This SiC sensor demonstrates a change in glucose levels as a shift in resonant frequency, which electrically translates as a change in blood permittivity and conductivity. To test glucose levels, measurements using synthetic body fluid, which is electrically equivalent to blood plasma, and pig blood was used to determine the RF resonance peak shift with increasing glucose level (Fig. 8.3B). For every 1 mg/dL change in blood glucose, resonance

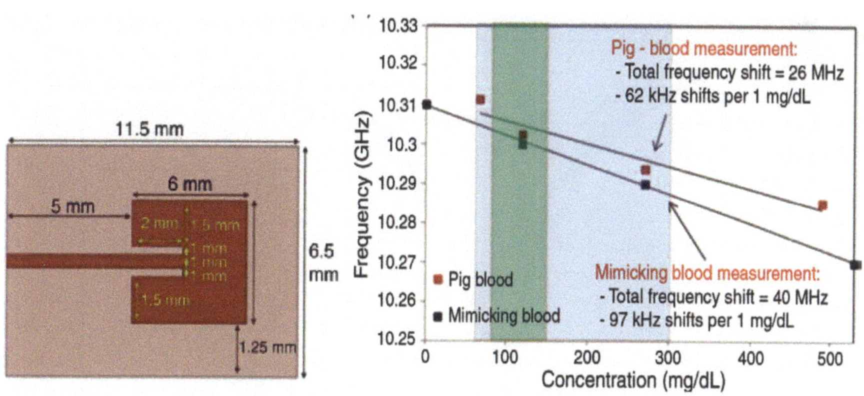

(a) (b)

Figure 8.3 (A) The pictorial representation of the SiC antenna-based glucose-sensing electrode operating at 10 GHz. (B) Graphical representation of glucose concentration versus resonance frequency. *(Reprinted with permission from Ref. [57].)*

frequency shifts of 97 and 62 kHz were recorded (Fig. 8.3B). Lower resonant frequency shifts were observed with an increase in glucose levels, showing a dose-dependent response to glucose concentration from 0 to 530 mg/dL, as shown in Fig. 8.4. The glucose-sensing process was based on the concentration of glucose in the blood with respect to a change in resonant frequency, which is caused by changes in blood permittivity and conductivity caused by glucose. Surprisingly, they did not require direct interaction with the liquid environment containing the analyte to work. For each 1 mg/dL change in blood glucose, resonance frequency shifts of 97 and 67 kHz were recorded. This cutting-edge SiC RF antenna was demonstrated to perform effectively across the glucose level range of medical interest, from normal clinical settings to critical health conditions such as hypoglycemia and hyperglycemia.

2.3 SiC electrode for DNA sensing

Several biomolecules have been detected with high sensitivity using biosensors that use SiC as an electrode or substrate material. Yang et al., for example, were the first to discover covalent attachment of DNA molecules on 3C–SiC films employed as electrochemical electrodes [58]. The surface of the 3C–SiC was first functionalized with diazonium ions, and then

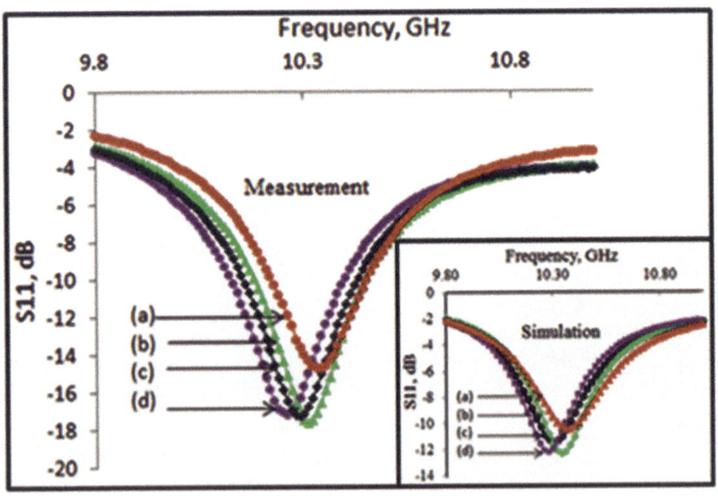

Figure 8.4 Simulated and measured S11 antenna response as function of glucose concentration change at 10 GHz: (A) 0 mg/dL (no glucose was added), (B) 120 mg/dL, (C) 270 mg/dL, (D) 530 mg/dL. Note resonance shift to lower frequency with increasing glucose level. *(Reprinted with permission from Ref. [57].)*

DNA molecules were bound to it. The CV curves of the ss-DNA and ds-DNA strands immobilized on the SiC-modified electrode surface are depicted in Fig. 8.5A submerged in a buffer solution were used to detect DNA hybridization. A redox center of ferrocene was tagged on the DNA probe. After hybridization of ss-DNA with complementary DNA, two redox waves of ferrocene that were present in the CV curve of ss-DNA vanished, producing a fingerprint of the DNA hybridization seen in Fig. 8.5B. A reduction in the redox current verified the qualitative detection of DNA.

2.4 SiC electrode for immunosensor

The characteristics of SiC nanostructures were developed to create specialized frameworks appropriate for biomolecule discovery. Yang et al. used uniform and widely scattered gold—silicon carbide nanocomposites, formulated through ascorbic acid assisted chemical reduction for label-free electrochemical immunosensing of human chorionic gonadotrophin (hCG) [25]. The device, which uses Au/SiC modified glassy carbon electrodes (GCE), has a limit of detection (LOD) of 0.042 IU/L, with a good linear response from 5 to 1000 IU/L and 0.1 to 5 IU/L as shown in Fig. 8.6C. The immunosensor demonstrated good selectivity as well as adequate stability and reproducibility, indicating that it might be used to detect hCG as shown in Fig. 8.6D. In another work silicon carbide with titanium dioxide nanohybrid was used to perform instantaneous electrochemical detection of bisphenol A (BPA) and hydroquinone (HQ) [25]. Palladium nanoparticles remained anchored on a GCE modified with a silicon carbide with titanium dioxide nanohybrid [25].

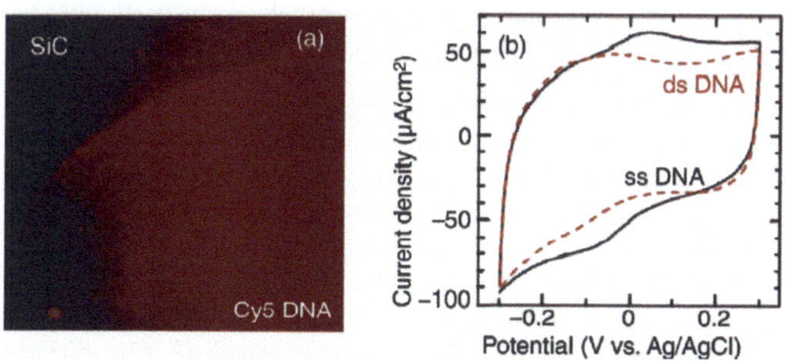

Figure 8.5 (A) Fluorescence microscopic image of ds DNA functionalized SiC electrode and (B) CV curve of DNA functionalized SiC electrode. The *solid-line* shows CV curve of electrode functionalized with ss DNA and *dashed-line* shows ds DNA. *(With permission from Ref. [58].)*

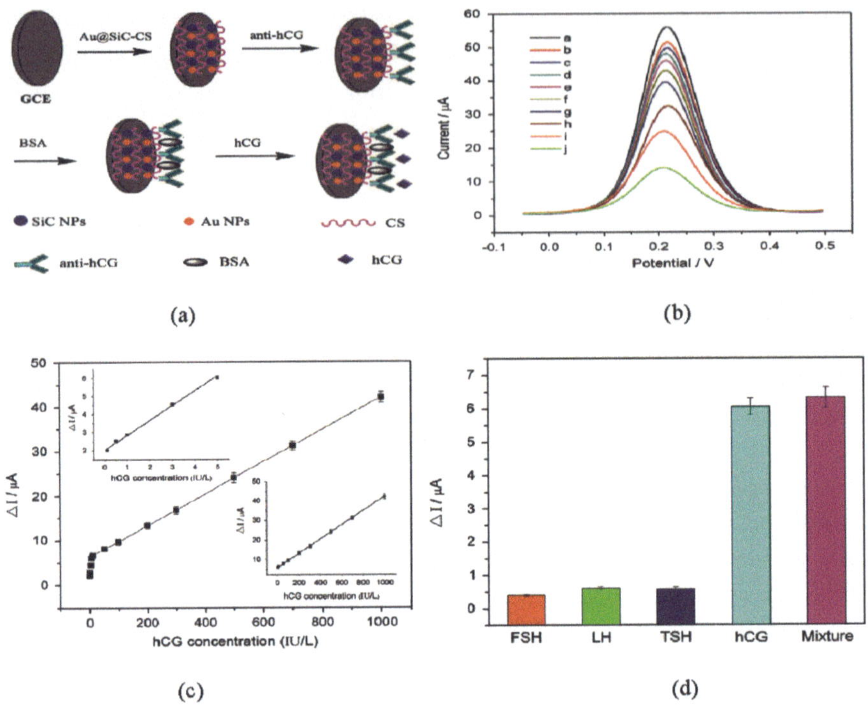

Figure 8.6 (A) Schematic illustration of the stepwise immunosensor fabrication process. (B) The immunosensor's DPVs were incubated with various doses of hCG standard solution. (C) Under ideal conditions, calibration plots of the reduction current change (I) vs hCG concentration. (D) Selectivity of the proposed immunosensor with FSH, LH, TSH, hCG, and hCG(5IU/L) containing the above mixture of three interferents with the same concentrations. *(Adapted from Ref. [25], with permission from Elsevier.)*

2.5 SiC electrode for electrochemiluminescence sensor

An electrochemiluminescence (ECL) biosensor shown in Fig. 8.7A used a composite film of SiC-tyrosinase-chitosan that was modified for adrenaline [60]. The adrenaline catalyzed the tyrosinase to produce hydrogen peroxide which was the basis for this ECL sensor's operation. The electrochemical reaction of numerous putative interferents, such as vitamin-C, DA, citric acid, and noradrenaline, was investigated to take a step toward real-world biomedical applications. Unfortunately, the ECL sensor response was not significantly enhanced in the presence of these species. Several metal ions, including Zn^{2+}, Fe^{3+}, Cu^{2+}, Pb^{2+}, Mg^{2+}, and Ca^{2+}, did not induce interference, indicating the ECL sensor's strong selectivity for adrenaline, with a signal-to-noise ratio of 3 and a detection limit of 0.5 nmol/L with the correlation coefficient R is 0.9928 as shown in Fig. 8.7B [60].

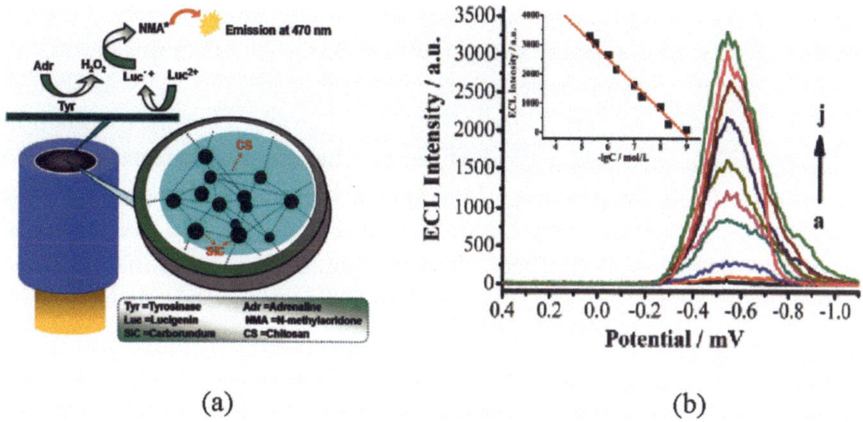

Figure 8.7 (A) The pictorial representation of ECL adrenaline assay sensor mechanism. (B) The ECL versus potential graphs at different adrenaline concentrations, inset graph shows the calibration curve of the ECL intensities versus adrenaline concentrations. *(With permission from Ref. [60].)*

3. SiCNPs-based electrochemical glucose sensor

There is a huge market need in the field of sensor innovation, growing at a compound annual growth rate (CAGR) of 7.9% over the next time frame, ending in 2026 [61]. There is a precipitous development of low power devices for biomedical applications on the rise, and there is a huge market need in the field of sensor innovation, growing from USD 15.6 billion in 2016 at a CAGR of 7.9%. For example, in the clinical field, there are several important factors: (1) a growing diabetic population, (2) a demand for scaled-down and low-power devices, and (3) a need for swift mechanical headways, all of which is driving market growth [62]. Because of the growing population of diabetic patients and the growing demand for point-of-care detection and diagnostics, glucose sensors have the largest market presence among biosensors.

Approximately 285 million people worldwide suffer from the consequences of diabetes, with that number expected to rise to 430 million by 2030. Diabetes, more specifically, is a disease caused by insufficient insulin release, and a large number of people suffer from the consequences of this problem, which can cause harm to the eyes, kidneys, nerves, and even death. One way to cope with this problem is to check for disease symptoms and, more specifically, the glucose level in a person's blood. For those with diabetes, monitoring and detecting glucose (sugar) levels in the blood are critical. One of the most well-known methods for detecting diabetes is to use biosensors to monitor glucose levels in the circulatory system. Glucose sensors are used to determine the glucose grouping of a patient's blood and are an important part of diabetic care management [63–67]. Nonetheless, to be truly beneficial, the glucose [2] sensor should be able to function properly for an extended period of time. The lifetime, affectability, and biocompatibility of a glucose sensor are all limited by the device's core properties. SiC is a biocompatible material that has been used in a variety of biomedical devices and has been used in clinical trials for bone implants, cardiac stents, and glucose sensors, demonstrating that these forms of SiC are biocompatible [68–71].

Because of higher catalyst immobilization, excellent electrical conductivity, better processability, observed electrochemical steadiness, dependability, and biocompatibility, poly(3,4-ethylenedioxythiophene):poly(styrene sulfonate) (PEDOT:PSS) have been currently used in biosensors compared with other CP materials [71–73]. The surface construction, in addition to the use of a conductive polymer substrate, contributes to the catalyst's effective immobilization. The use of electrospun nanofibrous structures is particularly compelling for this work because they provide a large surface area, high porosity, biocompatibility, and dimensionality benefits, resulting in better containment of the analyte within the cathode for efficient electron movement resulting in higher sensitivity [72–80].

The morphological, manufacturing, and electrochemical deployment and characterization of GO_x chemically entangled in PEDOT:PSS CP with SiCNPs electrospun in a nanofibrous-membrane matrix (ENFM) and as spin-coated thin film (SCTF)-based glucose-sensing electrodes are described in this work. In comparison to SiCNPs-SCTF-sensing electrodes, the SiCNPs-ENFM displayed a faster reaction time, better LOD, higher sensitivity, and longer duration. It has been shown that polymers could be directly used as a mediator for glucose detection. This is thought to be due to a direct electron transfer from glucose oxidase to the CP support, which is an oxygen-free site. This research looked at the viability of using SiCNPs-ENFM-sensing electrodes as an alternative to SiCNPs-SCTF-sensing electrodes for the manufacture of wearable glucose sensors [80].

3.1 Fabrication process of SiC-based glucose-sensing electrodes

The electrodes were constructed using PEDOT:PSS with 3.0%–4.0% in H_2O, high-conductivity grade and tested using D-Glucose with 180.16 g/mol subatomic weight and potassium ferricyanide with 329.26 g/mol subatomic load from Sigma Aldrich. SiCNPs from Sigma Aldrich with a subatomic burden of 40.1 g/mol and a molecular size of 45—65 nm were added to the electrodes. The SiCNPs-SCTF and SiCNPs-ENFM-sensing electrodes studied were made with glucose oxidase (without additional oxygen) from *Aspergillus niger*, tetrahydrofuran (THF), and polyvinylidene fluoride (PVDF) with a subatomic load of 534,000, all from Sigma Aldrich.

The electrolyte solution was made with deionized water, 5 mM potassium ferricyanide, and 5 mM glucose in a 1:1 ratio. Working and counter cathodes were made of shattered chromium (100 nm) and gold (100 nm) on glass substrates, with a reference anode of silver/silver chloride (Ag/AgCl) which were used in these electrochemical studies.

The manufacture of an electrospun leading polymer of PEDOT:PSS with SiCNPs was used to create a nanofiber-based glucose sensor involving the stages outlined in Fig. 8.8. PVDF (1.18 g) was dissolved in 2 mL of THF, 0.05 g of SiCNPs was added, followed by 0.22 g of PEDOT: PSS, which was then vigorously mixed for 1 h at 60°C. The following blend was electrospun using the following parameters: a single 18-measure needle spout with an applied voltage of 20 kV at a stream rate of 15 L per minute [80]. The distance between the tip and the gatherer plate was set at 32 cm. A rotating mandrel was used to create a globule-free stringy lattice, which aids in consistent filament conveyance on the anode surface. A gold-covered glass substrate was adhered to the mandrel surface, which was spinning at 54 RPM. The SiCNPs-ENFM cathode was dried at 70°C for 4 hours after the strands were formed on the gold surface space of 0.35 cm × 0.5 cm. The formation interaction of the SiCNPs-SCTF glucose-sensing terminal is shown in Fig. 8.9. A thin film SiCNPs-PEDOT:PSS was made by covering 0.05 g of SiCNPs with 0.0482 g of PEDOT in a turn-covering process: PSS at 490 RPM for 1.5 minutes on a 0.35 cm × 0.5 cm gold terminal with a thickness of 110 nm, followed by 4.5 hours of drying at 70°C. The 1.5 mg GO_x protein arrangement was dropped onto the nanofibrous film, with the twist covering the terminals. The cathodes were maintained at 4°C for 24 hours to ensure protein immobilization [80].

3.2 Morphological characterization of SiC-based glucose-sensing electrodes

The morphology of SiCNPs was observed using transmission electron microscopy (TEM) (50 nm scale bar) and energy-dispersive X-ray spectroscopy (EDX) as shown in Fig. 8.10A and B, respectively. The

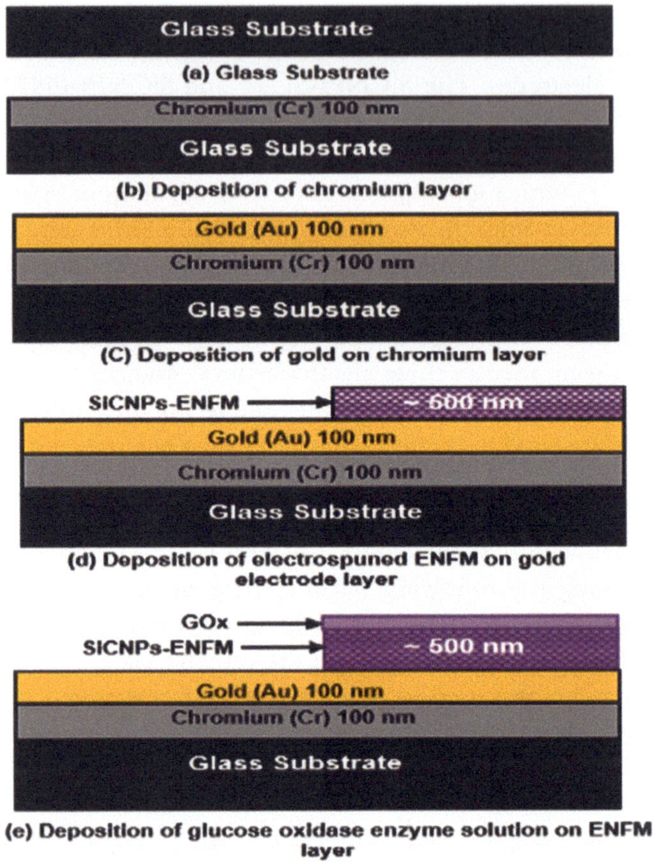

Figure 8.8 Fabrication process sequence of SiCNPs-ENFM-based glucose-sensing electrode.

morphology of the SiCNPs-ENFM and SiCNPs-SCTF films was characterized using a SEM. Fig. 8.10C displays SEM micrographs of the generated conductive polymer-based SiCNPs-ENFM without GO_x with a 25 kV beam accelerating voltage, 1100× amplification (10 μm scale bar). These images depict a structure with a sinewy morphology and a dimensional range of 110–140 nm. Fig. 8.10D displays SEM micrographs of firmly a pressed network-like construct that operated with increased GO_x surface inclusion of the nanofibrous framework. The larger surface area aided in the advancement of the GO_x compound limitation inside the cathode's stringy layer. Fig. 8.10E and F shows SEM images of SiCNPs-PEDOT:PSS SCTF surface with and without GO_x at a higher magnification of 15000X (2 μm scale bar). When the SCTF electrode was placed in an electrolyte, the

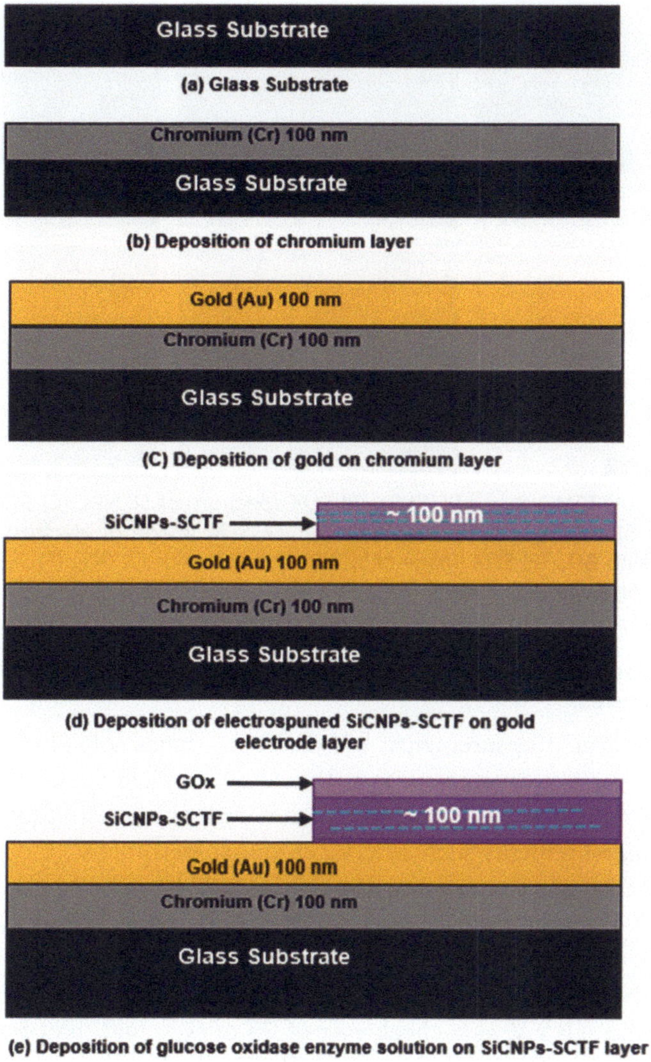

Figure 8.9 Fabrication process sequence of SiCNPs-SCTF-based glucose-sensing electrode.

nonuniform inclusion of chemical particles drains away quickly, affecting the detecting terminal's sensitivity, limit of detection, repeatability, and durability. SEM characterization revealed the distinct surface morphology of Au/SiCNPs-PEDOT:PSS (nanofibers) and Au/SiCNPs-PEDOT:PSS (nanofibers)/GO_x layers, with the twist covering Au/SiCNPs-PEDOT: PSS (film) and Au/SiCNPs-PEDOT: PSS (film)/GO_x layers [80].

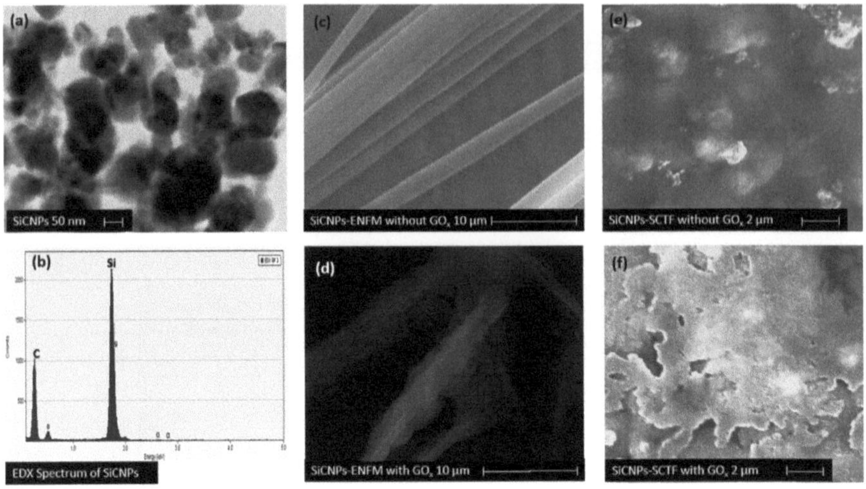

Figure 8.10 (A) TEM image of SiCNPs. (B) EDX spectrum of SiCNPs. (C) SEM image of electrospun SiCNPs nanofibers without GO_x. (D) SEM image of electrospun SiCNPs nanofibers with GO_x. (E) SEM image of SiCNPs thin film without GO_x. (F) SEM image of SiCNPs thin film with GO_x [80].

3.3 Electrochemical characterization of SiC-based glucose-sensing electrodes

Electrochemical measurements of the two types of glucose-sensing electrodes were conducted using a Princeton Applied Research analyzer in a three-terminal setup for electrochemical characterization. Electrochemical measurements such as CV, chronoamperometry (CA), and EIS were used to focus the examination of the SiCNPs-ENFM Au/SiCNPs-PEDOT:PSS(nanofibers)/GO_x and SCTF Au/SiCNPs-PEDOT:PSS (film)/GO_x-based glucose detecting electrodes. Fig. 8.11A shows the CV of SiCNPs-ENFM and SiCNPs-SCTF terminals with a potential range of +0.9 V to −0.9 V at a check rate of 75 mVs^{-1} with glucose concentration of 5 mM. The CV of the SiCNPs-ENFM based electrode exhibits an oxidation peak of +1.52 mA at +0.6 V and a reduction peak of −1.501 mA at - 0.4 V, whereas the SiCNPs-SCTF electrode shows a lower oxidation peak of +1.04 mA at +0.5 V and a reduction peak of −1.08 mA at −0.25 V.

The CA behavior of the SiCNPs-ENFM at +0.6 V and SiCNPs-SCTF at +0.5 V with 5 mM potassium ferricyanide for glucose focus move from 0.5 mM to 20 mM, as shown in Fig. 8.12B and C, respectively. At 60 seconds, the current reaction ranged between 41.1 $\mu A \pm 0.0010$ μA and

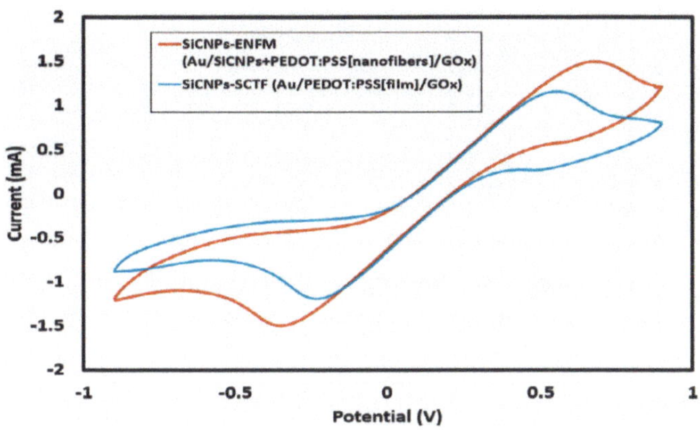

Figure 8.11 CV graphs of SiCNPs-ENFM (red) electrode exhibit an oxidation peak of +1.52 mA at +0.6 V and a reduction peak of −1.501 mA at −0.4 V, whereas the SiCNPs-SCTF (blue) electrode shows a lower oxidation peak of +1.04 mA at +0.5 V and a reduction peak of −1.08 mA at −0.25 V.

146.2 μA ± 0.0013 μA for SiCNPs-ENFM electrodes and 0.75 μA ± 0.002 μA–3.34 μA ± 0.0025 μA for SiCNPs-SCTF electrodes, respectively. The sensitivity and LOD of the SiCNPs-ENFM-sensing electrode were observed to be 30.75 μA/mM cm^2 and 0.56 μM, which is significantly better than the SiCNPs-SCTF electrode's 0.68 μA/mM cm^2 and 50 μM as shown in Fig. 8.12D.

EIS was performed at an amplitude of 20 mV over the frequency range from 0.1 Hz to 10 kHz at a glucose concentration of 5 mM. Equivalent circuit models using Nyquist plots for the SiCNPs-ENFM and SiCNPs-SCTF-sensing electrodes are shown in Fig. 8.13E. In comparison to the SiCNPs-SCTF electrode, which has a charge transfer (R_{WE}) and solution resistance (R_s) of 379.04 and 210.06 Ω, a Warburg impedance of 432.79 Ω/$\sqrt{s}$ and a double layer capacitance (C_{WE}) of 24.3 μF, the SiCNPs-ENFM-based sensing electrode had a lower charge transfer (R_{WE}) and solution resistance (R_s) of 28.58 and 196.08 Ω, respectively, with a Warburg impedance of 418.16 Ω/$\sqrt{s}$ and a double-layer capacitance (C_{WE}) of 2.78 μF [80].

The durability of the SiCNPs-ENFM electrode at +0.6 V and the SiCNPs-SCTF electrode at +0.5 V was estimated with a glucose concentration of 5 mM. Fig. 8.14F demonstrates that, over a 50-day time span, a 14% lower change in current reaction for SiCNPs-ENFM electrodes resulted compared to a 75% reduction for the SiCNPs-SCTF electrode.

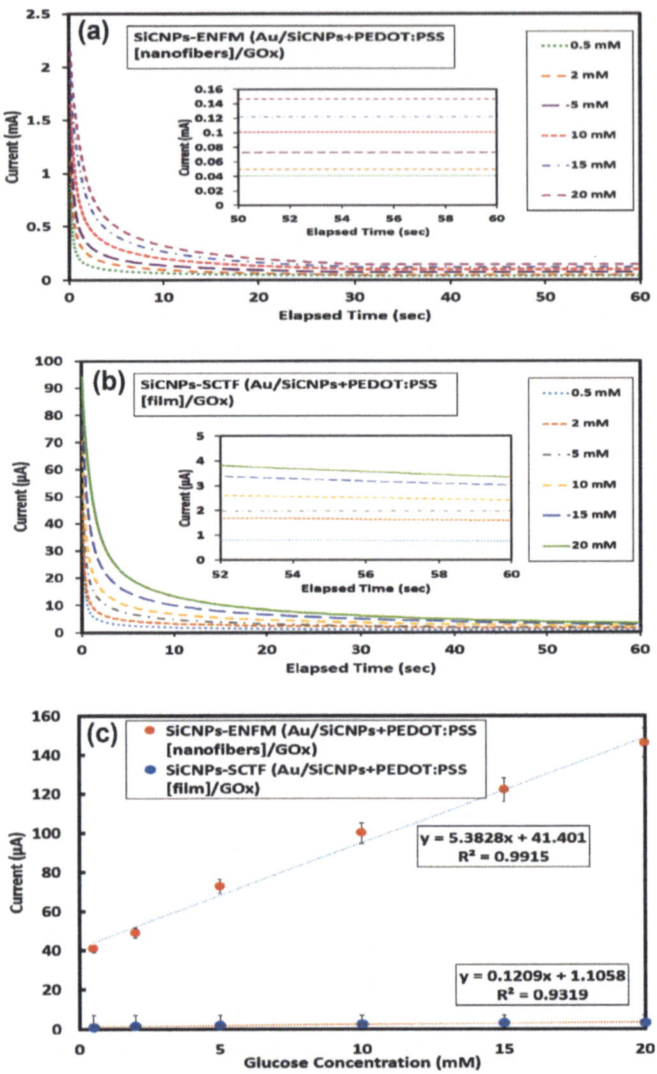

Figure 8.12 CA curves of (A) SiCNPs-ENFM electrode. (B) SiCNPs-SCTF electrode. (C) Calibration plots show that SiCNPs-ENFM (red) have better sensitivity and LOD compared to SiCNPs-SCTF (blue) electrodes.

GO_x compound atoms were trapped on the electrospun nanofibrous surface due to the permeable structure of the nanofibrous network. As shown in Fig. 8.15G, the selectivity of the SiCNPs-ENFM glucose sensor was confirmed through CA testing at +0.5 V under the interference of various components such as sodium chloride and potassium ferricyanide. The current increased only when the glucose was administered, indicating that

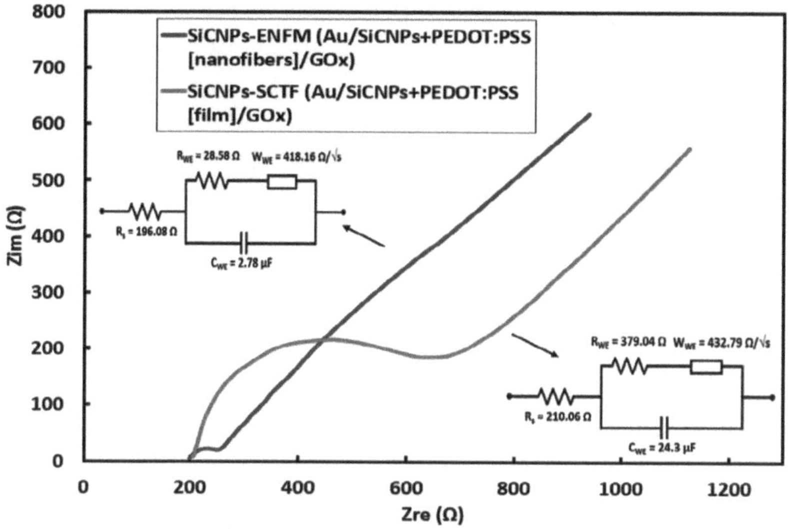

Figure 8.13 Nyquist graphs shows the comparative performance of SiCNPs-ENFM (red) and SiCNPs-SCTF (blue) electrodes [80].

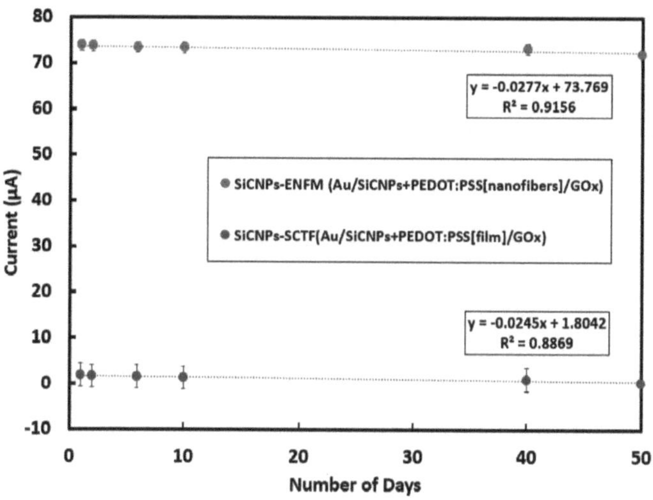

Figure 8.14 The comparative durability analysis of SiCNPs-ENFM (red) and SiCNPs-SCTF (blue) electrodes.

the SiCNPs-ENFM functions as a specific glucose sensor at a specific glucose level. When using SiCNPs-ENFM electrodes, these results are indicative of an adequate stability and selectivity through solid electrochemical processes, paving the way for the future use of SiC-based nanofibers in the development of prospective biosensors.

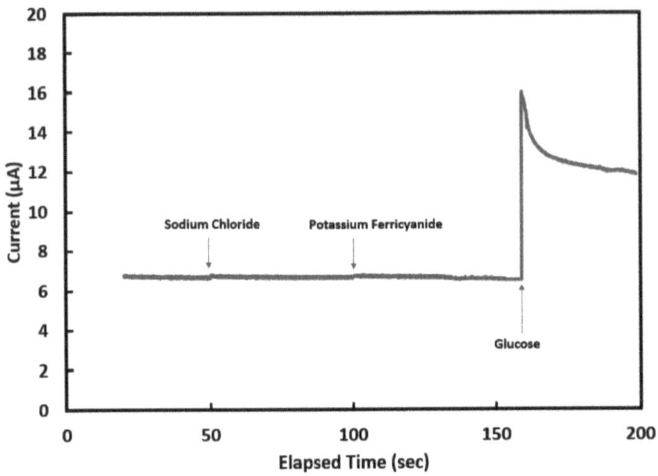

Figure 8.15 Selectivity test for the SiCNPs-ENFM-based glucose-sensing electrode. Note: negligible change in sensor current for two salt solutions whereas the sensor electrode rapidly responds to glucose.

3.4 Performance comparison

When compared to previously published state-of-the-art PEDOT conductive polymer-based glucose sensors [76,77], the SiCNPs-ENFM glucose sensor shows a considerable improvement in performance, with superior sensitivity, LOD, stability, and durability. Table 8.1 compares the performance and highlights the improved sensitivity, limit of detection, and performance period of the SiC-based glucose sensors reported here.

Table 8.1 Comparison of SiCNPs-ENFM sensor with PEDOT glucose sensors.

Reference	[76]	[77]	This work [78]
Sensing electrode	Pt/PEDOT-NFs/GO_x	NPG/PEDOT/GO_x	Au/SiCNPs-PEDOT:PSS/PVDF/GO_x
Sensitivity	9.2 μA/mM cm^2	7.3 μA/mM cm^2	30.75 μA/mM cm^2
Limit of detection	0.26 mM	10 mM	0.56 μM
Concentration range	0.1–25 mM	0.1–15 mM	0.5–20 mM
Number of days	30 days	7 days	50 days

4. Summary

In this chapter, the relative comparison of SiC-based enzymatic electrochemical glucose sensors (i.e., SiCNPs-ENFM and SiCNPs-SCTF), which can be conceivably utilized for checking the blood glucose level in diabetic patients, has been described. Electrochemical investigations showed that a SiCNPs-PEDOT:PSS ENFM electrode allows for a higher circulation and entanglement of GO_x, when contrasted with a SiCNPs-PEDOT:PSS SCTF electrode. Electrospun SiCNPs-CP nanofibers, utilized as a novel detecting grid, helped to speed up GO_x immobilization. The charge transport between the sensor electrode and GO_x enzyme was significantly enhanced when utilizing the conducting polymer PEDOT:PSS with SiCNPs to realize a nanofibrous film electrode. The SiCNPs-ENFM-based detection electrode displayed a glucose detection sensitivity of 30.75 μA/mM cm^2, the lowest LOD of 0.56 μM, and better durability for up to 50 days contrasted with the SiCNPs-SCTF electrode. This supports the possible utilization of nanofibrous layers for practical biosensing applications.

References

[1] N.L. Kazanskiy, S.N. Khonina, M.A. Butt, A. Kaźmierczak, R. Piramidowicz, State-of-the-art optical devices for biomedical sensing applications—a review, Electronics 10 (8) (April 2021) 973.

[2] J.L. Cano Perez, J. Gutiérrez-Gutiérrez, C. Perezcampos Mayoral, E.L. Pérez-Campos, M. del S. Pina Canseco, L. Tepech Carrillo, L.P.-C. Mayoral, M. Vargas Treviño, E.L. Apreza, R. Rojas Laguna, Fiber optic sensors: a review for glucose measurement, Biosensors 11 (3) (February 2021) 61.

[3] S.E. Saddow, Silicon Carbide Biotechnology: A Biocompatible Semiconductor for Advanced Biomedical Devices and Applications, Elsevier Science, Netherlands, 2012.

[4] K. Puttananjegowda, M. Ababneh, S. Thomas, The Design of High Efficiency Voltage Mode Integrated Converter for Glucose Monitoring Systems. IEEE 12th Annual Computing and Communication Workshop and Conference (CCWC), IEEE, 2022, pp. 649–653, https://doi.org/10.1109/CCWC54503.2022.9720789.

[5] K. Puttananjegowda, Y. Cao, M. Green, DC-DC Boost Converter for Wireless Power Transfer Systems, in: IEEE 12th Annual Ubiquitous Computing, Electronics & Mobile Communication Conference (UEMCON), IEEE, 2021, pp. 661–665, https://doi.org/10.1109/UEMCON53757.2021.9666551.

[6] U. Starke, W.Y. Lee, C. Coletti, S.E. Saddow, R.P. Devaty, W.J. Choyke, SiC pore surfaces: surface studies of 4H-SiC (-1102) and 4H-SiC (-110 -2), Applied Physics Letters 88 (3) (2006) 031915.

[7] A.A. Burk Jr., L.B. Rowland, The role of excess silicon and in situ etching on 4HSiC and 6H-SiC epitaxial layer morphology, Journal of Crystal Growth 167 (1996) 586–595.

[8] J. Botsoa, V. Lysenko, A. Géloën, O. Marty, J.M. Bluet, G. Guillot, Application of 3C-SiC quantum dots for living cell imaging, Applied Physics Letters 92 (2008) 173902.
[9] S. Dhar, O. Seitz, M.D. Halls, S. Choi, Y.J. Chabal, L.C. Feldman, Chemical properties of oxidized silicon carbide surfaces upon etching in hydrofluoric acid, Journal of the American Chemical Society 131 (2009) 16808−16813.
[10] P. Kavyashree, et al., The design of low noise amplifiers in nanometer technology for WiMAX applications, International Journal of Scientific and Research Publications 3 (10) (October 2013).
[11] P. Kavyashree, S.S. Yellampalli, The design of ultra low power CMOS CGLNA in nanometer technology, in: 2014 Fifth International Symposium on Electronic System Design, 2014, pp. 15−19.
[12] P. Kavyashree, S.S. Yellampalli, The design of ultra low power RF CMOS LNA in nanometer technology, in: M. Sharma, et al. (Eds.), Design and Modeling of Low Power VLSI Systems, IGI Global, 2016, pp. 229−251.
[13] P. Kavyashree, S.S. Yellampalli, The design of ultra low power differential CGLNA for IEEE 802.15.4 applications, in: 2015 IEEE International RF and Microwave Conference (RFM), 2015, pp. 54−56.
[14] K. Puttananjegowda, S. Thomas, A detailed review on physical unclonable function circuits for hardware security, in: 2018 IEEE 9th Annual Information Technology, Electronics and Mobile Communication Conference (IEMCON), 2018, pp. 609−612.
[15] A. Bolz, M. Schaldach, Artificial heart valves: improved blood compatibility by PECVD a-SiC:H coating, Artificial Organs 14 (4) (1990) 260−269.
[16] C. Coletti, Silicon Carbide Biocompatibility, Surface Control and Electronic Cellular Interaction for Biosensing Applications (Graduate theses and dissertations), 2007, https://scholarcommons.usf.edu/etd/676.
[17] S. Thomas, B. Seufert, W. Garcia, M. Devisetty, R. Khan, K. Puttananjegowda, N.A. Alcantar, book chapter "Eco-friendly, Biodegradable, and Biocompatible Electrospun Nanofiber Membranes and Applications". Sustainable Nanotechnology: Strategies, Products, and Applications, Subthemes: Nanotechnology and Eco-Friendly Bio based products, Wiley, April 2022.
[18] C. Harder, A. Rzany, M. Schaldach, Coating of vascular stents with antithrombogenic amorphous silicon carbide, Progress in Biomedical Research 4 (1999) 71−77.
[19] N.G. Wright, A.B. Horsfall, SiC sensors: a review, Journal of Physics D: Applied Physics 40 (2007) 6345−6354.
[20] S. Santavirta, M. Takagi, L. Nordsletten, A. Anttila, R. Lappalainen, Y.T. Konttinen, Biocompatibility of silicon carbide in colony formation test in vitro, Archives of Orthopaedic and Trauma Surgery 118 (1998) 89−91.
[21] M. Mahmoodi, L. Ghazanfari, Fundamentals of biomedical applications of biomorphic SiC, in: Properties and Applications of Silicon Carbide, INTECH Open Access Publisher, Rijeka, Croatia, 1999, pp. 297−345.
[22] D.N. Hume, I.M. Kolthoff, The silicon carbide electrode, Journal of the American Chemical Society 63 (10) (1941) 2805−2806.
[23] N. Aghdassi, D. Dulson, S. Linden, L.Q. Li, L.F. Chi, H. Zacharias, Very large-bandgap insulating monolayers of ODS on SiC, Applied Surface Science 258 (2012) 7280−7285.
[24] J. Bouclé, N. Herlin-Boime, A. Kassiba, Influence of silicon and carbon excesses on the aqueous dispersion of SiC nanocrystals for optical application, Journal of Nanoparticle Research 7 (2005) 275−285.
[25] L. Yang, H. Zhao, S. Fan, S. Deng, Q. Lv, J. Lin, C. Li, Label-free electrochemical immunosensor based on gold−silicon carbide nanocomposites for sensitive detection of human chorionic gonadotrophin, Biosensors and Bioelectronics 57 (2014) 199−206.

[26] R. Gomez, A. Ivorra, R. Villa, P. Godignon, J. Millan, I. Erill, et al., A SiC microdevice for the minimally invasive monitoring of ischemia in living tissues, Biomedical Microdevices 8 (2006) 43–49.
[27] M. Saki, M. Kazemzadeh Narbat, A. Samadikuchaksaraei, H.B. Ghafouri, F. Gorjipour, Biocompatibility study of a hydroxyapatitealumina and silicon carbide composite scaffold for bone tissue engineering, Yakhteh Medical Journal 11 (2009) 55–60.
[28] S. Iannotta, A. Romeo, P. D'Angelo and G. Tarabella, SiC Biosensing and Electrochemical Sensing: State of the Art and Perspectives Chapter 5 in [3].
[29] D.M. Brown, et al., Silicon carbide photodiode sensor for combustion control, IEEE Sensors Journal 5 (2005) 983–988.
[30] M.A.A. Tabrizi, M. Shamsipur, A. Mostafaie, A high sensitive label-free immunosensor for the determination of human serum IgG using overoxidized polypyrrole decorated with gold nanoparticle modified electrode, Materials Science and Engineering: C 59 (2016) 965–969.
[31] S.K. Mishra, R. Pasricha, A.M. Biradar, Zns-nanocrystals/polypyrrole nanocomposite film based immunosensor, Applied Physics Letters 100 (2012).
[32] Z. Matharu, G. Sumana, S.K. Arya, S.P. Singh, V. Gupta, B.D. Malhotra, Polyaniline Langmuir-Blodgett film based cholesterol biosensor, Langmuir 23 (2007) 13188–13192.
[33] P. Humpolicek, V. Kasparkova, P. Saha, J. Stejskal, Biocompatibility of polyaniline, Synthetic Metals 162 (2012) 722–727.
[34] Y. Kim, et al., A glucose sensor based on an organic electrochemical transistor structure using a vapor polymerized poly(3,4-ethylenedioxythiophene) layer, Japanese Journal of Applied Physics 49 (2010).
[35] F. Yana, J. Li, S. Man Mok, Highly photosensitive thin film transistors based on a composite of poly(3-hexylthiophene) and titania nanoparticles, Journal of Applied Physics 106 (2009) 074501.
[36] P. Lorwongtragool, E. Sowade, N. Watthanawisuth, R.R. Baumann, T. Kerdcharoen, A novel wearable electronic nose for healthcare based on flexible printed chemical sensor array, Sensors 14 (2014) 19700–19712.
[37] J. Rivnay, R.M. Owens, G.G. Malliaras, The rise of organic bioelectronics, Chemistry of Materials 26 (2014) 679–685.
[38] P. Lin, F. Yan, Organic thin-film transistors for chemical and biological sensing, Advanced Materials 24 (2012) 34–51.
[39] G.G. Malliaras, Organic bioelectronics: a new era for organic electronics, Biochimca Biophysica Acta – General Subjects 1830 (2013) 4286–4287.
[40] X. Cui, D.C. Martin, Electrochemical deposition and characterization of poly (3,4-ethylenedioxythiophene) on neural microelectrode arrays, Sensors and Actuators B: Chemical 89 (2003) 92–102.
[41] C. Liao, F. Yan, Organic semiconductors in organic thin-film transistor-based chemical and biological sensors, Polymer Reviews 53 (2013) 352–406.
[42] J.C. Scott, L.D. Bozano, Nonvolatile memory elements based on organic materials, Advanced Materials 19 (2007) 1452–1463.
[43] K. Puttananjegowda, A. Takshi, S. Thomas, Silicon carbide nanoparticles fibrous membrane for implantable glucose sensor integrated with chronoamperometric potentiostat, US Patent App.17/335,276 (Jun 2021).
[44] T.J. Fawcett, J.T. Wolan, A.L. Spetz, M. Reyes, S.E. Saddow, Thermal detection mechanism of SiC based hydrogen resistive gas sensors, Applied Physics Letters 89 (2006).
[45] A. Ellison, B. Magnusson, N.T. Son, L. Storasta, E. Janzén, High temperature CVD growth of SiC, Materials Science and Engineering B 61 (62) (1999) 113–120.

[46] A. Oliveros, et al., Silicon carbide: a versatile material for biosensor applications, Biomedical Microdevices 15 (2) (2013) 353–368.
[47] C.R. Deeken, M.J. Cozad, S.L. Bachman, B.J. Ramshaw, S.A. Grant, Characterization of bionanocomposite scaffolds comprised of amine-functionalized single-walled carbon nanotubes crosslinked to an acellular porcine tendon, Journal of Biomedical Materials Research A 96 (3) (March 1, 2011) 584–594, https://doi.org/10.1002/jbm.a.33014. Epub 2011 Jan 10. PMID: 21254390.
[48] S.E. Saddow, et al., SiC for biomedical applications, Materials Science Forum 858 (2016) 1010–1014.
[49] J.M. Hsu, P. Tathireddy, L. Rieth, A.R. Normann, F. Solzbacher, Characterization of a-SiC(x):H thin films as an encapsulation material for integrated silicon based neural interface devices, Thin Solid Films 516 (2007), pp. 34–4.
[50] C. Hehrlein, Stent passivation with silicon carbide as a possible alternative to Drugeluting stents - a comprehensive review of pre-clinical and clinical results, Interventional Cardiology Review 4 (2009) 60–63.
[51] M. Jorfi, J.L. Skousen, C. Weder, J.R. Capadona, Progress towards biocompatible intracortical microelectrodes for neural interfacing applications, Journal of Neural Engineering 12 (2015) 011001.
[52] W.-C. Wu, H.-W. Chang, Y.-C. Tsai, Electrocatalytic detection of dopamine in the presence of ascorbic acid and uric acid at silicon carbide coated electrodes, Chemicals Communications 47 (2011) 6458–6460.
[53] Z. Guo, S. Dong, Electrogenerated chemiluminescence determination of dopamine and epinephrine in the presence of ascorbic acid at carbon nanotube/nafion-Ru(bpy) composite film modified glassy carbon electrode, Electroanalysis 17 (2005) 607–612.
[54] Y. Zhao, Y. Gao, D. Zhan, H. Liu, Q. Zhao, Y. Kou, Y. Shao, M. Li, Q. Zhuang, Z. Zhu, Selective detection of dopamine in the presence of ascorbic acid and uric acid by a carbon nanotubes-ionic liquid gel modified electrode, Talanta 66 (2005) 51–57.
[55] S. Singh, R.C. Buchanan, SiC-C fiber electrode for biological sensing, Materials Science and Engineering C 27 (2007) 551–557.
[56] S. Afroz, A Biocompatible SiC RF Antenna for In-Vivo Sensing Applications (Doctoral dissertation), University of South Florida, 2013.
[57] F. Araujo Cespedes, S. Thomas, S. Afroz, S.E. Saddow, Chapter 6 - SiC RF antennas for in vivo glucose monitoring and WiFi applications, in: S.E. Saddow (Ed.), Silicon Carbide Biotechnology, second ed., Elsevier, 2016, pp. 179–205.
[58] N. Yang, et al., Nanocrystalline 3C-SiC electrode for biosensing applications, Analytical Chemistry 83 (2011) 5827–5830.
[59] R. Ghavami, et al., SiC nanoparticles-modified glassy carbon electrodes for simultaneous determination of purine and pyrimidine DNA bases, Biosensors and Bioelectronics 26 (2011) 3864–3869.
[60] H. Ye, H. Xu, X. Xu, C. Zheng, X. Li, L. Wang, X. Liu, G. Chen, An electrochemiluminescence sensor for adrenaline assay based on the tyrosinase/SiC/chitosan modified electrode, Chemical Communications 49 (2013) 7070–7072.
[61] A. Sun, T. Wambach, A.G. Venkatesh, D.A. Hall, A low-cost smartphone-based electrochemical biosensor for point-of-care diagnostics, in: IEEE Biomedical Circuits and Systems Conference: Healthcare Technology: [proceedings], 2014, pp. 312–315, https://doi.org/10.1109/BioCAS.2014.6981725.
[62] M. M Ababneh, A. Qaroot, K. Puttananjegowda, S. Perez, S. Thomas, Optimized power management circuit for implantable rectenna for in-body medical devices, IEEE International Conference on Power Electronics and Drive Systems (2017) 30–34.
[63] G. Cappon, Wearable continuous glucose monitoring sensors: a revolution in diabetes treatment, Electronics 6 (65) (2017) 1–16.
[64] K. Puttananjegowda, S. Thomas, A CNTFET based multi-stage transimpedance amplifier for blood glucose monitoring systems, in: IEEE Information Technology, Electronics and Mobile Communication Conference, Vancouver, Canada, 2018, pp. 383–388.

[65] K. Puttananjegowda, S. Thomas, A low-power low-noise multi-stage transimpedance amplifier for amperometric based blood glucose monitoring systems, Analog Integrated Circuits and Signal Processing Journal 102 (2020) 659–666. Springer.
[66] K. Puttananjegowda, M. Ababneh, S. Thomas, The design of ultra low noise CMOS transimpedance amplifier for biosensing applications, in: 2017 IEEE 8th Annual Ubiquitous Computing, Electronics and Mobile Communication Conference (UEMCON), 2017, pp. 16–19, https://doi.org/10.1109/UEMCON.2017.8248971.
[67] K. Puttananjegowda, S. Thomas, Cascode Common Source Transimpedance Amplifiers for Analyte Monitoring Systems, US Patent App. 16/008,864, April 2019.
[68] M.M. Ababneh, M. Jasim, K. Puttananjegowda, S. Perez, S. Afroz, S. Thomas, Design of a SiC implantable rectenna for wireless in-vivo biomedical devices, IEEE Annual Ubiquitous Computing, Electronics and Mobile Communication Conference (2017) 254–257.
[69] S.E. Saddow, C. Coletti, C.L. Frewin, N. Schettini, A. Oliveros, M. Jarosezeski, Single-crystal silicon carbide: a biocompatible and hemocompatible semiconductor for advanced biomedical applications, Materials Research Society Symposium Proceedings 12 (46) (2010) 193–198.
[70] X. Li, X. Wang, R. Bondokov, J. Morris, Y.H. An, T.S. Sudarshan, Micro/nanoscale mechanical and tribological characterization of SiC for orthopedic applications, Journal of Biomedical Materials Research Part B: Applied Biomaterials 72 (2) (2005) 353–361.
[71] U. Kalnins, A. Erglis, I. Dinne, I. Kumsars, S. Jegere, Clinical outcomes of silicon carbide coated stents in patient with coronary disease, Medical Science Monitor 2 (2002) 16–20.
[72] K. Puttananjegowda, A. Takshi, S. Thomas, Electrospun nanofibrous membrane based electrochemical glucose sensor, IEEE Sensors Letters 4 (2) (2020) 1–4.
[73] K. Puttananjegowda, A. Takshi, S. Thomas, Electrospun nanofibrous structures for electrochemical enzymatic glucose biosensing: a perspective, Journal of the Electrochemical Society 167 (3) (2020) 1–6.
[74] S.W. Thomas, R.R. Khan, K. Puttananjegowda, W. Serrano-Garcia, Conductive polymers and metal oxide polymeric composites for nanostructures and nanodevices, Advances in Nanostructured Materials and Nanopatterning Technologies (2020) 243–271.
[75] R.K. Pal, A.A. Farghaly, C. Wang, M.M. Collinson, S.C. Kundu, V.K. Yadavalli, Conducting polymer-silk biocomposites for flexible and biodegradable electrochemical sensors, Biosensors Bioelectronics 81 (Jul. 2016) 294–302.
[76] Y. Aleeva, et al., Amperometric biosensor and front-end electronics for Remote glucose monitoring by crosslinked PEDOT-glucose oxidase, IEEE Sensors Journal 18 (12) (2018).
[77] X. Xiao, M. Wang, H. Li, P. Si, One-step fabrication of bio-functionalized nanoporous gold/poly(3,4-ethylenedioxythiophene) hybrid electrodes for amperometric glucose sensing, Talanta 116 (2013) 1054–1059.
[78] K. Puttananjegowda, A. Takshi, S. Thomas, Silicon carbide nanoparticles electrospun nanofibrous enzymatic glucose sensor, Biosensors and Bioelectronics 186 (11385) (2021) 1–4.
[79] K. Puttananjegowda, Electrospun Nanofibrous Membrane Based Glucose Sensor with Integration of Potentiostat Circuit (Doctoral dissertation), Electrical Engineering, University of South Florida, Tampa, Florida, USA, 2020.
[80] K. Puttananjegowda, A. Takshi, S. Thomas, Silicon carbide nanoparticles based nanofibrous membrane in comparison with thin-film enzymatic glucose sensor, IEEE Transactions on NanoBioscience 20 (4) (2021) 577–580.

CHAPTER 9

Manufacturable biosensors based on graphene films

Sukanya Pal, Amy Peters, Karthik Nagareddy and Alton Horsfall
Department of Engineering, University of Durham, Durham, United Kingdom

Contents

1. Introduction

The isolation of free-standing graphene in 2004 initiated an explosion in research that covers the full range from materials modeling, through to the inclusion of graphene flakes in concrete. One of the areas that have emerged from the raft of potential applications is the realization of sensors, with reports covering electrochemical, gas, electronic, optical, mechanical, and chemical detection available. The interest in biological sensing using graphene and graphene-based materials has resulted in the publication of thousands of research papers annually, with over 100,000 listed in the field to date. The unique physical structure of graphene, a single layer of sp^2 bonded carbon atoms, makes it ideally suited for use in the realization of sensors. The high surface area to volume ratio of graphene gives it a

Silicon Carbide Technology for Advanced Human Healthcare Applications
ISBN 978-0-323-90609-8
https://doi.org/10.1016/B978-0-323-90609-8.00013-2

sensitivity to the surroundings that is unsurpassed in conventional bulk materials, such as silicon. This property has driven the interest in sensing using graphene but is also responsible for challenges in the manufacture and realization of sensors.

The exceptional physical and electronic properties of graphene have been well documented, with a surge of interest in developing devices including high-speed field-effect transistors (FETs) [1,2], chemical sensors, and high-frequency amplifiers [3,4]. Many of these properties, however, are true only of pristine, uncontaminated graphene. Generally, the electronic properties of graphene are degraded due to a number of limiting factors such as contaminants on the surface, choice of substrate, and overall quality of the graphene layer. For example, device fabrication by standard lithography exposes the hydrophobic graphene surface to organic resist residues that cannot be removed using standard solvents. These residues can act as external scattering sites on the surface that degrade the transport properties [5]. Thermal annealing is often used to remove residues and restore the graphene surface; however, residues will remain in areas covered by metal contacts. As such, the development of fabrication techniques that reduce contamination and damage of the graphene film is critical for the realization of high-performance graphene devices with a high yield.

On the other hand, even though pristine graphene has many outstanding electronic properties, several issues need to be addressed before the full potential of graphene can be realized. For example, unlike conventional semiconductors graphene does not possess a bandgap and, hence, the graphene-based field-effect transistor cannot be turned off completely [3,6,7], limiting its use in digital electronic applications, where high ON/OFF ratios are critical. Additionally, the highly hydrophobic nature of the graphene surface results in weak metal electrode adhesion, leading to metal delamination [8]. Furthermore, as graphene is chemically inert, chemical sensors made of pristine graphene typically suffer from weak sensing responsivity, poor selectivity issues, and extremely long recovery times due to the lack of polar functional groups on the surface [9,10]. The absence of these polar groups also makes interfacing graphene with other chemical moieties extremely challenging, thereby limiting its use in biological applications.

Hence, surface functionalization of graphene is essential to enhance its capabilities and promote chemical reactivity on its surface to support a range of applications from chemical and biological sensing to the manufacture of high-performance transistors. Data to demonstrate the characteristics of oxygen functionalized epitaxial films using e-beam generated plasmas are presented and discussed. In addition, as the use of functionalized graphene films in device applications inevitably requires metal contacts, data to demonstrate the influence of oxygen at the metal—graphene interface on the device's electrical characteristics are presented.

However, to be able to control the surface of graphene using functionalization techniques, it is necessary to manufacture graphene with a pristine surface, especially at the wafer level. Hence, the first section of the chapter describes the fabrication of large-area graphene films with high yield to realize devices with carrier mobilities similar to unprocessed films. The first portion of the chapter describes the use of a sacrificial metal layer during the processing of graphene films, and how the selection of the metal influences the graphene surface and the chemical processes required to achieve this. The later sections then discuss the potential of functionalization using low power plasma techniques and how this influences the ability of the graphene to act as a resistometric sensor. The chapter then concludes with a summary of how functionalized graphene films have been demonstrated for use as biological sensors.

2. The use of copper-based sacrificial layers

Standard lithographic processing typically used in microelectronic device fabrication presents a number of challenges when applied to graphene. Photoresist residues contaminate the graphene surface, resulting in the degradation of electronic properties and, ultimately, poor device performance. Additionally, the low surface adhesion results in graphene detachment from the substrate when using standard solvents including tetramethylammonium hydroxide (TMAH), a common ingredient in photoresist developers. This generally results in a low device yield and significant variability in device performance across the wafer. E-Beam lithography is a popular technique to minimize sample contact with organic solvents; however, it has low throughput and, as such, is not scalable for high volume, wafer-scale device manufacturing [11,12]. Fig. 9.1 shows optical micrographs of graphene films patterned using standard lithographic processing. Clearly visible are graphene films exhibiting signs of wrinkling and detachment from the substrate. This is particularly evident in the right-hand image with the lighter blue area shown being the graphene film that is only partially covering the desired pattern. The left-hand image also shows areas of residue on the unpatterned areas of the substrate

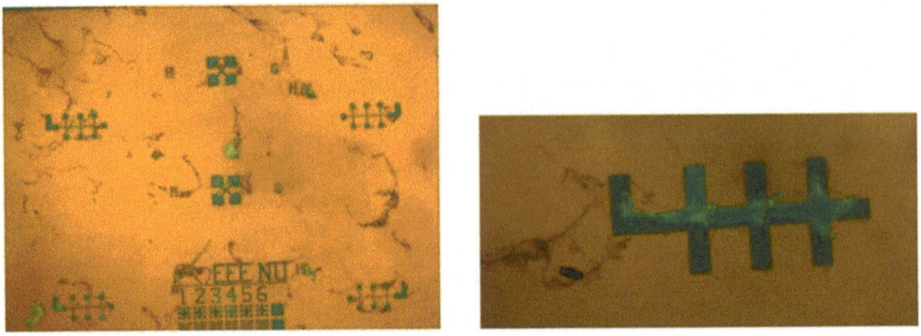

Figure 9.1 Optical micrographs of devices fabricated on CVD graphene without the use of a metal sacrificial layer [13].

that is graphene film residue that has detached from the patterned areas and redeposited on other regions of the wafer.

One solution to reduce this issue is to deposit a metal sacrificial layer onto the graphene surface before exposure to any organic contaminants. Nickel (Ni) has been proposed as a suitable metal [14]. However, the Ni–Gr interface is based on a chemisorption reaction (rather than a physisorption interaction) and, as such, forms a nickel carbide that disturbs the electronic structure of the graphene film in the area underneath the metalized region [15]. This in turn leads to the degradation of the electronic and transport properties that are fundamental to achieving optimal device characteristics. Aluminum (Al) is also a popular choice of the metal sacrificial layer and is, in fact, recommended by many chemical vapor deposition (CVD) graphene suppliers as part of their fabrication processes. While the use of Al does reduce detachment in comparison to conventional fabrication methods, Al is etched by TMAH-based developers [16] and, as such, the graphene film is not fully protected with partial detachment still occurring at the edges of the desired pattern, resulting in a degradation of the electronic properties. To identify a suitable alternative, the interaction of metals when in contact with the graphene film needs to be considered.

The data in Table 9.1 show the work function of different metals and the work function of graphene when in contact with these metals. Changes in the graphene work function when in contact with the metal film result in charge transfer and unintentional doping of the graphene layer [17]. It is thus important to choose a metal that causes a minimal shift in work function to preserve the electronic properties of the graphene film. Of the metals listed, Cu results in the smallest shift in graphene work function,

Table 9.1 Metal (*WM*) and graphene (*WG*) work function versus metals suitable as a sacrificial layer [17].

	Gr	Ni	Cu	Al	Au
W_M (eV)	—	5.01	5.22	4.08	5.54
W_G (eV)	4.48	3.66	4.40	4.04	4.74

$\Delta W_G = -0.08$ eV. Studies reported in the literature for the growth of CVD graphene on a Cu catalyst demonstrate that Cu has minimal interaction with the graphene film and the solubility of carbon in copper is low [18,19]. There have been several studies into the behavior of the Cu–Gr interface, as this is a fundamental consideration for the CVD growth of graphene on Cu films. Previous studies have shown that Cu is a favorable catalyst for this process because of the low carbon solubility and lack of a chemical-based interaction with the graphene surface. Additionally, the chemicals used to chemically remove excess copper during wet transfer processes, including ammonium persulphate (APS), have been shown to cause little or no damage to the material and electronic properties of the graphene film [20,21]. Considering these factors, a hypothesis that a thin Cu film deposited on the graphene surface would make a more suitable metal sacrificial layer in comparison to either Al or Ni was explored.

Nine (9) commercial CVD graphene samples on SiO_2/Si substrates were investigated to enable the direct comparison of three (3) fabrication approaches: no sacrificial layer, an Al sacrificial layer, and a Cu sacrificial layer. Twelve (12) eight-terminal Hall structures of varying width, six (6) identical Van der Pauw structures, and four (4) transfer length method (TLM) structures were fabricated onto each sample to enable the extraction of the electronic material properties. For the fabrication processes that utilized a sacrificial metal layer, a 50-nm metal film was deposited onto the surface of the graphene using e-beam evaporation. Subsequently, conventional photolithographic patterning using S1813 positive resist was performed to define the physical dimensions of the graphene channels. The unwanted metal film was then etched using a 0.1 M solution of APS for Cu and TMAH for Al, followed by a reactive-ion-etch (RIE) process to remove the excess graphene. The residual photoresist was then removed using acetone. A second photolithography step was then performed to define windows for the deposition of the metal contacts to the graphene. After the removal of the unwanted metal film using APS and TMAH, deposition of Ni/Au (5 nm/100 nm) films were performed using e-beam evaporation, before lift-off to define the pattern in warm acetone. The metal film protecting the surface of the graphene in the active device was subsequently removed. A schematic representation of the process flow using a Cu sacrificial layer is shown in Fig. 9.2. For devices fabricated using no sacrificial layer, steps 2, 5, 10, and 13 were not involved in the process.

2.1 AFM analysis

Atomic force microscopy (AFM) measurements of the graphene surface were obtained using a Park AFM system operating in noncontact mode. The measurements were taken across each of the nine wafers with the largest flake on each sample that allowed for a full 10 × 10 μm image to be captured to enable a direct comparison between the surface morphology of the different fabrication methods. Typical topographic images of the as-received graphene films are shown in Fig. 9.3A. The existence of residue on the graphene film can be seen from the image, which can be observed as the bright areas. These are likely to originate from the transfer of the graphene film to the SiO_2/Si substrate by the commercial supplier of the

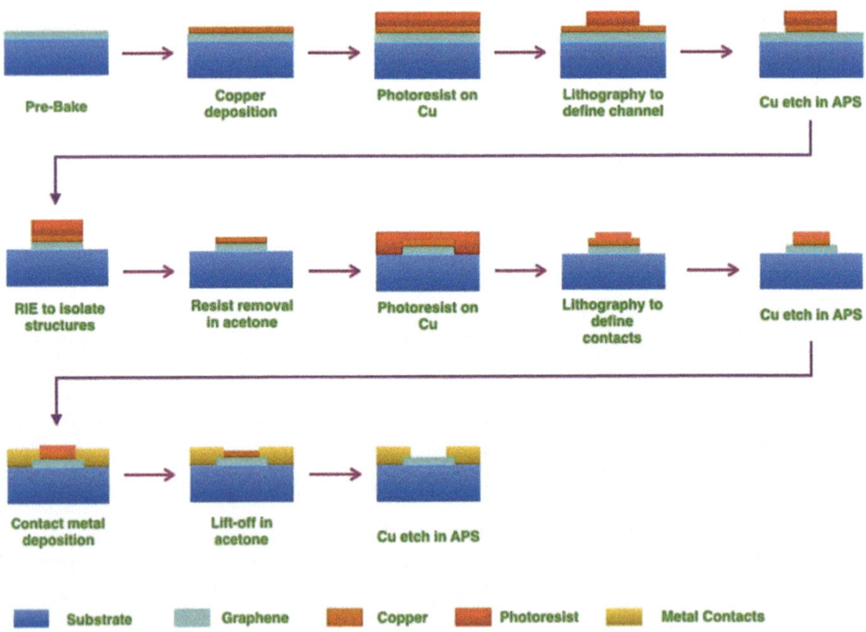

Figure 9.2 10 × 10 μm AFM topography of (A) as-received graphene films, (B) graphene films processed with no sacrificial layer, (C) Al sacrificial layer, and (D) Cu sacrificial layer [13].

graphene film. The image also shows that the film has the appearance of being continuous over the length scale investigated here, which agrees with the typical domain size for commercial CVD-grown graphene, which is typically 20 μm. The average root mean square (RMS) surface roughness across the as-received films was 2.5 ± 0.5 nm. The images in Fig. 9.3B–D show the topography of the surfaces for samples fabricated using conventional fabrication methods, an Al sacrificial layer and a Cu sacrificial layer, respectively. Considering the surface topology for the samples fabricated without a sacrificial layer, it can be seen that the majority of the graphene film has detached from the substrate, as the image shows large areas where the surface is dominated by SiO_2. The bottom right of the image shows evidence of graphene that has remained on the sample, and it shows an increase in RMS roughness of the graphene to 15.5 ± 0.6 nm. This represents an increase in roughness of over 500% in comparison to the as-received films. Fig. 9.3C shows the AFM topography of samples

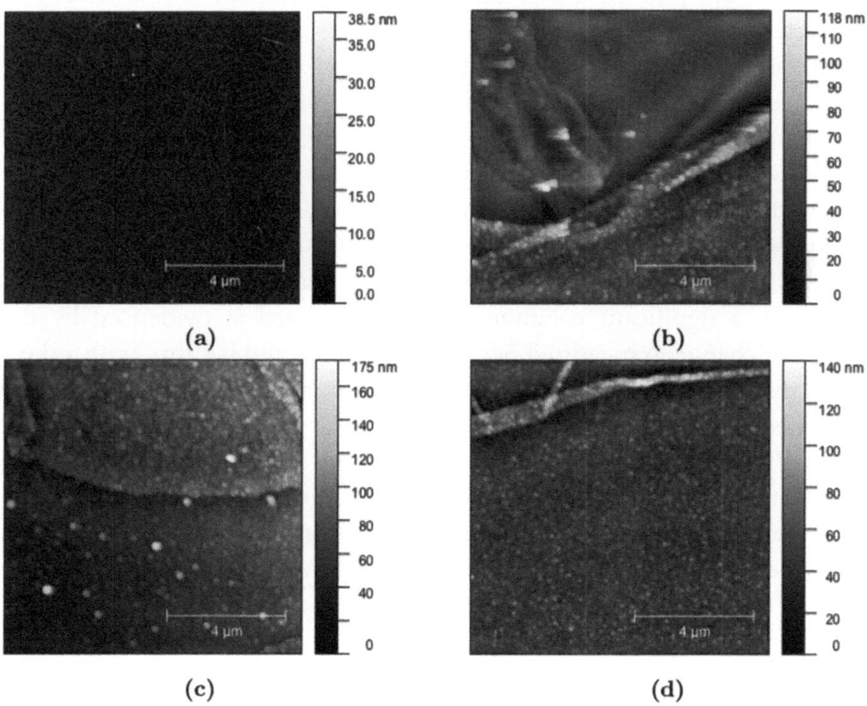

Figure 9.3 10 × 10 μm AFM topography of (A) as received graphene films, (B) graphene films processed with no sacrificial layer, (C) Al sacrificial layer, and (D) Cu sacrificial layer.

fabricated using an Al sacrificial layer; it can be seen that while this layer has reduced detachment of the graphene film, it has folded in some regions, which results in a noncontinuous film. The AFM image shows significant residue on the surface, as evidenced by the high concentration of bright features, suggesting that the Al layer has not been completely removed by the TMAH etch process. The average RMS surface roughness of the films processed using the Al sacrificial layer is found to be 17.3 ± 0.4 nm, a significant increase over the as-received film and an increase of 11.6% over the samples fabricated using conventional lithography without a sacrificial layer.

In contrast, the samples fabricated using a Cu sacrificial layer have an average surface roughness of 8.8 ± 0.2 nm, which is a significant reduction in comparison to the values reported for the no sacrificial layer and Al sacrificial layer films. The topography of the sample surface can be seen in Fig. 9.3D, with the film shown to be mostly continuous. There is still some minor cracking present in the graphene film in the upper left portion of the image; however, there is no detachment of the film from the substrate. The low density of bright features on the surface of the graphene film indicates that there are little to no copper or resist-based residues remaining on the graphene film after the removal of the copper sacrificial layer.

The corresponding height profiles of the AFM images seen in Fig. 9.3 are shown in Fig. 9.4. The data show the variation in height along a line across a 10 μm wide area of the continuous graphene films. Considering the height profile for the as-received graphene films, shown in Fig. 9.4, it can be seen that the height profile is consistent across the measured area. However, a significant roughness can be observed as evidenced by the repetitive change in measured height between 0.2 and 0.7 μm, with a short lateral displacement period. In contrast, the height profile of graphene films fabricated using no sacrificial layer and an Al sacrificial layer, shown in Fig. 9.4B and C, respectively, exhibit an overall trend in the height profile along the line of measurement. This trend is not observed in the underlying SiO_2 film in either case, so the observed behavior must arise from the graphene film, rather than the substrate. This trend may have arisen due to a number of factors, which include tears in the graphene film, a large number of residues on the surface, or nonuniform removal of the metal sacrificial layer. Finally, the height profile of samples fabricated using a Cu sacrificial layer is shown in Fig. 9.4D. It can be observed from the data that the sample shows a significant reduction in the height variability along the 10 μm line in comparison to those fabricated with either no sacrificial layer or an Al

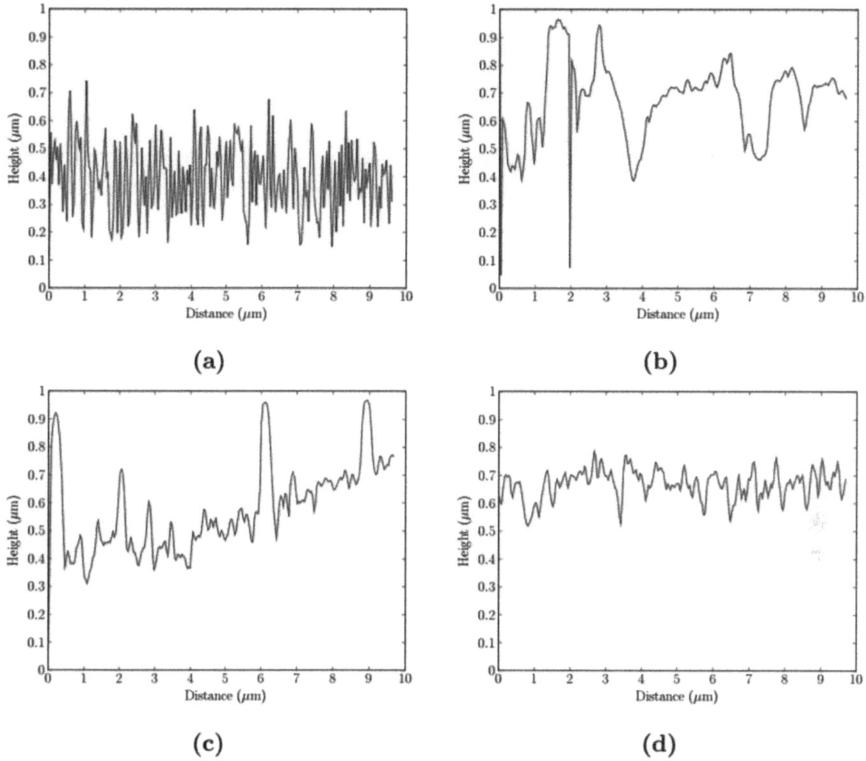

Figure 9.4 10 × 10 μm AFM topography of (A) as-received graphene films, (B) graphene films processed with no sacrificial layer, (C) Al sacrificial layer, and (D) Cu sacrificial layer [13].

sacrificial layer. Taking this into account, alongside the reduced RMS surface roughness previously described, suggests that the use of a Cu sacrificial layer results in a graphene film with a smoother surface and more continuous layer in comparison to alternative methods.

2.2 Raman spectroscopy

In addition to chemical contaminants observed on the surface during AFM analysis, exposure to the chemicals required for device fabrication can result in unwanted structural damage to the graphene film. As such, it is advantageous to be able to measure the mechanical strain in the graphene film using techniques such as Raman spectroscopy, which also allows for the mapping of strain distribution across a film. The ability to measure the mechanical strain alongside the chemical composition of the surface enables the determination as to whether a shift in Raman characteristics is due to mechanical strain in the graphene film or doping of the surface. The most prominent features of the Raman spectra for graphene are the G peak, observed at 1580/cm, and the 2D peak at 2670/cm. The Raman spectra of disordered graphene exhibit additional D and D′ peaks at approximately 1350/cm and 1620/cm, respectively. The concentration of defects in the graphene film can be determined by analyzing the ratio of the intensities of the D and G peaks, via measurement of the D/G peak ratio. The intensity of the D peak is known to increase with defect density. In addition, the ratio of the 2D to G peak intensities can be analyzed to determine the number of graphene layers, while any shifts in these peaks can be used to extract the doping of the graphene film from contaminants on the surface.

The data in Fig. 9.5 show the Raman spectra of the as-received and after device fabrication graphene films. Initially, considering the spectra of the as-received films, it can be seen that the characteristic 2D and G peaks are present at 2690/cm and 1593/cm, respectively, similar to those observed in CVD graphene films [22]. The 2D/G peak ratio of 1.1 ± 0.1 is lower than expected for high-quality monolayer graphene. In general, the intensity of the 2D peak is higher for mono-layer graphene, with values of the 2D/G ratio in excess of 2.0 typically observed in CVD graphene [22]. The spectra show evidence of an additional D peak that is located at 1350/cm, which is indicative of defects or impurities on the graphene surface. These impurities are likely left over from the wet transfer processes commonly used to transfer the CVD-grown graphene film from a catalytic metal to an insulating substrate. This process generally involves the use of organic chemicals, such as polymethylmethacrylate (PMMA), to support the graphene film during the transfer [23].

Lorentzian fitting was applied to the D peaks of the spectra and is shown in Fig. 9.6 to enable a direct comparison between the data sets to examine the influence of the different fabrication techniques on the defect density. Initially, comparing Fig. 9.6A and B, the D peak intensity extracted from this data is found to be approximately 11.5 ± 0.12 for as-received samples and 97.04 ± 0.43 for devices fabricated using no sacrificial layer, resulting in an increase in the D/G ratio from 0.03 for the as-received films, to 0.2 for devices processed using no sacrificial layer. This significant increase in the D/G ratio indicates that fabrication has introduced further defects in the graphene film, likely due to the fact that when no sacrificial layer is used, photoresist comes into direct contact with the graphene film. This results in organic contaminants on the surface that remain after the use of acetone for

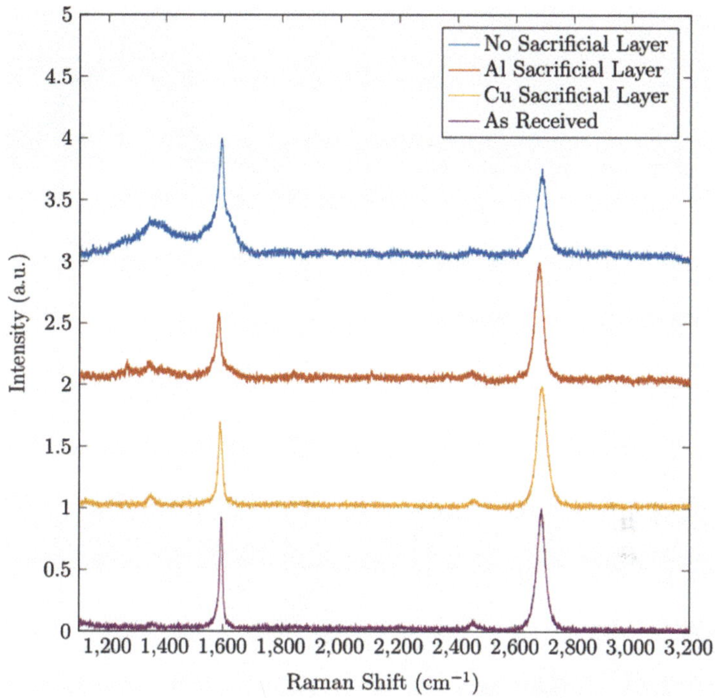

Figure 9.5 Raman spectra of as received films (*purple trace*), devices fabricated using conventional lithography (*red trace*), Al sacrificial layer (*yellow trace*), and Cu sacrificial layer (*blue trace*) [13].

photoresist removal. These contaminants introduce external scattering sites into the graphene film, which are expected to increase the transfer doping of the film and reduce the carrier mobility [24]. Additionally, it can be seen that the G peak has been red shifted from 1593/cm in the as-received film to 1591/cm. This red shift typically occurs due to the uniaxial strain in the graphene layer [25]. The origin of uniaxial strain in the sample processed using conventional photolithography is likely to be physical tears in the graphene film, resulting in the weakening of carbon bonds [26].

The Raman spectra for the graphene film processed using a Cu sacrificial layer showed a decrease in the D peak intensity in comparison to those processed using no sacrificial layer, resulting in a D/G ratio of just 0.07. In contrast, the D peak intensity for the samples that were fabricated using an Al sacrificial layer has increased to 147.6 ± 0.93, giving a D/G ratio of 0.22, similar to that of samples fabricated using no sacrificial layer. This high D/G ratio can be interpreted as an increased defect density in the graphene,

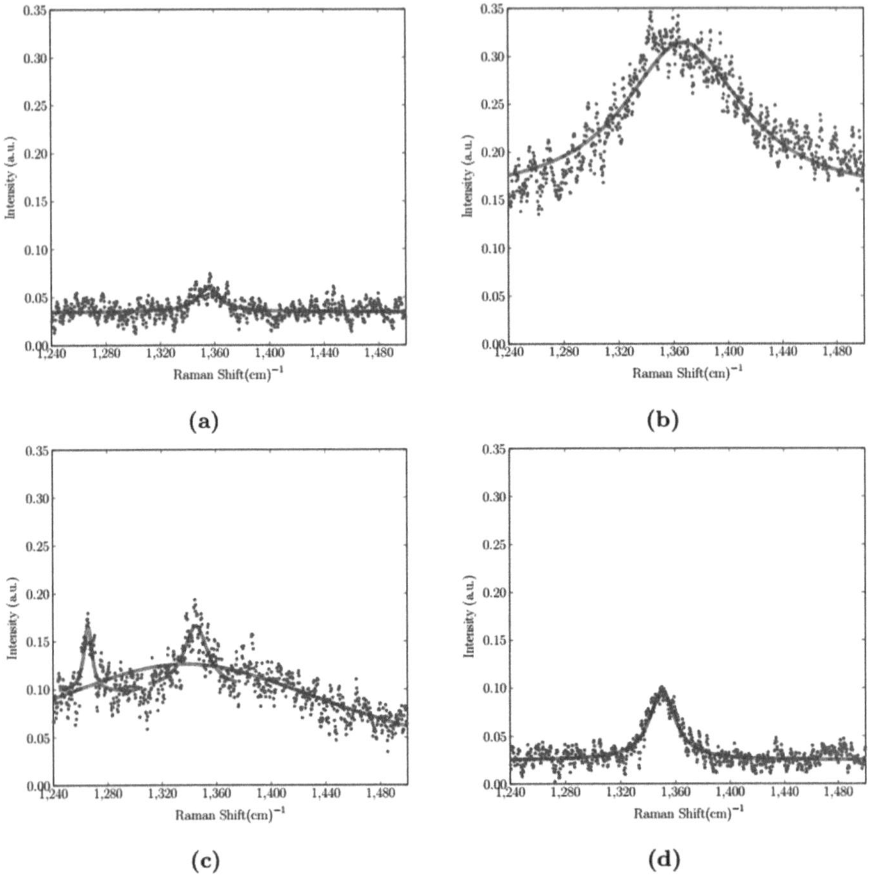

Figure 9.6 Isolated Raman D peak spectra intensity of (A) as-received films, (B) devices fabricated with no sacrificial layer, (C) Al sacrificial layer, and (D) Cu sacrificial layer.

indicating that an Al sacrificial layer either does not provide sufficient protection against resisting contaminants, or the Al layer is introducing defects to the surface, which correlates with the AFM data presented in the previous section. The data in Fig. 9.6C also show the existence of a further peak, located at around 1260/cm, which is only present in samples fabricated using an Al sacrificial layer. While it has not been possible to identify the chemical composition of this peak from reports in the literature, it is highly likely that this originates from residual Al-based species that are chemically bound to the graphene surface, most likely at defects [27]. The data show that the use of a Cu sacrificial layer significantly reduces the concentration of defects and contaminants on the graphene surface, with a

D/G ratio of 0.07, which is comparable to that of as-received graphene, which is 0.03. This suggests that, unlike the Al sacrificial layer, Cu protects the surface from organic contaminants as a result of the photolithography process and that the ammonium persulphate etch process results in negligible Cu residue on the graphene film at the conclusion of the fabrication process. The ratio of the 2D to G peak intensities is often used as a parameter to determine the number of graphene layers, with values in excess of one often being obtained for monolayer graphene films [28]. However, it is also dependent on surface doping and, as such, cannot be used as a definitive method. Nevertheless, the full width half maximum (FWHM) of the 2D peak and shift of the centroid can be used to give a more complete picture of both the number of layers in the graphene film and of the surface doping. The 2D peaks for the samples can be seen in the data in Fig. 9.7. The 2D/G ratio for the samples processed with an Al sacrificial layer is found to be 1.69 ± 0.08, while for the Cu-based samples it is 1.51 ± 0.02. For samples fabricated with no sacrificial layer, this is found to be reduced to a value of 0.73 ± 0.03. The reduction in the 2D/G peak ratio is therefore unexpected; however, studies into the Raman spectroscopic characterization of graphene have found that the 2D/G ratio is also dependent on doping of the graphene layer by the substrate or surface contaminants. Previous reports in the literature have identified that for this reason it can be difficult to accurately determine the number of graphene layers when the film has been deposited on or transferred to an insulating substrate [26].

Das et al. [29] presented data that showed the impact of hole and electron doping on the 2D/G ratio, the result of which is shown in Fig. 9.8. Correlating the extracted shifts in 2D/G ratio to this data, it is possible to estimate the shift in sheet dopant concentration. Using the 2D/G ratio of as-received films (taken to be 1.1 as a starting point), it is estimated that when using no sacrificial layer the carrier concentration is shifted by approximately $1.5 \times 10^{13}/cm^2$. This could be either an increase or decrease in the carrier concentration depending if the dopant is n- or p-type. This shift is reduced to approximately $1.0 \times 10^{13}/cm^2$ when using an Al sacrificial layer and even further to $0.6 \times 10^{13}/cm^2$ when using a Cu sacrificial layer. This suggests that the use of a Cu sacrificial layer reduces doping of the surface by approximately 60% in comparison to devices fabricated using no sacrificial layer. As the 2D/G ratio is heavily influenced by doping in the graphene film, the FWHM of the 2D peaks can also be evaluated to accurately determine the number of graphene layers. This metric has been

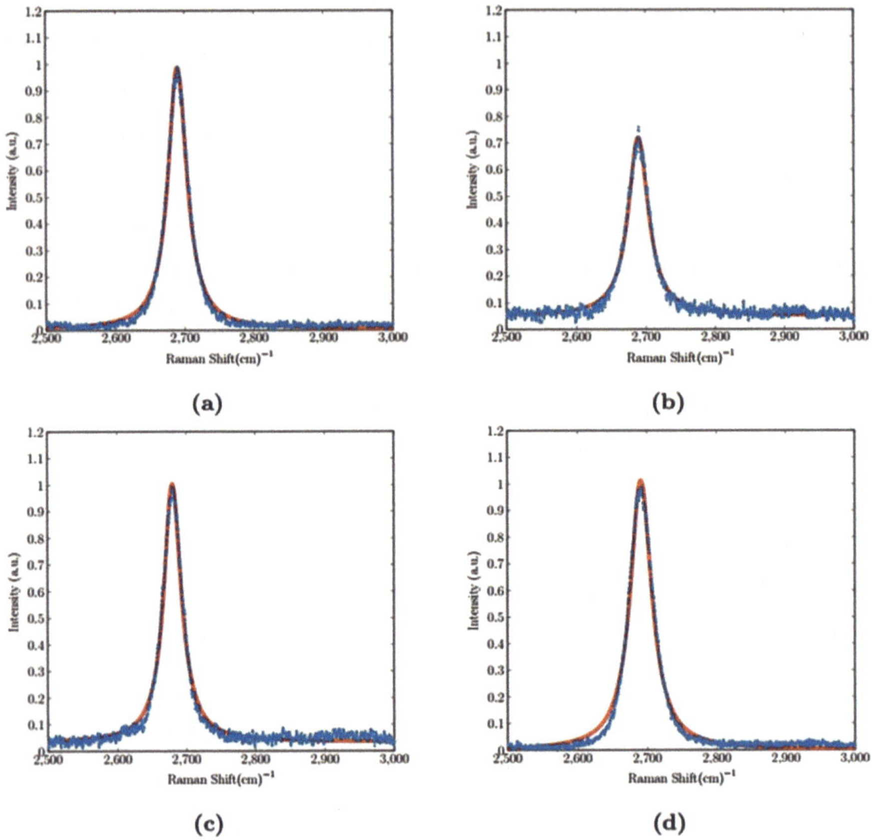

Figure 9.7 Isolated 2D peak intensity of (A) as-received films, (B) devices fabricated with no sacrificial layer, (C) Al sacrificial layer, and (D) Cu sacrificial layer [13].

shown to increase by a factor of two when the graphene transitions from single to bilayer form [30]. The isolated 2D peak intensities are shown in Fig. 9.7 with the FWHM of the peaks subsequently extracted from this data. The extracted FWHM for the as-received graphene yields a value of 37.00 ± 0.30/cm. For graphene devices fabricated using standard lithography this value increases to 39.00 ± 0.37/cm, for the Al sacrificial layer it reduces to 34.00 ± 0.03/cm, and for the Cu sacrificial layer it remains the same at 37.00 ± 0.03/cm. This suggests that the number of layers remains consistent across the samples, with the variation in the 2D/G ratio likely due to doping effects.

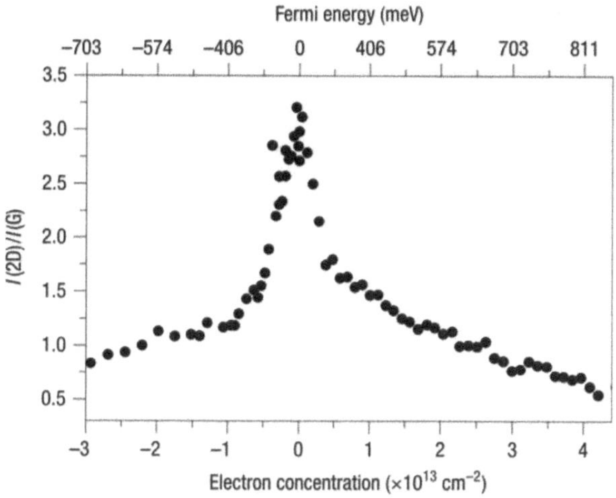

Figure 9.8 The influence of electron doping on the 2D and G peak intensity of graphene films [29].

2.3 Electrical characterization

Two-terminal measurements have been used to determine the variation in graphene sheet resistance versus process conditions on two-terminal test structures. The resulting current–voltage characteristics are shown in Fig. 9.9. For devices fabricated using conventional lithography, it can be seen that the channel is highly resistive in comparison to that of pristine graphene that typically has resistance values in the 100–200 Ω/□ range [31].

This is likely due to surface contaminants and a noncontinuous graphene film. Comparatively, devices fabricated using Al and Cu sacrificial layers have a significantly reduced resistance, although the *I–V* characteristics of the Al devices are shown to be nonlinear. This could be due to residues on the surface that unintentionally dope the graphene layer [32,33], or an unusually high contact resistance that is common in graphene devices fabricated using optical lithography [34].

The explanation of unintentional doping of the graphene layer is supported by the Raman spectroscopy results shown in Fig. 9.5, with the increased defect density, observed with the Al device results correlating with the suggestion that there is residue present on the graphene surface. Two terminal measurements alone, however, are not an accurate method for determining the sheet resistance across the graphene film as these

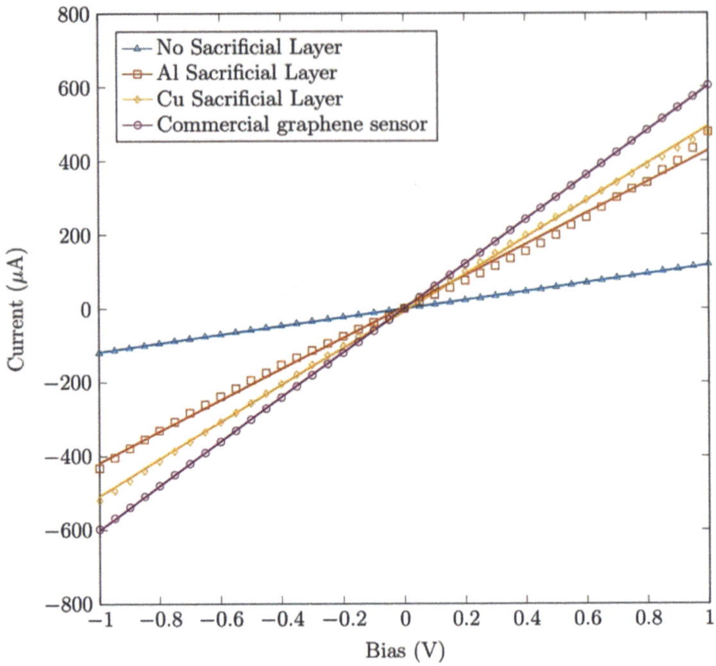

Figure 9.9 *I*—*V* characteristics of four terminal Hall structures of as-received commercial devices, along with those fabricated using no sacrificial layer, Al sacrificial layer, and Cu sacrificial layer [13].

measurements do not remove the influence of the contact resistance, with the total resistance given by Ref. [35]:

$$R_T = R_{Gr} + 2R_C \tag{9.1}$$

where R_{Gr} is the resistance of the graphene film in Ohms and R_C is the contact resistance in Ohms.

The TLM is a two-probe technique that is commonly used to extract the contact resistance, sheet resistance, and the transfer length characteristics of metal interfaces. A TLM test structure consists of a series of metal electrodes patterned in a resistor network, as can be seen in Fig. 9.10A. These electrodes are separated by a varying channel length, L_{Ch}, with the width (W) and length (L) of each contact remaining fixed. The total resistance is then measured between adjacent metal contacts and can be described by

$$R_T = R_{Sh}(L_{Ch} / W) + 2RC \tag{9.2}$$

where R_{Sh} is the sheet resistance of the graphene film in $\Omega/\square$, L_{Ch} the channel length in μm, and W the contact width in μm.

By plotting the measured total resistance as a function of the channel length, both R_C and R_{Sh} can be extracted from the resulting linear fit of the experimental data. An example of such a plot is shown in Fig. 9.10. It can be seen that R_{Sh} can be extracted from the slope of the linear fit while RC can be extracted from the y-intercept. However, this method relies on the assumption that the sheet resistance underneath the contact is equal to the value between the contacts. In graphene, this is not the case with carrier concentration in the film underneath the contact typically dependent on the type of contact metal used. This can lead to a different density of states underneath the metal contact in comparison to that of the channel areas resulting in a significant variation in sheet resistance [36]. This often results in nonlinear behavior, and the low repeatability of measurements meaning an accurate value of sheet and contact resistance is difficult to quantify.

TLM measurements were initially carried out on samples using both no sacrificial layer and an Al sacrificial layer. However, due to the low yield and damage to the TLM structures that occurred during processing, a representative dataset could not be extracted. TLM measurements shown were therefore extracted from samples fabricated using a Cu sacrificial layer only. These results, however, show the difficulty of using TLM structures to isolate the contact and sheet resistance in 2D materials. The data in Fig. 9.11 show the resulting TLM plot from measurements on Cu sacrificial layer devices. The nonlinearity of the extracted total resistance as a function of channel length is evident from these results. In addition to the issues with TLM measurements in 2D materials described previously, such as the different density of states underneath the contact area, the nonuniform

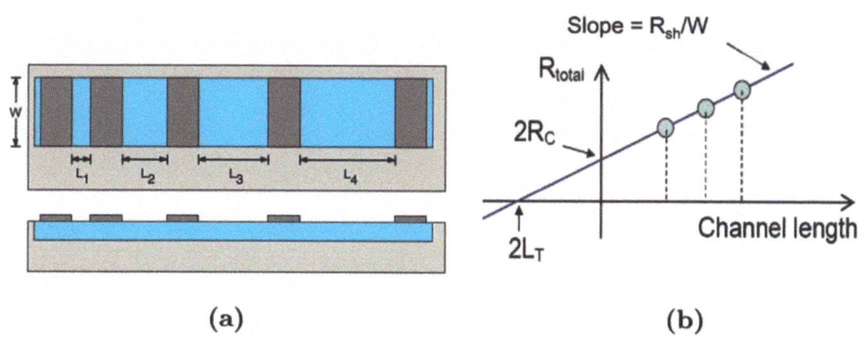

Figure 9.10 (A) Schematic diagram of a typical TLM test structure and (B) TLM plot of total resistance as a function of channel length [9].

quality of the graphene layer across the channel described in previous sections can also contribute to this nonlinearity.

Nonetheless by excluding the data point at 40 μm as an outlier, there is a linear region present between 20 and 45 μm, which allows for the extraction of both contact and sheet resistance. Extrapolation of this line gives a value of 29 Ω for the contact resistance and 1.63 kΩ/□ for the sheet resistance. Initially, the sheet resistance value extracted appears accurate. However, the contact resistance value extracted from this is lower than expected although it has been reported with Ni electrodes on graphene previously [36]. Unfortunately, the small number of data points available for extrapolation in the linear region makes it difficult to assess the validity of these results. This also represents an issue when it comes to result in reproducibility, with extracted values varying significantly across a wafer. Due to the difficulties encountered in separating the contact resistance from sheet resistance, Van Der Pauw (VDP) structures were employed to extract more accurate sheet resistance values. While this does not allow for the

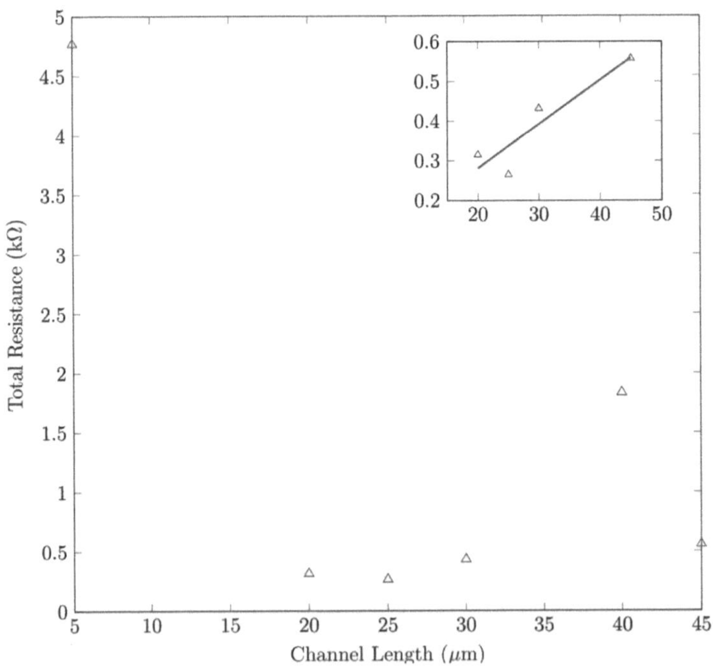

Figure 9.11 TLM plot of devices fabricated using a Cu sacrificial layer showing total resistance as a function of channel length with the linear region shown in the inset [13].

separation of contact resistance from the sheet resistance, this method minimizes the influence of metal contacts on the measured resistance value allowing for a more accurate determination of overall sheet resistance and any electrical parameters extracted. The resulting sheet resistances extracted using this method are summarized in Table 9.2.

2.4 Hall effect measurements

Hall measurements were performed on fabricated devices to extract critical electrical parameters including sheet carrier density and carrier mobility. They also give a good indication of how the sensor performs in comparison to commercial devices. Schematic diagrams of the Hall structures used to perform these measurements are shown in Fig. 9.12.

The data in Fig. 9.13A show the normalized Hall resistance (R_{Hall}-$R_{Hall(0)}$) as a function of magnetic field for devices fabricated using no sacrificial layer, an Al sacrificial layer, and a Cu sacrificial layer with a fixed current of 3 mA. The sensors are shown to demonstrate highly linear behavior with an R^2 value of >0.99, comparable to graphene devices reported in the literature and even that of commercially available devices [37]. The Hall resistance is normalized as a function of the Hall resistance at zero fields to demonstrate the impact of offset shifting on device characteristics, with devices fabricated using a Cu sacrificial layer showing the highest level of offset shifting. The current-related sensitivity can additionally be extracted from the gradient of Fig. 9.13B, which shows the Hall voltage as a function of the magnetic field. It is defined as the ratio of the change in Hall voltage to the change in the multiple of magnetic field and current bias, given by the equation: $S_I = V_H/BI$.

As shown by the data in Fig. 9.13B, devices fabricated using both no sacrificial layer and an Al sacrificial layer are shown to exhibit a similar magnitude of response in the region of 20–40 mV, although devices fabricated using no sacrificial layer have a slightly increased current related sensitivity (32 V/AT in comparison to 17 V/AT for devices fabricated using an Al sacrificial layer). Comparatively, devices fabricated using a Cu sacrificial layer exhibit a significantly increased magnitude of response, with a current related sensitivity of 165 V/AT. Extracted current-related sensitivities for devices fabricated using the Cu sacrificial layer are also shown to be increased over that of commercially available CVD graphene devices tested in this study (58 V/AT) although they still remain lower than that of graphene devices previously reported in the literature [38–40]. These

Table 9.2 Electrical properties of graphene devices compared to commercial devices.[a]

	R_{SH} (Ω/□)	n_s (cm^{-2})	SI (V/AT)	μ ($cm^2V^{-1}s^{-1}$)	Yield (%)
No sacrificial layer	1100 ± 2200	$1.9 \pm 0.38 \times 10^{13}$	32.4 ± 6.4	1200 ± 240	12
Al sacrificial layer	1300 ± 455	$7.0 \pm 2.5 \times 10^{13}$	17 ± 5.9	1022 ± 358	25
Cu sacrificial layer	800 ± 80	$3.8 \pm 0.38 \times 10^{12}$	165 ± 16.5	2057 ± 206	82
Commercial devices	1200 ± 180	$1.0 \pm 0.15 \times 10^{13}$	58 ± 8.7	1290 ± 194	75

[a]Data extracted from Fig. 9.31.

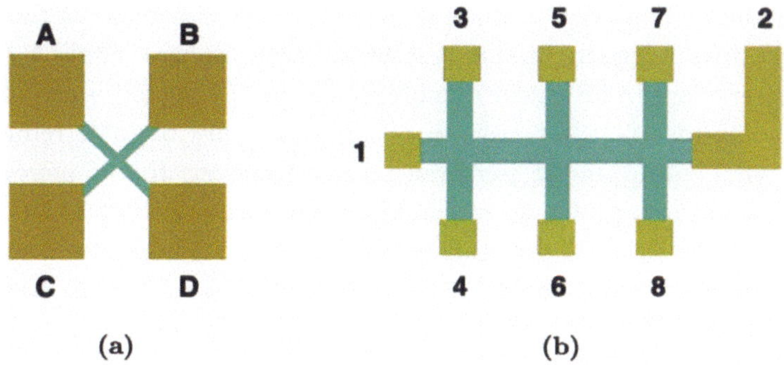

Figure 9.12 Schematic diagrams of (A) four terminal Hall structures and (B) eight terminal Hall structures used in this study [13].

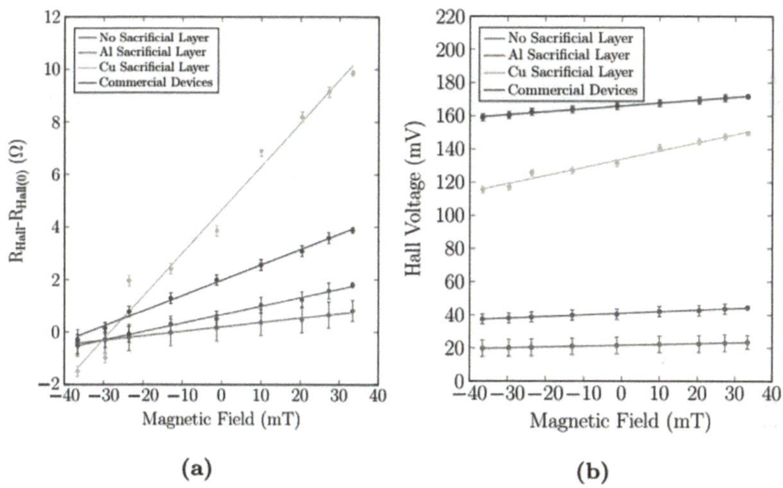

Figure 9.13 Hall effect measurements showing (A) Hall resistance normalized by the offset and (B) Hall voltage as a function of the magnetic field with a fixed current bias of 3 mA for commercial devices, devices fabricated using no sacrificial layer, Cu sacrificial layer, and Al sacrificial layer [13].

devices have reported sensitivities of >1000 V/AT. However, this is largely due to the external biasing of the graphene film to allow for Dirac point operation. As such it is expected that through external gate biasing the sensitivity limit of devices fabricated in this study can be explored further. Comparatively, Hall effect devices available commercially are typically limited to sensitivities of <100 V/AT [41].

Offset shifting at zero applied field is the potential difference exhibited in the graphene film with electric current flow in the absence of an external magnetic field. This offset is undesirable as it limits the ability of the sensor to detect low magnetic fields. Offset shifting at zero applied field is exhibited in Fig. 9.13B, most notably in devices fabricated with no sacrificial layer with an offset voltage of approximately 39 mV, reduced to 21 mV when using an Al sacrificial layer. However, this is increased to 120 mV when using a Cu sacrificial layer and even further to 160 mV for commercial devices. This could be attributed to the increased current-related sensitivity exhibited in these devices. As such, it is important to use these parameters to extract the offset equivalent magnetic field for a more accurate comparison of device performance. The offset equivalent magnetic field, defined as the ratio of offset voltage to absolute sensitivity, can be determined using equations:

$$S_A = V_H/B \text{ and } B_{off} = V_{off}/S_A, \tag{9.3}$$

where B_{off} is the offset equivalent magnetic field in Tesla, V_{off} the offset voltage in Volts, and S_A the absolute sensitivity of the Hall structure in V/T.

This is a critical parameter to consider as reducing the offset equivalent magnetic field leads to improvements in device sensitivity and result reproducibility [42]. This yields values of 0.39 and 0.42 T, respectively, for devices fabricated using no sacrificial layer and an Al sacrificial layer. Both fabrication methods are shown to be comparable with regards to magnetic field offset, with the resulting uncertainty being too large to determine whether devices with lower current-related sensitivity (those fabricated using Al sacrificial layer) do, in fact, exhibit a larger offset equivalent magnetic field. To investigate this further, samples fabricated using a Cu sacrificial layer were investigated.

The offset equivalent magnetic field is found to be reduced by approximately 40% to 0.24 T for samples fabricated using a Cu sacrificial layer despite having a larger offset voltage, largely due to the higher current-related sensitivity. Commercial devices, however, exhibit an anomalously high offset magnetic field of 0.9 T, the origin of this offset is not evidentially clear but it is often described in the literature as being a direct result of contact misalignment [43]. To investigate this further, it is pertinent to consider other critical electronic properties of the fabricated graphene films. These can also be extracted from the data in Fig. 9.13A with the resultant parameters shown in Table 9.2. Both the sheet carrier density and carrier mobility can be further extracted from Fig. 9.13B according to equations:

$$\mu = R_H / R_{SH} \tag{9.4}$$

and

$$R_H = 1/ne \tag{9.5}$$

where R_H is the Hall coefficient in m^2/C^{-1}, which can be extracted by converting the current related sensitivity from mks to cgs units ($\times$ 10^4) and R_{SH} the sheet resistance in $\Omega/\square$, where e is the charge of an electron (1.6×10^{-19} C).

These data are summarized in Table 9.2 alongside the sheet resistance data extracted using the VDP method described previously. A key trend that can be seen from these data are that higher carrier mobility and reduced sheet carrier density result in an increase in the current-related sensitivity of devices. The sheet resistance is also reduced in devices with higher current-related sensitivity. It can be seen that this occurs when devices are fabricated using a Cu sacrificial layer. The reduced carrier mobility exhibited when fabricating devices with no sacrificial layer, and an Al sacrificial layer suggests that these processes have introduced scattering sites into the graphene film, limiting mobility. Remarkably, fabrication of devices through the use of a Cu sacrificial layer is shown to provide not only an improvement in electrical characteristics over those fabricated with no sacrificial layer and an Al sacrificial layer but over those fabricated commercially. The most notable difference in results is the dramatic increase in device yield when using a Cu sacrificial layer—increasing from just 12% when using no sacrificial layer to 82%. This is particularly advantageous in the use of wafer-scale processing as it significantly reduces the cost of the final sensor. The use of an Al sacrificial layer does slightly increase yield to approximately 25%; however, this is still not high enough for wafer-scale processing using this technique to be viable. It should be noted that, in this study, a working device is defined as a Hall sensor that produces a potential difference across two terminals when a current bias is applied to the adjacent terminals and is also responsive to changes in a magnetic field.

In addition to the significant increase in yield, a critical parameter to consider when fabricating devices is reproducibility. In graphene processing, this is a particular issue due to the sensitivity of the graphene film to contaminants introduced during lithographic processing. The variability of devices fabricated has been quantified by extracting the sheet resistance of devices across each 1 × 1 cm die. The data in Fig. 9.14 show a box plot of device sheet resistances for devices fabricated using a Cu sacrificial layer, an Al sacrificial layer, and no sacrificial layer. From these data, it can be seen that devices fabricated using an Al sacrificial layer exhibit the largest variability (approximately 40% spread) in characteristics across a wafer whereas the variability across Cu sacrificial layer devices is significantly reduced to as low as 10%. The variability of devices fabricated using a Cu sacrificial layer is also shown to be slightly reduced to that of commercially available graphene devices that exhibit a spread in characteristics of 15%. This corresponds to the data previously shown that the use of a Cu sacrificial layer improves the protection of the surface during fabrication and reduces the introduction of dopants during these processes.

Overall, both the surface analysis and electrical characterization of graphene devices fabricated in this section strongly suggest that the use of a Cu sacrificial layer offers an improved surface quality of the graphene film and enhances the electrical characteristics of the final device. While devices fabricated using a Cu sacrificial layer are found to be comparable to that of commercially available bulk semiconductor and graphene devices, the current-related sensitivity and mobilities observed remain lower than that of some graphene devices described in the literature.

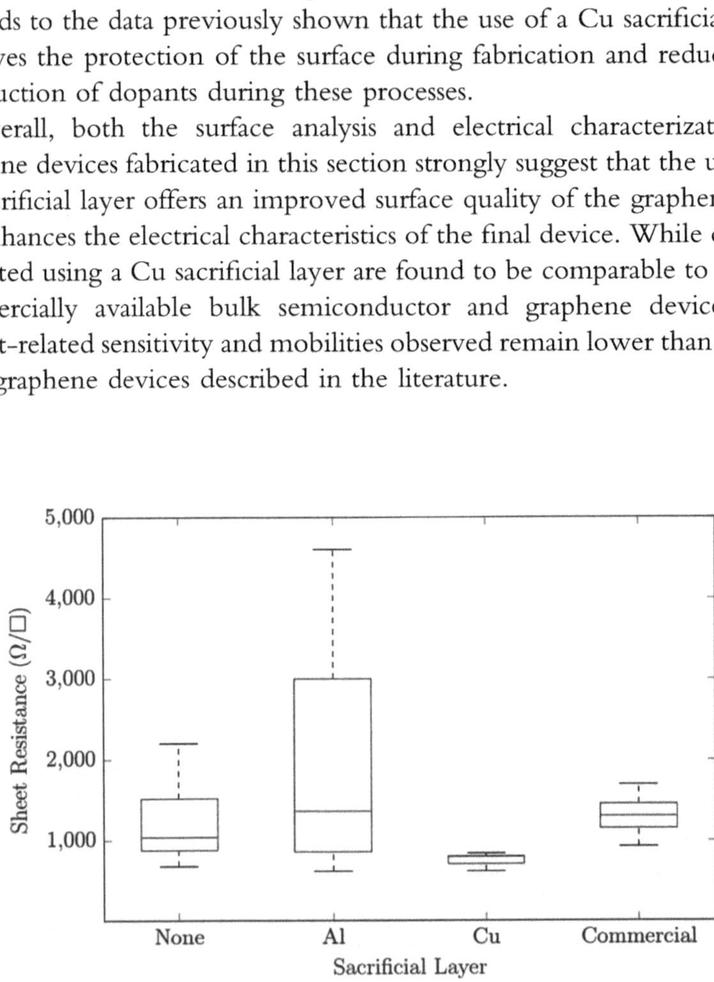

Figure 9.14 Variability of sheet resistance across a wafer for devices fabricated using no sacrificial layer, an Al sacrificial layer, a Cu sacrificial layer, and as-received commercial devices.

3. Surface functionalization

The surface functionalization of graphene basal planes is challenging. This is because each carbon atom in graphene has a p_z orbital in the direction perpendicular to the basal plane, forming a self-passivating π-conjugated system with a highly delocalized network [44]. Attaching functional species to such a thermodynamically stable and chemically inert structure requires controlled modification techniques with high-energy reactants that can break the carbon—carbon π bonds and distort the surrounding lattice without damaging the carbon—carbon σ bonds of graphene. In principle, graphene can be functionalized using two approaches: (a) noncovalent functionalization and (b) covalent functionalization [45—48]. Noncovalent functionalization offers the possibility of attaching functional groups without disrupting the structural properties of graphene [49,50]. Here, the adsorbed molecules interact with the π-electrons of graphene, resulting in a change in electronic and chemical properties of the graphene due to the charge transfer process [50]. The nature of the charge transfer, or the doping magnitude, depends on the electronic nature of the graphene surface and the chemical nature of the analyte being tested. For instance, negative surface charges on epitaxial graphene are expected to attract positive-charged poles of molecules, which strongly adsorb to graphene. This strong interaction leads to charge transfer between the adsorbed analyte and graphene, which greatly affects its charge carrier concentration depending on the analyte type [48,51]. Although this noncovalent functionalization approach preserves the structural properties of graphene, the long-term stability of adsorbed functional groups is an important issue [52] where, due to their weak binding nature with the graphene surface, these physisorbed functional groups desorb when the graphene device is operated under high bias or operated continuously for several cycles. In contrast, covalent functionalization is relatively more stable due to the strong bonding of functional groups with the graphene surface [49,52]. Highly reactive species such as hydrogen, fluorine, chlorine, and oxygen are commonly used for covalent functionalization [47,53,54], which have sufficient energy to overcome the kinetic and thermodynamic barriers associated with the covalent chemical reactions on the graphene basal plane. To make covalent bonding possible, the carbon atoms in graphene change their hybridization from sp^2 to sp^3 as shown in Fig. 9.15 [55], which leads to the opening of a band gap [56,57]. This transformation not only affects the sp^3 carbon atom that undergoes the reaction but also creates geometric distortion that extends over multiple lattice positions [55]. While hydrogenation, fluorination, and chlorination of graphene exhibit interesting chemical and electrical properties, oxidation of graphene is particularly attractive for a wide range of applications. For example, oxygen functionalization can induce strong photoluminescence behavior in single-layer graphene [58], which could be utilized for realizing graphene-based optoelectronic devices. In addition, oxygen functionalization induces p-type doping in graphene due to the highly electronegative nature of oxygen (3.5), in comparison to carbon (2.3), leading to charge transfer from graphene to the adsorbed oxygen species. This is significant because the as-grown epitaxial graphene on the Si-face of SiC is highly n-doped and, to reduce this intrinsic n-type character, oxygen functionalization is necessary. Apart from changing the polarity, oxygen functional groups were also found to induce a band gap in single-layer graphene [59,60]. The DFT simulations in Fig. 9.16 show the change in Density of States (DOS) for Single Layer Graphene (SLG) and Bi-Layer Graphene (BLG) with epoxy and hydroxyl configurations [59]. It is known that SLG is a zero-bandgap semiconductor with vanishing DOS at E_F. However, the chemisorption of oxygen atoms strongly affects the electronic structure of SLG, in which the increase in epoxy functional group density creates a bandgap of ~1.5 eV [59,60]. This bandgap increases with the increasing concentration of epoxy functional groups and reaches 3.2 eV at 50% oxygen coverage. In contrast,

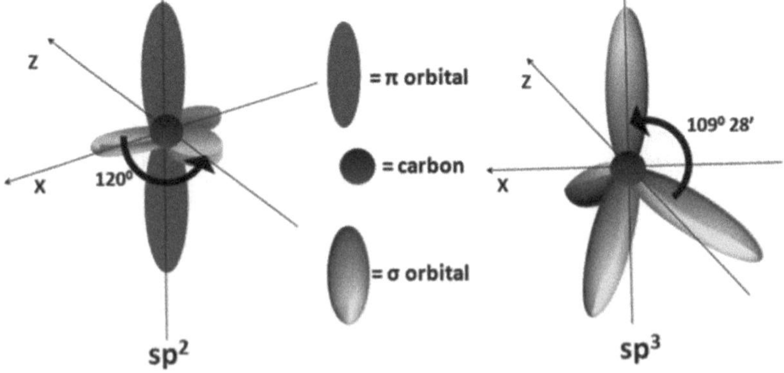

Figure 9.15 Transformation of sp^2 hybridization to sp^3 hybridization upon functionalizing graphene with reactive chemical species [55].

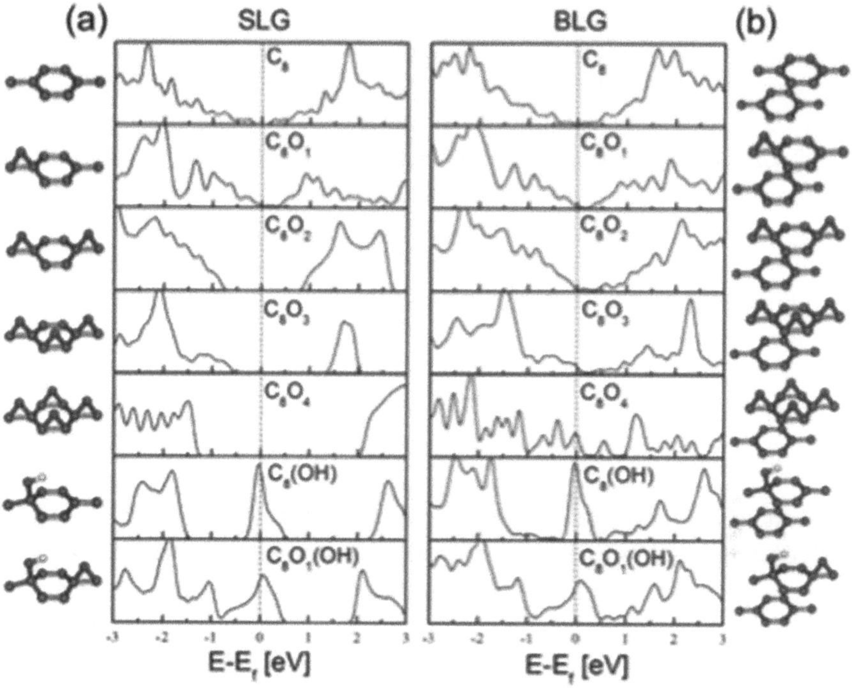

Figure 9.16 Evolution of the band structures of (A) SLG and (B) BLG with surface O-functional groups [59].

as shown in Fig. 9.16, O-functionalization did not induce a bandgap in BLG and, hence, retains its characteristic semimetallic behavior.

The presence of polar oxygen functional groups converts the highly hydrophobic nature of graphene to more hydrophilic in character [8]. Fig. 9.17 summarizes the contact angle measurements of graphene under different conditions. Firstly, the contact angle of water on 6H–SiC before graphene growth was measured as 69.3 degrees. After the growth of epitaxial graphene, the contact angle increased to as high as 92.5 degrees,

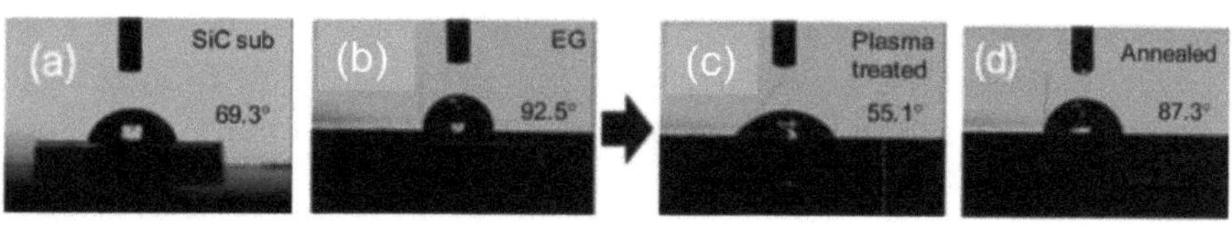

Figure 9.17 Contact angle measurements of (A) 6H–SiC substrate, (B) epitaxial graphene on SiC, (C) oxygen plasma-treated epitaxial graphene, and (D) after annealing plasma-treated graphene [8].

indicating the hydrophobic nature of as-grown graphene. However, immediately after oxygen functionalization the contact angle decreased to 55.1 degrees, demonstrating the change in the hydrophobic nature of graphene to more hydrophilic in character. Such hydrophilic behavior is crucial for the wetting of metal films on graphene, where oxygen functional groups significantly improve the adhesion strength of deposited metal contacts, thereby eliminating metal delamination issues [8]. It was also shown that by annealing this O-functionalized sample at 300°C in ultrahigh vacuum (UHV) for 30 min, the intrinsic hydrophobic nature of graphene can be recovered with a contact angle of 87.3 degrees, indicating no significant damage to the graphene occurred as a result of the O-functionalization process [10]. It was further reported that the presence of oxygen at the metal—graphene interface significantly enhances the thermal transport across the metal—graphene interface, enabling efficient heat transport to the surrounding device architecture [61].

Three main experimental routes have been developed to oxidize graphene. The first method involves direct oxidation of graphene using strong oxidants such as concentrated sulfuric acid, nitric acid, and potassium permanganate [62]. The second method is the most popular and commonly employed approach using aggressive acidic solutions based on the modified Hummer's method [63], where the graphite layers are oxidized first, followed by exfoliation into two-dimensional graphene oxide (GO). The third approach is the oxygen plasma technique [64], which involves exposing graphene to energetic oxygen radicals at either room or high temperatures for covalent attachment of O-functional groups onto the graphene surface.

Although synthesizing GO using wet-chemical methods is relatively easy and inexpensive, the resultant GO material is chemically inhomogeneous, electrically insulating, and structurally defective due to the extensive use of harsh acidic treatments [65,66]. To reduce the insulating nature of GO, strong acids and/or several hours of high-temperature thermal annealing are commonly employed to reduce the concentration of O-functional groups on the graphene surface [65].

Nevertheless, these reduced GO (rGO) films still suffer from inferior electrical properties due to the destruction of graphene lattice as a result of harsh treatment conditions. Fig. 9.18 shows high-resolution X-ray Photoelectron Spectroscopy (XPS) spectra of the evolution of the surface chemical composition of GO when subjected to high temperature annealing in UHV [65]. It is therefore very challenging to control the type

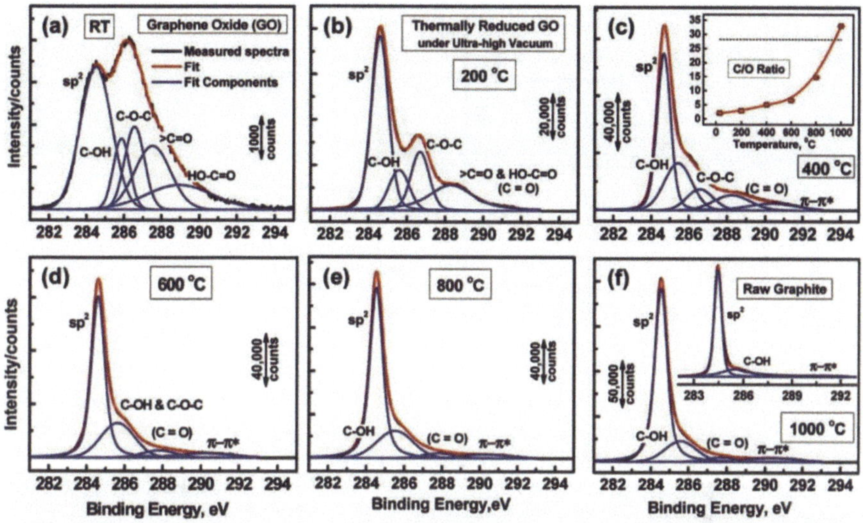

Figure 9.18 XPS C1s spectra of (A) as-synthesized GO, (B) thermally reduced GO in UHV at 200°C (C), and (D), (E), and (F) reduction of oxygen functional groups with the increasing annealing temperature to up to 1000°C [65].

and concentration of functional group(s) present on the graphene surface using wet chemical functionalization techniques.

Although plasma functionalization, to be discussed later in this chapter, is a promising approach for the selective modification of graphene surfaces, the aggressive nature of plasmas usually results in the etching of the graphene film [67,68]. For instance, as shown in Fig. 9.19, even for an extremely low plasma power (5 W) and very short exposure time (5 s) time, a significant increase in the defect peak (D-peak) was observed along with a new D′ peak as a shoulder to G peak. After 80 s of exposure, the 2D-peak, which represents the sp^2 bonding in graphene, has completely vanished, indicating etching of the graphene film. This irreversible damage to the graphene lattice is enhanced by the presence of higher energy ions such as $O^{+}{}_2$ that can sputter carbonaceous material. The destruction in the graphene lattice was further confirmed by the electrical characteristics of the graphene film, in which the sheet resistance increased by more than three orders of magnitude for just 20 s of plasma exposure, making it highly insulating in character. For electronic applications, specifically electronic sensor applications that rely on the changes in resistivity of the graphene film, low sheet resistances along with no appreciable damage to the graphene lattice are required.

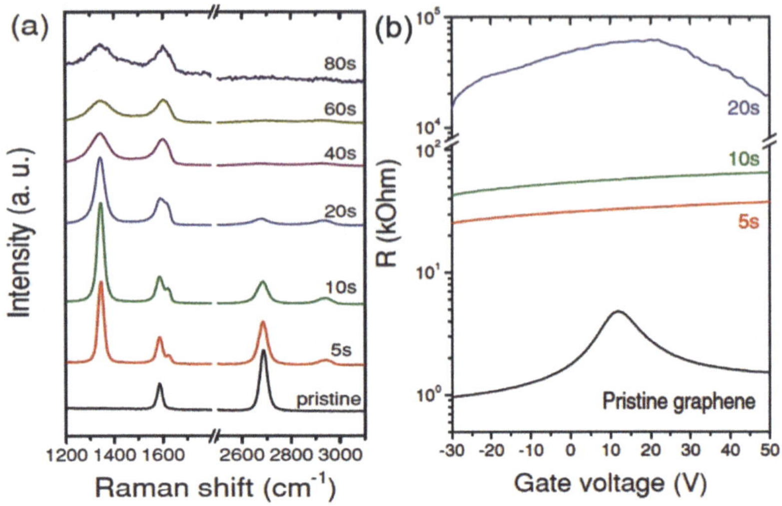

Figure 9.19 (A) Evolution of the Raman spectra of single-layer graphene upon oxygen functionalization with varying functionalization times. (B) The corresponding electrical characteristics of the functionalized graphene [67].

Hosseini et al. [69] demonstrated that the etching of graphene films can be significantly suppressed by performing functionalization in a UHV atmosphere with thermally cracked atomic oxygen instead of plasmas. In this study, epitaxial graphene grown on 6H–SiC (0001) was exposed to atomic oxygen species, which resulted in homogeneous coverage of only one type of functional group (epoxide), bonded to the graphene surface. This was observed by scanning tunneling microscopy (STM) imaging, which showed a random distribution of chemisorbed oxygen species that appeared as bright protrusions in Fig. 9.20B and C and was further confirmed by Auger and XPS. Such protrusions are characteristic of epoxy oxygen atoms lying out of the graphene plane as depicted in Fig. 9.20D. These chemisorbed epoxy functional groups are completely reversible by thermal annealing the sample at 260°C as shown in Fig. 9.20E and F, without significantly disturbing the intrinsic graphene lattice structure [69].

Various studies have been performed to modify the intrinsic chemical, electronic, and optical properties of graphene, using reactive species such as hydrogen, fluorine, oxygen, and chlorine [31,70–72]. Oxygen functionalization has attracted enormous attention because of its rich and complex chemical reactions with graphene that results in the formation of multiple covalent carbon–oxygen chemical bonds, transforming its hydrophobic

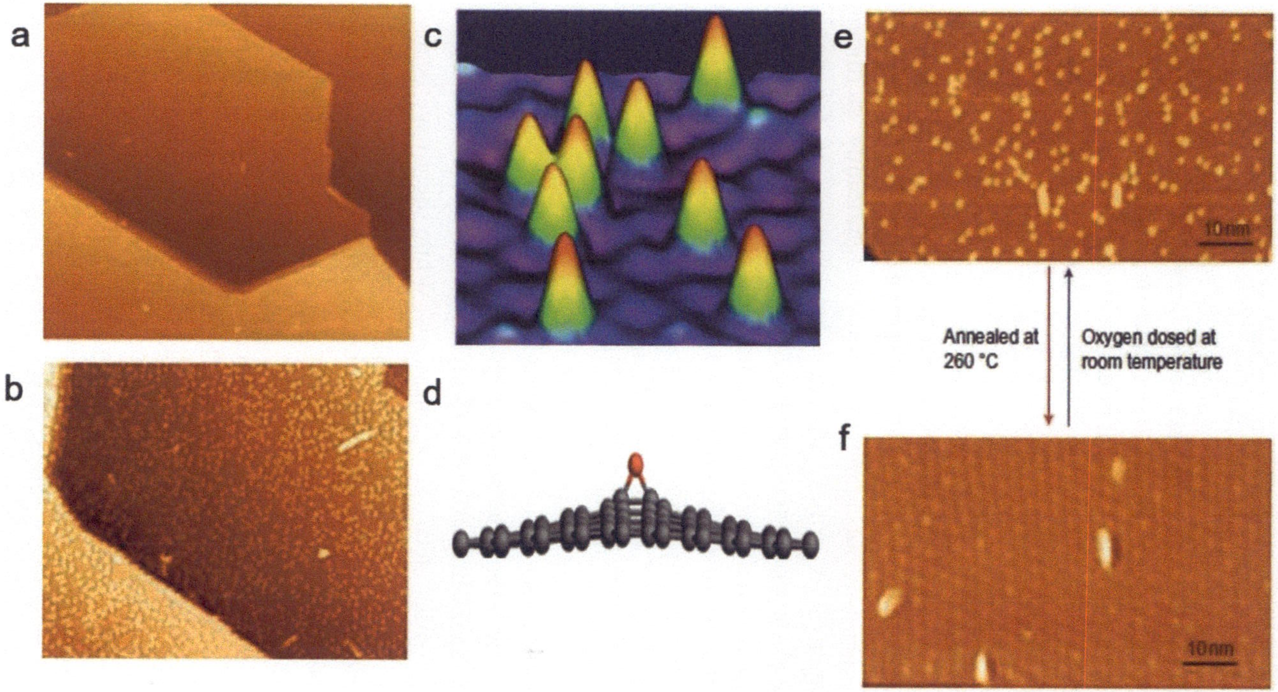

Figure 9.20 STM topography image of epitaxial graphene (A) before and (B) after oxygen functionalization; (C) STM protrusions showing the epoxy-functional groups. (D) Schematic illustration of the epoxy-functional group bonded to the graphene surface (E) and (F) functionalization and the annealing induced recovery of the graphene [36,69].

nature to more hydrophilic in character. Such oxygen functionalized graphene surfaces were shown to be highly promising for chemical and biological sensing [73,74], nonvolatile memories [75], and optoelectronic applications [68]. As discussed, the functionalization process also significantly degrades the intrinsic properties of graphene due to the reactive nature of O-functional groups. For example, it was shown that O-functionalization increases the graphene sheet resistance by several orders of magnitude, while the mobility decreases by three orders of magnitude even for mild functionalization conditions [68,70].

As graphene-based applications, such as chemical sensors, rely on the change in electrical resistance induced by adsorbed analyte molecules, maintaining low sheet resistance is crucial for maximizing the sensor response. Hence, identifying functionalization techniques that can modify the surface chemistry of graphene without significantly sacrificing its intrinsic properties is critical for the development of functionalized graphene-based electronic applications. Also of great interest is the effect of functionalization on the electrical characteristics of metal/graphene interfaces. As the use of O-functionalized graphene films in electronic applications inevitably requires metal contacts, it is critical to understand the electrical properties of metal/O-functionalized graphene interfaces. The performance of electronic devices greatly depends upon the nature and quality of metal contact interfaces. Poor interface quality can result in high contact resistance, R_C, and can degrade the performance of a device significantly. Therefore, understanding the characteristics of metal/O-functionalized graphene interfaces is an important aspect of contact engineering for potential electronic applications. While there have been many studies on the interaction of metals with pristine graphene, a detailed study on the electrical characterization of metal/O-functionalized graphene interfaces has not been reported.

The findings from a systematic study on the effect of O-functionalization on the electrical characteristics of epitaxial graphene/metal contact interfaces are reported here. Two functionalization approaches were investigated: for the first approach, O-functionalization was performed on as-grown blanket graphene films, followed by device fabrication (herein after referred to as method-A) and, for the second approach, device fabrication was performed first, followed by O-functionalization (herein after referred to as method-B). By employing such approaches, metal—graphene contact interfaces were created with oxygen atoms present primarily underneath the metal electrodes (method-A case) and at the metal contact edge sites (method-B case). To monitor the changes in chemical and structural properties of graphene, XPS and Raman spectroscopy were used.

Fig. 9.21 shows the schematic illustration of process steps used for method-A and method-B samples, respectively. For both methods, as-grown graphene films were precleaned in Hydrofluoric Acid (HF) solution (48%) for 2 min to remove any residual oxides from the graphene surfaces. After this cleaning procedure, the sample used for method-A was immediately functionalized with an Ar/O_2 plasma, exposing the blanket graphene film to reactive oxygen species. This O-functionalized graphene sample was then lithographically patterned into mesa structures by reactive-ion-etching and subsequently metalized with Ti/Au to complete the device fabrication process. For the method-B sample, the blanket graphene film was first patterned into mesa structures, followed by metallization and N_2/H_2 annealing at 400°C for 30 min. Here, the annealing step was necessary to remove photo-resist residues from the graphene surface after lithographic processing. Finally, this patterned graphene sample was functionalized with an Ar/O_2 plasma. Note, apart from the additional annealing step used in method-B, similar device fabrication procedures and functionalization conditions were followed for both methods.

3.1 XPS analysis

To characterize the surface chemical composition of these samples, XPS analysis was performed both before and after functionalization. As the functionalization was performed on blanket (method-A) and patterned (method-B) graphene films, the bonding mechanism of O-functional groups is expected to differ between these two methods due to the presence of dangling bonds at the patterned graphene edges. Fig. 9.22A shows the high-resolution C1s spectra of the method-A sample taken immediately after HF treatment and just before O-functionalization, while Fig. 9.22C shows the spectra of the method-B sample taken after N_2/H_2 annealing and just before O-functionalization. Fitting the C1s spectra with mixed Gaussian–Lorentzian functions revealed three characteristic peaks at ~283.1, ~283.9, and ~ 284.6 eV for both samples, corresponding to the 6H–SiC substrate, C–C (graphene), and the interfacial layer, respectively. The relative concentration of these peaks corresponds to 33.5%, 38.6%, and 27.6%, respectively. In addition to these peaks, a shoulder peak was observed at 285.2 eV (2.03%) in the C1s spectrum of the method-B sample,

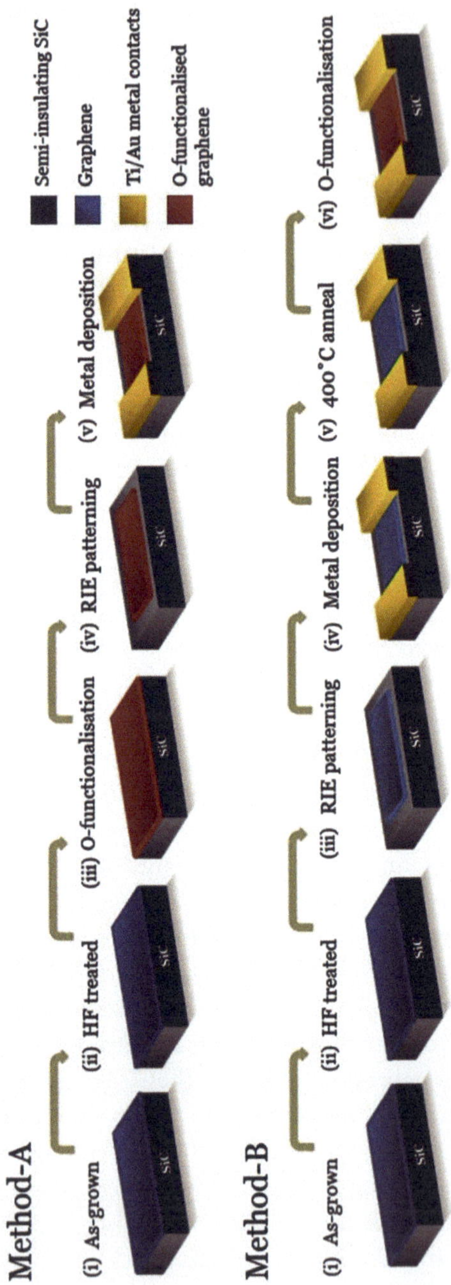

Figure 9.21 Schematic cross-section of process steps followed for samples functionalized using method-A (top) and method-B (bottom) approaches [76].

representing hydroxyl groups. The presence of this peak is consistent with previous studies, where it was shown that graphene attracts residual oxygen species from the ambient atmosphere after annealing. More importantly, no peaks related to photoresist residues were observed, indicating clean graphene surfaces after the thermal treatment.

Upon exposure to O-plasma, a clear change in the surface chemistry of both the method-A and method-B samples was observed with an increased FWHM of the C1s spectra along with shoulder peaks appearing at higher binding energies (Fig. 9.22B and D), representing different carbon-oxygen functional groups. However, the extent of surface modification and the polarity of O-functional groups varied markedly between method-A and method-B samples. For example, as shown in Table 9.3, the concentration of sp^2 C—C bonds in the method-A sample reduced significantly from 38.6% to 25.8% after functionalization, indicating a substantial modification to the graphene film. In contrast, the method-B sample showed only a

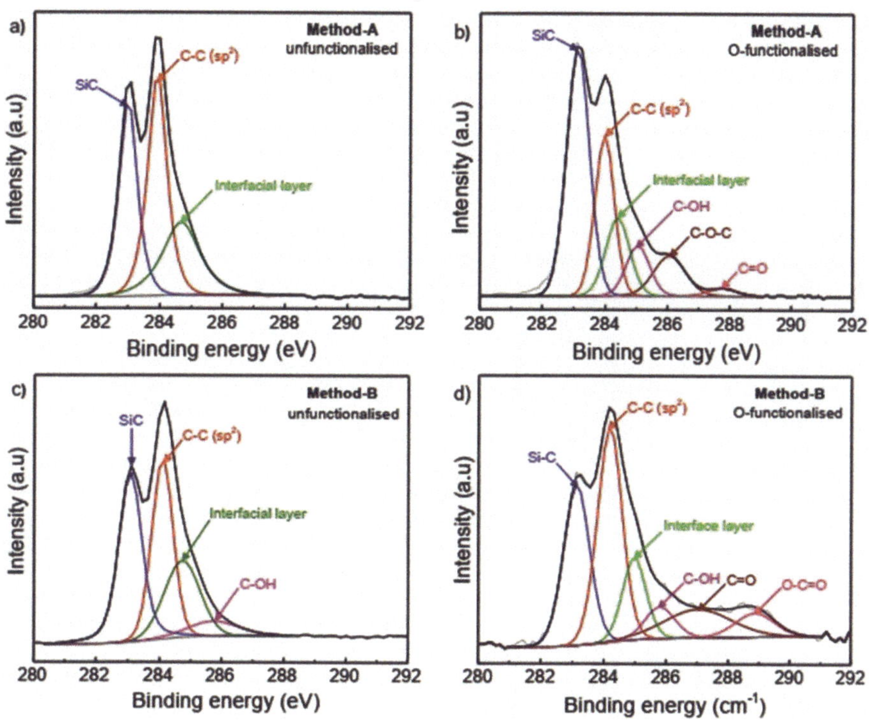

Figure 9.22 High-resolution XPS C1s spectra of epitaxial graphene taken before and after oxygen plasma functionalization using method-A and method-B, respectively [76].

Table 9.3 Differences in relative concentration of O-functional groups on graphene [76].

Functional group	Method-A			Method-B		
	BE (eV)	FWHM (eV)	Concentration (%)	BE (eV)	FWHM (eV)	Concentration (%)
Si–C	283.10	0.84	42.25	283.13	0.96	27.14
C–C (sp^2)	284.02	0.73	25.84	284.18	0.92	34.95
IF layer	284.41	0.92	14.31	284.97	0.88	12.80
C–OH	285.05	0.79	6.04	285.79	1.12	5.42
C–O–C	286.08	1.20	9.92	N/A	N/A	N/A
C=O	287.79	1.06	1.64	287.02	2.53	12.61
O–C=O	N/A	N/A	N/A	288.86	1.50	7.08

small reduction in concentration (34.95%) of sp^2 C−C bonds, implying minimal impact of O-plasma on the graphene lattice.

The deconvoluted C1s spectrum of the method-A sample (Fig. 9.22B) showed three O-functional peaks at 285.5 eV, 286.3, and 287.6 eV, attributed to C−OH (hydroxyl), C−O−C (epoxy), and C=O (carbonyl) groups, respectively. As shown by the data in Fig. 9.8b and in Table 9.1, the most favorable configuration of these O-functional groups was found to be epoxy groups with 9.92% of the total oxygen coverage, followed by hydroxyls and carbonyls with 6.04% and 1.64%, respectively. The chemical composition of the carbon-oxygen functional groups observed here is in agreement with previous studies, where, using nuclear magneto resonance spectroscopy, Lerf et al. [77] and Cai et al. [78] have demonstrated that the basal planes of oxidized graphene are predominantly decorated with epoxy and hydroxyl groups, while the edge sites or vacancies in the graphene film form exclusive adsorption sites for carbonyl and carboxyl species. The limited number of carbonyls and the absence of carboxyl functional groups in the C1s spectrum of the method-A sample indicate a negligible number of edge sites present in the as-grown blanket graphene film, thereby restricting the rise of carbonyl or carboxyl species and therefore resulting in an epoxy and hydroxyl rich graphene surface.

In contrast, for the method-B sample, the deconvoluted C1s spectrum (Fig. 9.22D) showed three peaks representing C−OH, C=O, and O−C=O (carboxyl) groups at 285.7 eV, 286.7, and 287.0 eV, respectively. Table 9.1 shows the chemical state of the method-B sample surface, in which carbonyls constitute the majority of oxygen functional groups present on the graphene surface with a relative concentration of 12.61%, while carboxyl and epoxy groups account for 7.33% and 5.15% each. The high concentration of carbonyl and carboxyl groups indicates the presence of edge sites, which is expected for patterned graphene structures. It is well known that the edge sites of graphene with dangling bonds are more reactive than the basal planes, enabling the formation of double (C=O) or triple bonds (OC=O) that are more favorable, in comparison to single bonds (C−OH or C−O−C) that are typically seen in homogeneous/blanket graphene films. Here, the presence of carboxyl groups is of particular interest because they are commonly used as anchoring sites for attaching DNA and other biomolecules for chemical and biological sensors [79], making the method-B sample highly attractive for sensing applications.

To validate the distribution of carbon-oxygen functional groups observed here, high-resolution O1s core level spectral analysis was performed. For the method-A sample, the O1s spectrum was fitted with six components (Fig. 9.9A), located at 530.1 eV, 530.8 eV, 531.7 eV, 532.5, and 533.0 eV. By reference to C1s peak shifts, these binding energies were assigned to carbonyl, epoxy, hydroxyl, silicon—oxycarbide, and silicon—oxide bonds, respectively. As it can be seen in Fig. 9.23A, epoxy functional groups clearly dominate the O1s spectrum, which is in excellent agreement with the concentration of carbon—oxygen functional groups found in the C1s spectrum of method-A sample. Fig. 9.23B shows the O1s spectrum of the method-B sample, also fitted with six major peaks at 530.1, 530.8, 531.7, 532.5, and 533.0 eV, corresponding to carboxyl, carbonyl, hydroxyl, silicon-oxycarbide, and silicon-oxide bonds, respectively. In addition to these peaks, a new component has been observed at 534.9 eV, which is assigned to residual H_2O bonds. Carboxyls were found to be the dominant functional species followed by carboxyls and epoxy groups, consistent with the finding in the C1s spectrum of the method-B sample shown earlier. This shows that the surface chemistry of graphene is greatly dependent upon the ordering of the functionalization step during the device fabrication, in which an epoxy rich surface can be created by functionalizing the graphene film immediately after growth and before device fabrication (method-A), while a carbonyl rich surface can be realized by functionalizing graphene after the final device fabrication step (method-B).

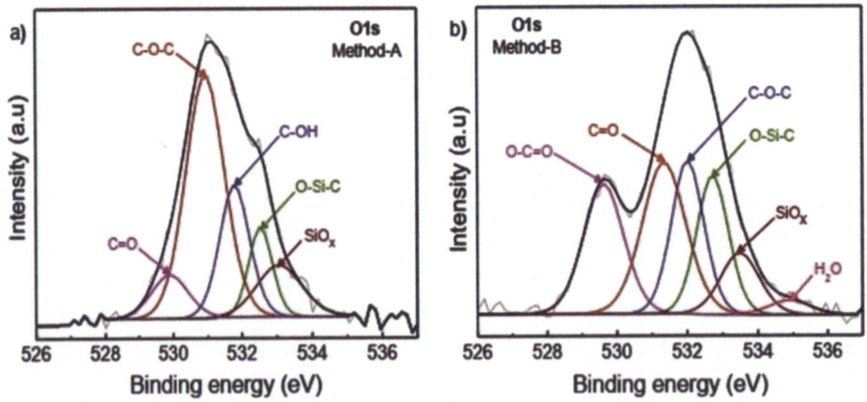

Figure 9.23 High-resolution XPS O1s spectra of (A) method-A and (B) method-B sample [76].

3.2 Raman analysis

Raman spectroscopy was used to verify the effect of O-plasma treatment on the structural characteristics of epitaxial graphene. Fig. 9.24 shows the typical Raman spectrum of an unfunctionalized graphene film along with the spectra of method-A and method-B functionalized samples. The position and the FWHM of the G and 2D peaks that were taken before and after functionalization are summarized in Table 9.4. The unfunctionalized graphene Raman spectrum showed G and 2D peaks at ~1599/cm and ~2739/cm, respectively, with no visible D peak, indicating the high crystalline quality of graphene films. The FWHM of the G peak was measured as 19/cm, while it was recorded as 34/cm for the 2D peak. Here, the FWHM (2D) indicates that the thickness of the graphene film for the probed area is a single layer, which was further confirmed by fitting the 2D peak with a single Lorentzian function. The ratio of the intensity of 2D peak (I_{2D}) to the intensity of the G peak (I_G), that is, I_{2D}/I_G was calculated as 1.15.

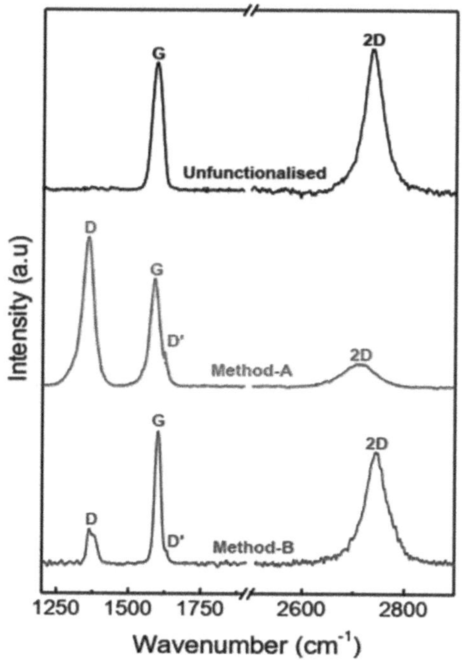

Figure 9.24 Raman spectra of unfunctionalized graphene and O-functionalized graphene using method-A and method-B approaches [76].

Upon exposure to an O-plasma, significant changes to the G and 2D peaks were observed along with the presence of a new disorder-induced D-peak in the Raman spectrum of both method-A and method-B functionalized samples, indicating structural modifications to the graphene film. The activation of the D-peak is attributed to the covalent attachment of oxygen functional groups to the graphene surface, which structurally disrupts the planar sp^2 symmetry of graphene by forming out-of-plane chemical bonds and resulting in sp^3 hybridization. Note that an additional peak has been observed at 1625/cm as a shoulder to the G peak for both methods, representing another defect-activated peak (D′). This D′-peak is due to intravalley resonant Raman scattering events, where the defect provides the missing momentum to satisfy momentum conservation during the Raman scattering process. Here, the extent of structural modification to the graphene film depends on the functionalization method used. For example, functionalizing graphene using the method-A approach resulted in a significant increase in the intensity of the D peak (I_D). The I_D/I_G ratio, which is used as a footprint for measuring the concentration of covalent defect sites in graphene, was calculated as 1.33. Interestingly, when the graphene was functionalized using the method-B approach, only a small rise in I_D was observed with an I_D/I_G ratio of 0.27. From this ratio, the average distance between the defect sites, L_D, can be calculated using [80]:

$$L_D^2(nm^2) = (1.8 \pm 0.5) \times 10^{-9} \lambda_{laser}^4 (I_D/I_G)^{-1} \tag{9.6}$$

where λ is the excitation laser wavelength in *nm*. For the method-A functionalized sample, L_D was measured as 10.2 nm, while for the method-B sample it was calculated as 27.5 nm. This shows that the concentration of O-functionalization-induced defects significantly varies, depending on the functionalization approach used. The average defect density, n_D, in the graphene film can be estimated by using [80]:

$$n_D(\mathrm{cm}^{-2}) = \frac{(1.8 \pm 0.5) \times 10^{12}}{\lambda_{laser}^4} (I_D / I_G) \tag{9.7}$$

The resultant n_D for the method-A sample was calculated as $1.5 \times 10^{11}/\mathrm{cm}^2$, while it was recorded as $4.3 \times 10^{11}/\mathrm{cm}^2$ for the method-B sample. Such a variation in the concentration of defect sites was also reflected in the intensity of the 2D peak, where a strong reduction in I_{2D} was observed for the method-A sample, while only a moderate decrease in I_{2D} was seen for the method-B sample. It is known that the intensity of the 2D peak is

Table 9.4 Raman data for method-A functionalized sample [76].

Probed area	ω_D (cm^{-1})	ω_G (cm^{-1})	ω_{2D} (cm^{-1})	FWHM D (cm^{-1})	FWHM G (cm^{-1})	FWHM 2D (cm^{-1})	I_D/I_G
Basal plane - Before functionalization	N/A	1599.1	2738.8	N/A	19.3	48.3	N/A
Basal plane - After functionalization	1356.1	1588.6	2709.6	41.9	38.6	75.7	1.40
Edge site - After functionalization	1357.3	1587.3	2797.3	45.3	36.2	79.6	1.47

proportional to the electron/hole inelastic scattering rate. As the O-functional groups adsorbed onto the graphene surface act as defect sites as well as introduce doping, an increase in the probability of scattering events occurs and, therefore, the intensity of the 2D peak decreases. As the intensity of the G peak (I_G) shows negligible dependence on doping-related effects, the I_{2D}/I_G ratio can be used as a sensitive parameter to monitor doping in the graphene film, where the I_{2D}/I_G ratio decreases with increasing doping concentration, irrespective of the dopant type. Here, the average I_{2D}/I_G ratio for the unfunctionalized graphene was calculated as 1.15, which reduced significantly to 0.15 when functionalized with the method-A approach, whereas it reduced only to 0.85 when functionalized using the method-B technique. This shows that the magnitude of doping, or the doping induced charge carrier scattering, is substantially higher when the blanket graphene is functionalized, in comparison to patterned graphene films. The decrease in I_{2D}/I_G was followed by an increase in the FWHM of the 2D peak, where an increase from 34/cm to 80/cm was observed for the method-A sample, while it was increased to 50/cm for the method-B sample, respectively. Despite this increase, the 2D peak can still be fitted with a single Lorentzian function, implying the thickness of the graphene film has not been altered during the functionalization process.

In addition to the change in peak intensity and FWHM, functionalization also shifted the position of G (ω_G) and 2D (ω_{2D}) peaks as shown in Table 9.4. There are several origins for the shift of Raman peaks, including the effects of doping and strain. Depending on the initial position of the Fermi level (E_F), G either red shifts or blue shifts upon exposure to the O-plasma. For example, the G peak displays the smallest energy value when the E_F of graphene is closer to the Dirac point, while it shifts to higher energies when E_F is far away from the Dirac point due to either n or p doping [49]. In contrast, the *2D* peak does not show major changes for low doping levels, but it increases with increasing hole doping concentration and decreases for increasing electron concentration [49]. Nevertheless, the relative shift of the G peak is usually greater than the relative shift of the 2D peak, that is, $\Delta\omega_G >> \Delta\omega_{2D}$. Here, $\Delta\omega_{2D}$ and $\Delta\omega_G$ are relative shifts in peak positions with respect to ω_{2D} and ω_G of unfunctionalized graphene. Apart from doping-induced shifts, ω_G and ω_{2D} are also strongly influenced by strain-related variations [81].

As an example, it was shown that both ω_G and ω_{2D} blue shift when the graphene was subjected to compressive strain, while the tensile strain results in their red shift [50]. It was found that for strain-induced variations, the relative shift of the G-peak is always lower than the relative shift of the 2D-peak, that is, $\Delta\omega_G << \Delta\omega_{2D}$. Here, for the sample functionalized using the method-A approach, ω_G red shifted from 1599 ± 1/cm to 1588 ± 1/cm ($\Delta\omega_G = 10 \pm 1$/cm), while ω_{2D} also red shifted from 2739 ± 1/cm to 2012 ± 1/cm ($\Delta\omega_{2D} = 27 \pm 1$/cm). As can be seen, $\Delta\omega_{2D}$ is larger than $\Delta\omega_G$, implying that strain plays a major role in the shift of these Raman peaks [76]. Here, the red shift of the G and 2D peaks can be understood on the basis of the stretching/elongation of the C–C bonds, which weakens the bond strength and therefore lowers their vibrational frequency. For example, as O-functionalization was performed on the blanket graphene film that has a negligible amount of edge sites or vacancies, the resultant surface chemistry consists of a high concentration of epoxy and hydroxyl functional groups (see XPS data above), which induces significant distortion to the graphene lattice by pulling the carbon atoms out of the graphene basal plane [14]. To adapt to this tetrahedral sp^3 geometry, stretching of C–C bonds occurs around the epoxy and hydroxyl defect sites. As epitaxial graphene grown on 6H–SiC is already compressively strained (−0.42%) due to the variation in thermal expansion coefficients between SiC and graphene, this oxygen-induced stretching of the C–C bonds results in strain relaxation in the graphene lattice, thereby reducing the native compressive strain present in graphene to −0.26%. It should be noted that although O-functionalization induces strain relaxation in epitaxial graphene, it also results in significant doping (as evidenced by the reduction in 2D-peak intensity). Nevertheless, strain-related variations dominate the doping-induced changes to the graphene film for the method-A functionalized sample.

Similar to the method-A approach, functionalization using the method-B approach also resulted in a red shift of ω_G from 1599 ± 1/cm to 1597 ± 1/cm ($\Delta\omega_G = 4 \pm 1$/cm), while no noticeable change was observed for ω_{2D} ($\Delta\omega_{2D} \leq 1$/cm), indicating doping is the main cause for the observed changes. As O-functionalization was performed on the patterned graphene film that contains edge sites or dangling bonds, the reactive nature of these unterminated bonds enables the formation of carbonyls and carboxyls more favorable than hydroxyl or epoxy species. It was shown before that both carbonyls and carboxyls maintain the planar sp^2 structure of graphene and do not have the same structural influence as hydroxyl or epoxy groups. This is because, unlike inner carbon atoms (i.e., basal planes), edge carbon atoms can adapt to a tetrahedral configuration more freely without causing extra strain, making the doping-induced changes more visible in the Raman peak shifts (Fig. 9.25).

It is well known that the graphene grown on 6H–SiC (0001) is electron doped (n-type) due to the charge transfer from the SiC substrate with EF located at around 0.35–0.4 eV above the Dirac point. The red shift in the G peak observed here after functionalization implies that E_F is now located closer to the Dirac point due to the change in charge carrier density in the graphene film. Interestingly, a higher reactivity was observed at the edges of graphene where the peak shift was more pronounced than the basal plane areas. For example, as shown in Fig. 9.11, $\Delta\omega_G$ was found to be 12/cm when probed near the edge of the graphene, in comparison to 4 cm^{-1} observed at the central regions. Similarly, $\Delta\omega_{2D}$ showed 4/cm change near the edge sites, in comparison to less than 1/cm change seen at the basal plane areas. This clearly shows that the doping near the graphene edge sites is significantly higher than the basal plane regions. Moreover, after O-plasma treatment, the I_D/I_G ratio at the edge sites of graphene was calculated as 1.18, whereas it was only measured as ~0.35 at the graphene basal planes. The higher I_D/I_G ratio suggests higher reactivity of carbon atoms close to the edges than in the bulk plane. This indicates that functionalization induced distortion to the graphene lattice can be significantly minimized by choosing patterned graphene films for functionalization, where the reactive graphene edge sites with dangling bonds form exclusive adsorption sites for derivative O-functional groups, thereby reducing the

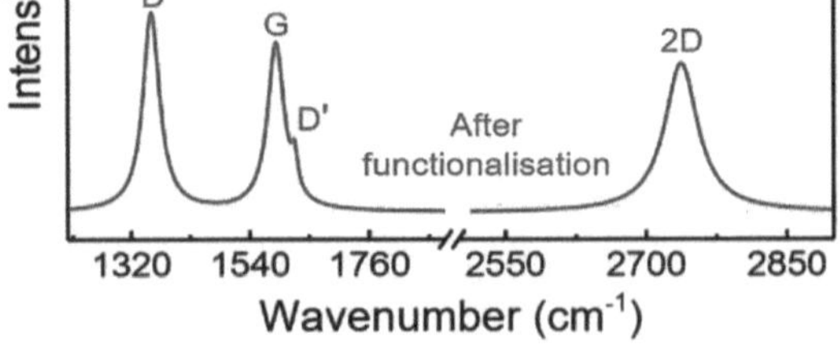

Figure 9.25 Raman spectra of method-B sample taken at patterned graphene edge before and after functionalization, showing significant doping. Solid lines indicate Lorentzian fittings [76].

structural impact on graphene lattice. Fig. 9.26 and Table 9.5 further verify the differences between edge sites and basal planes of the method-B functionalized sample.

4. Plasma functionalization

Owing to its exceptional material properties, graphene has been extensively studied for applications such as interconnects [82,83], thermal management in nanoelectronic circuits [83–85], flexible electronic displays [86], photodetectors [87,88] and as electrodes for solar cells [89], light-emitting diodes [90], and memory devices [91]. However, the same intrinsic structure of graphene that provides many of the desired properties also results in poor wettability and low chemical reactivity due to its structural homogeneity and highly delocalized electronic structure. This limits the suitability of graphene for other important applications. For example, chemical sensors made of pristine graphene typically suffer from weak sensing responses, poor selectivity issues, and extremely long recovery times due to the lack of polar functional groups on the surface [9,92]. The absence of these polar

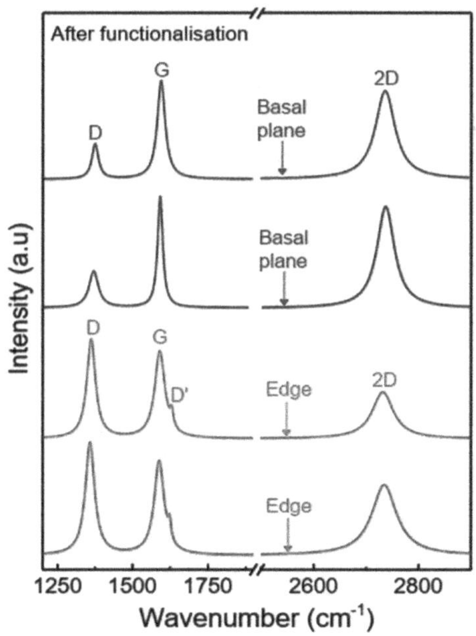

Figure 9.26 Raman spectra of method-B sample showing the magnitude of doping at basal plane areas and at patterned graphene edge sites. Solid lines indicate Lorentzian fittings [76].

Table 9.5 Raman data of method-B functionalized sample taken from different areas of the sample [76].

Probed area	ω_D (cm^{-1})	ω_G (cm^{-1})	ω_{2D} (cm^{-1})	FWHM D (cm^{-1})	FWHM G (cm^{-1})	FWHM 2D (cm^{-1})	I_D/I_G	I_{2D}/I_G
Basal plane unfunctionalized	N/A	1597.5	2738.4	N/A	34.7	47.2	N/A	0.97
Basal plane 1	1372.6	1597.7	2737.7	31.0	20.9	48.6	0.24	0.84
Basal plane 2	1376.5	1596.7	2737.6	26.1	28.7	45.5	0.89	0.84
Basal plane 3	1374.5	1597.9	2737.8	38.1	21.0	41.3	0.32	0.85
Edge site unfunctionalized	1357.3	1587.3	2797.3	45.3	36.2	79.6	1.47	
Edge site 1	1358.0	1588.3	2733.2	37.4	37.4	44.2	1.18	0.62
Edge site 2	1362.3	1589.7	2732.4	34.8	40.3	51.98	1.14	0.53
Edge site 3	1358.0	1588.3	2734.3	37.4	39.8	57.6	1.19	0.65

groups also makes interfacing graphene with other chemical moieties extremely challenging, thereby limiting its use in biological/biomedical applications. Moreover, the highly hydrophobic nature of pristine graphene surfaces inhibits uniform deposition of ultrathin (2–10 nm) high k-dielectric layers [93–95], further impeding the development of graphene-based electronics for high-frequency applications. Here, the hydrophobicity of graphene is due to the lack of polar functional groups on its surface, which leads to the chemically inert nature of graphene. To overcome these issues, functionalization of graphene is essential to enhance its capabilities and promote chemical reactivity on its surfaces.

As discussed earlier, there have been many studies in the past demonstrating the chemical modification of graphene using highly reactive species such as hydrogen, fluorine, chlorine, oxygen, and other organic functional groups [31,59,70,71,95–100]. These reactants were shown to not only change the surface chemistry of graphene but also greatly alter the hybridization state of carbon atoms, charge carrier type, and density, resulting in the transformation of graphene from a semimetal to a semiconductor or a strong insulator [101,102]. Among these functional species, oxygen is of particular interest, because of the advantages it offers for a diverse range of applications. For example, unpaired electrons of oxygen make it highly reactive to surface adsorbates and allow the derivative oxygen functional groups to act as anchoring sites for the attachment of designated molecules or enzymes, making it attractive for chemical [103–105] and biosensor applications [74,106,107]. Oxygen functional species also reduce the hydrophobicity of graphene and make the surface more hydrophilic [8,108]. This change in surface wettability significantly increases the adhesion strength of metal contacts on graphene, which otherwise suffer from metal delamination issues [108–110]. In addition, it has also been demonstrated that O-plasma treatment increases the thermal transport across the metal/graphene interface, enabling efficient heat transport to the surrounding device architecture [61]. Furthermore, it was shown that O-functionalization creates a band-gap of over 1 eV [60] and induces a strong photoluminescence behavior in graphene [58], which could pave the way toward developing graphene-based electronic and optoelectronic devices.

As discussed, a wide variety of techniques have been proposed for functionalizing graphene with oxygen species, including exposure to ozone [111,112], wet solution of strong acids [63,103–106], oxygen plasma [59,60,67,70,113], and photochemical oxidation [114,115]. Among these techniques the most popular and commonly employed approach is using aggressive acidic solutions based on the modified Hummer's method, where the graphite layers are oxidized first, followed by exfoliation into two-dimensional GO. However, the resultant GO material is chemically inhomogeneous, electrically insulating, and structurally defective due to the extensive use of harsh acidic treatments. While the reduction of GO (i.e., reduced graphene oxide, rGO) by strong acids and several hours of thermal annealing was shown to partially recover the structural characteristics of graphene [116–119], these rGO films still suffer from inferior electrical properties that also lead to inevitable contamination by unwanted functional groups during the reduction process. Moreover, accommodation of such oxidation/reduction steps involving toxic chemicals and/or multiple annealing cycles into a Complimentary Metal Oxide Semiconductor (CMOS) process flow is highly undesirable.

Alternatively, plasma treatment is attractive because plasmas are extensively used in the semiconductor fabrication process and are also capable of modifying material surfaces with nanoscale precision [120]. Moreover, plasma processing has advantages of shorter reaction times, a solvent-free, nonpolluting process, and provides a wider range of functional groups depending on parameters such as power, treatment time, gases used, and operating pressure. Plasma functionalization is an efficient method to modify the physical, chemical, and electrical properties of large-area graphene films. Different types of plasma functionalization approaches have been reported to date, including capacitively [121] or inductively coupled plasma [70], radio frequency plasma [122], microwave plasma [123], and RIE plasma techniques [124]. In these techniques, plasmas are usually produced by supplying energy to electrons through an external electric field generated by a power supply and applied to a low-pressure gas. This external electric field heats plasma electrons to a temperature of several eV, which results in ionization, excitation, and other collision processes. The resultant plasmas, therefore, contain chemically active species such as neutral radicals and atoms/molecules in excited states, ions, electrons, and photons. The highly reactive nature of these plasmas strongly interacts with the graphene and break the carbon–carbon sigma bonds of the lattice, creating active sites for binding different functional groups, thereby modifying the chemical and physical properties of the graphene film. Unfortunately, the high ion-energies produced using these plasma approaches often cause irreversible damage to the graphene due to the ion-induced etching of the film [67]. In contrast, electron beam (ebeam) generated plasmas were demonstrated to be inherently well suited for functionalizing ultra-thin materials such as graphene [125,126], because they offer high plasma densities in the range of $10^{10}-10^{11}$ cm^{-3}, along with low electron temperatures (<1 eV) [125,127]. Such low electron temperatures are due to the use of high-energy electron beams to drive the plasma production rather than external electric fields. In noble gas atmospheres such as Ar, the elastic scattering and the ambipolar electrostatic cooling are the main energy loss mechanisms, which limit electron temperatures at around 1 eV [127]. In the presence of molecular gases, the inelastic collision between electrons and gas molecules leads to a further reduction in electron temperature to less than 0.3 eV. As a consequence, large fluxes of low energy (3−5 eV) ions are delivered to the material surface. Such ion-energies are crucial in preserving carbon basal planes from ion-induced etching, due to the low energy thresholds for vacancy creation (7.44 eV) and displacement (35 eV) in graphite [128].

The relevance of e-beam generated oxygen plasmas for the functionalization of epitaxial graphene films is described in terms of the sensitivity to incident chemical species. The functionalization of graphene that is described here was performed at room temperature in a plasma reactor system, enclosed by magnetic field coils to produce a uniform magnetic field within the chamber, as shown schematically in Fig. 9.27. The vacuum chamber consists of a hollow cathode e-beam source, a slotted anode, an e-beam termination anode, and a sample holder. E-beam generated plasmas were produced by injecting a 2 keV e-beam into a mixture of Ar and O_2. This beam passes through the anode slot in a grounded anode and terminates at a grounded termination anode. The resulting e-beam plasma is magnetically confined by applying a magnetic field of 150 G to minimize the spreading, thereby producing a large area (60 × 25 cm^2) sheet-like plasma as shown in Fig. 9.27B and C. For this work, the operating pressure was varied between 25 and 90 mTorr, by controlling by the total gas flow rate (75−180 sccm). For all conditions, the reactive gas (O_2) was introduced at 5% of the total flow rate with argon as the remainder gas to dilute the impact of the oxygen plasma functional species on the graphene surface. Note that unlike other plasma exposure techniques, the e-beam generated plasmas do not directly interact with the sample surface. For instance, as shown in Fig. 9.27, the epitaxial graphene samples on the sample holder are placed 2.5 cm from the electron-beam axis, thus avoiding direct contact with the energetic plasma.

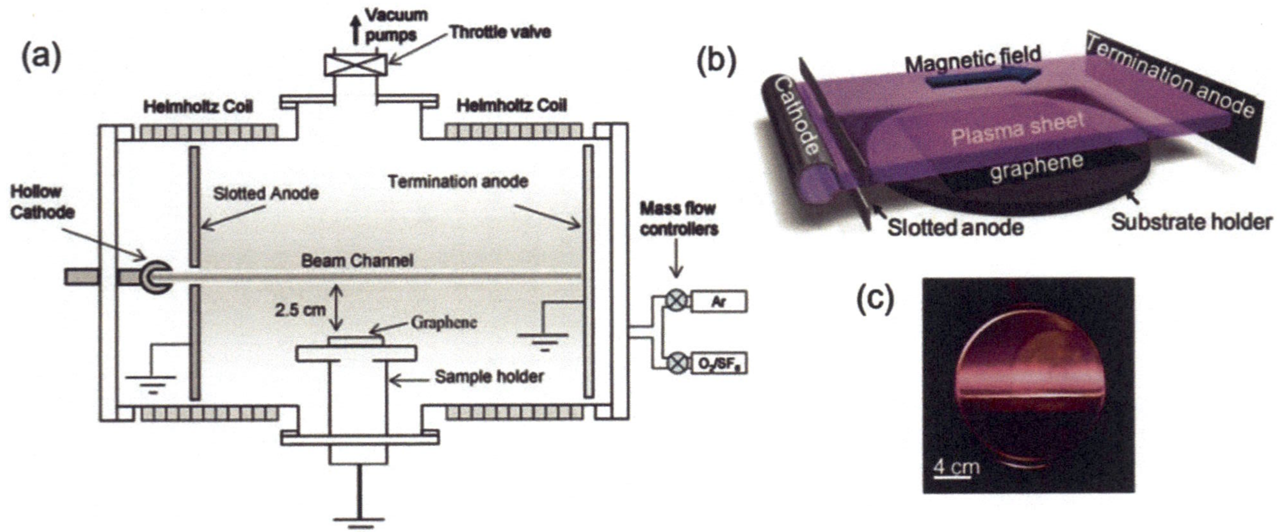

Figure 9.27 (A) Schematic view of the e-beam plasma reactor used for oxygen functionalization process. (B) Schematic illustration of the plasma during the exposure and (C) real-time digital image of the sheet-like plasma produced during the functionalization process [128].

The selective modification of epitaxial graphene films using electron-beam generated Ar/O_2 plasmas at room temperature was studied to allow enhanced control over the concentration of functional groups present on the graphene surface while maintaining compatibility with the state-of-the-art silicon fabrication process capabilities. Importantly, the functionalization process does not result in appreciable etching of graphene films due to the unique nature of e-beam plasmas. Here, we briefly discuss the effect of e-beam plasma treatment on the morphological and electronic characteristics of epitaxial graphene films, from initial to advanced oxidation stages using atomic force microscopy (AFM) and Hall measurements, respectively.

4.1 AFM analysis

AFM was used to examine the surface morphological changes to epitaxial graphene films as a result of the plasma functionalization process. The data in Fig. 9.28 (top) show the topographic images of as-grown and as-functionalized graphene samples at 90 mTorr. As can be seen, no obvious changes to the graphene surface morphology were observed even at the highest oxidation pressure within the instrument resolution. Nevertheless, the AFM surface roughness of the epitaxial graphene before and after functionalization shown in Fig. 9.28 (bottom), reveals an increase in surface roughness, which is attributed to the out-of-plane chemical bonding of oxygen functional groups, particularly epoxy and hydroxyl species. In addition, the RMS roughness of all functionalized graphene samples plotted as a function of the plasma pressure showed a small increase in the surface roughness with the increasing pressure as shown by the data in Fig. 9.29. This implies that the functionalization does not have a detrimental effect on the epitaxial graphene film quality.

4.2 Hall measurements

Hall measurements were performed on all functionalized samples to analyze the effect of O-functionalization on the electrical properties of graphene. As-grown films showed intrinsic n-type character with average sheet carrier densities of $7 \pm 2 \times 10^{12}/\text{cm}^2$ due to the induced charge transfer from the underlying unsaturated Si-bonds near the SiC/graphene interface. The average sheet conductivities and mobilities of as-grown graphene films were measured as $10{,}834 \pm 26$ S/cm and 850 ± 80 $\text{cm}^2/\text{V/s}$, respectively.

After functionalization, the electronic properties of the graphene films changed considerably. For example, all functionalized samples showed p-

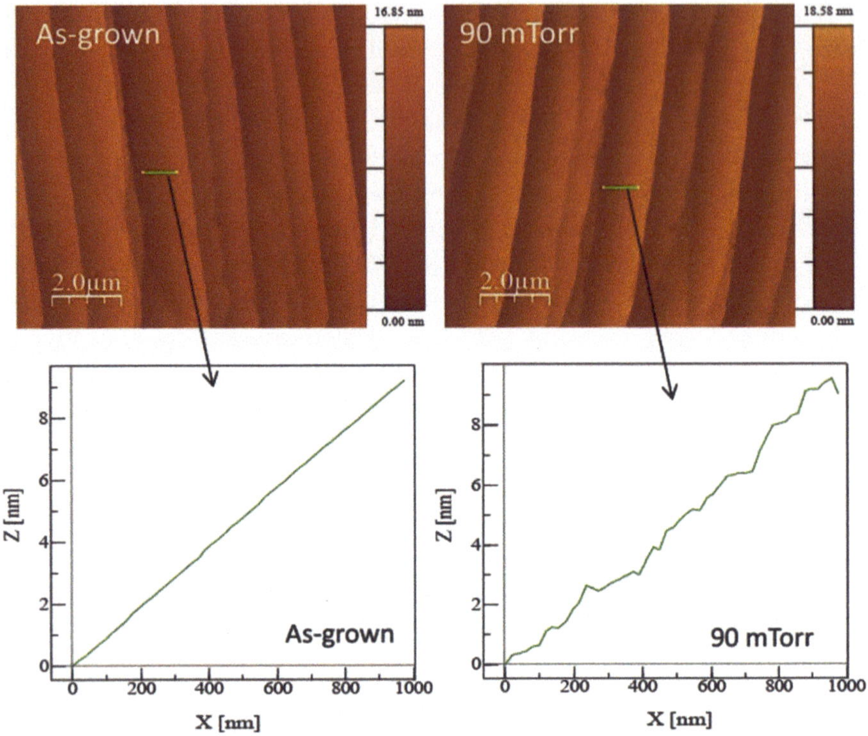

Figure 9.28 (Top) AFM topographic images of the graphene surface before and after oxygen functionalization. (Bottom) corresponding surface roughness measured on the sample step terraces [76].

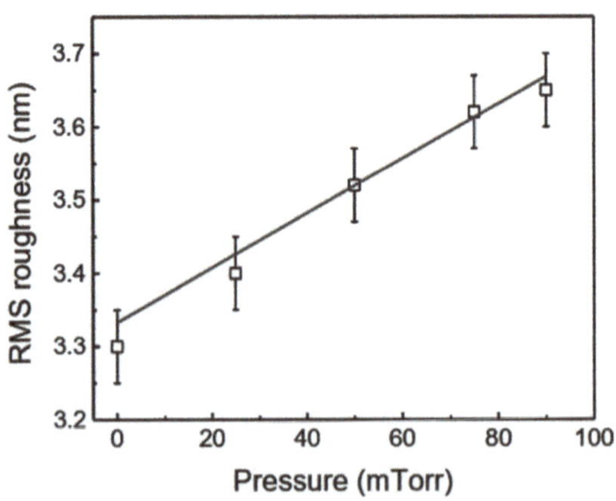

Figure 9.29 RMS roughness of functionalized graphene with the increasing pressure. Solid line is a guide to the eye only [76].

type conduction, due to the electron extracting nature of oxygen, which changes the intrinsic n-type character of graphene by shifting the Fermi level (E_F) below the Dirac point (E_D) as depicted in Fig. 9.30. The hole density in these functionalized films increased linearly with increasing plasma pressure as shown in Fig. 9.31 and reached $5 \times 10^{14}/cm^2$ at 90 mTorr, which is more than one order of magnitude larger than previously reported values $\sim 4 \times 10^{13}/cm^2$ for O, F, or N-functionalized graphene [129–131]. An increase in carrier density with increasing pressure is expected because the charge transfer between the adsorbed molecule and the graphene can grow with the concentration of adsorbed molecules.

The increase in carrier density resulted in a considerable decrease in Hall mobility along with a decrease in sheet conductivity due to the presence of sp^3 scattering sites produced by the oxygen functional groups. At 90 mTorr, the mobility and conductivity were measured as 15 $cm^2/V/s$ and 416 S/cm, respectively. The observed decrease in conductivity with plasma pressure is consistent with the increasing defect density observed in the Raman spectra [76]. Nevertheless, the sheet conductivities measured here are significantly better than previously reported oxygen plasma functionalized graphene studies [132] and comparable/better than that of commonly reported values on highly reduced graphene oxide films (see Ref. [76]). It should be noted that the reduction methods used for reducing GO films involve several hours of exposure to strong acids and/or multiple high-temperature

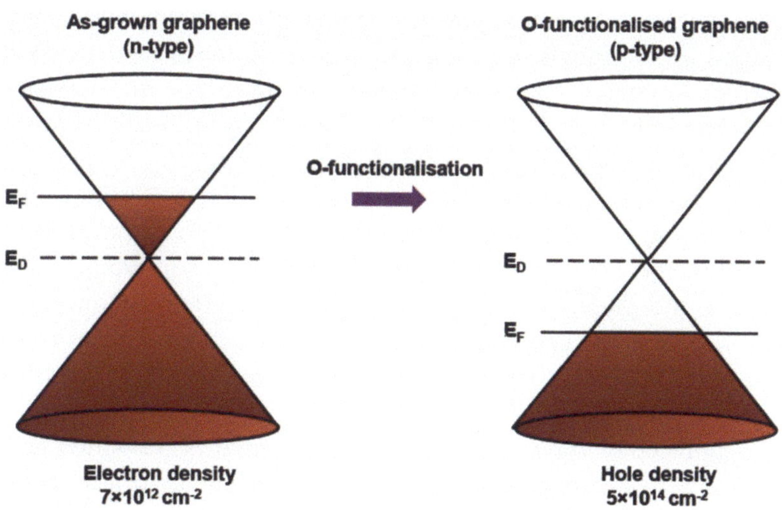

Figure 9.30 Schematic energy diagrams showing the effective hole doping of epitaxial graphene after O-functionalization at 90 mTorr pressure [76].

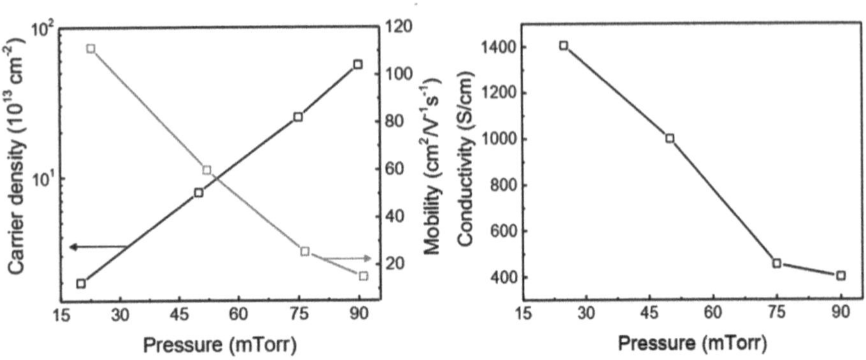

Figure 9.31 Plot showing the change in carrier density and mobility as a function of plasma pressure. Decrease in conductivity of functionalized epitaxial graphene films with the increasing functionalization pressure [76].

annealing cycles, which do not offer any degree of control over reduction in the concentration of specific functional group(s). In contrast, the e-beam plasma processing technique used here is relatively clean (no wet chemical or thermal processing required) and is extremely fast in comparison to other functionalization techniques.

4.3 Biological sensing

As outlined earlier, the large surface area to volume ratio of graphene makes it ideally suited for the realization of high sensitivity biological sensors. The low optical attenuation of the graphene film also opens up opportunities in the realization of combined optical and electronic measurements. While a number of biological sensing techniques are linked to the detection of specific chemicals, such as glucose [133], the interest in the direct detection of biomolecules using graphene sensors is significant.

Graphene-based sensors have been used to detect a wide range of biological systems, including dsDNA, *E. coli*, and Zika, as well as an incredible range of graphene-inspired sensors, such as carbon/graphene composites and graphene/polyaniline composites. Here, a summary of a suitable selection of sensors and the technology related to the detection mechanism is presented, rather than a complete review of the field, which can be found in a range of review articles, including [134].

The bioreceptor (which includes molecules such as antibodies and enzymes) needs to be chemically attached to the graphene surface. Enzymes are generally physisorbed, similar to gas and solvent molecules on unfunctionalized graphene surfaces, while antibodies are more commonly attached using a chemical-based functionalization technique involving 1-ethyl-3-(3-dimethylaminopropyl) carbodiimide hydrochloride and N-hydroxysuccinimide, the so-called EDC/NHS reaction [135]. It can be hypothesized that prior functionalization of the graphene surface will facilitate the reaction, which is water based, due to the removal of the hydrophobic nature of a clean graphene surface. In addition to the functionalization of the graphene surface with biological target receptors, patterning with metal nanoparticles has enabled the detection of a wide range of biological materials, including Salmonella (silver) [136], Hepatitis C (silver) [137], Avian Influenza H7 (Gold) [138], Alzheimer's (magnetic) [139], and Cancer (iron-based magnetic) [140]. These decorated systems offer detection limits an order of magnitude lower than graphene films, with cancer detection for the Fe_3O_4 decorated surface able to detect femtograms of cancerous material.

Proteins are known to bind to the graphene surface using $\pi-\pi$ interactions, which leads to changes in the doping in the graphene film, in a manner similar to that observed for the detection of polar protic solvents outlined earlier [141]. However, the complex nature of the protein means that the sensor response can also contain influences from the different charges, amino acid composition, and the orientation of the protein with the graphene surface, and so the simple interpretation of the data is more complex than for the gas sensor case. The shift in the doping with the protein interaction has been used to identify the n-type doping that is induced in graphene when exposed to DNA, which contains negative charges on the helix. This effect was found to dominate over the changes to the impurity screening or field effect that has been described under similar conditions.

The detection of individual cells has been developed using nano-wire structures; however, the two-dimensional nature of graphene opens up new possibilities. Because cell membranes are a two-dimensional structure, which comprises a 5-nm thick lipid bilayer, the graphene surface can intimately interact with the cell, which contrasts with the local curvature that results in the membrane from the nano-typographic features. As an example, CVD grown graphene has been used to detect *E. coli* in solution, with the surface of the graphene functionalized using *E. coli* antibodies and the use of a passivation layer to suppress the attachment of other bacteria species [142]. In contrast to the direct doping shift observed for the protein-based detection outlined earlier, the graphene parameters were shifted by means of the field effect, resulting from the negatively charged bacterial

Table 9.6 Summary of graphene-based electrochemical sensors materials.

Sensor type	Materials used	Targeted analyte	Detection range	Reference
Electrochemistry	Graphene—Antibody	Cystatin C	0.1–1000 ng/L	[144]
Electrochemistry	Graphene oxide—Fe_3O_4	Glucose	0.05–50 μM	[145]
Photoluminescence	Graphene oxide	Rotavirus	105 PFU/mL	[105]
Electrochemistry	Graphene oxide	Cardiovascular diseases	–	[146]
Electrochemical	Reduced Graphene oxide	Hormones	10 pg/mL	[147]
Electrochemical	Graphene/PMMA	Anti *E. coli* O157:H7 antibody	10 CFU/mL	[148]
Electrochemical	Reduced Graphene oxide	Generic *E. coli* antibody	10^3 CFU/mL	[149]
Electrochemical	Graphene oxide—MB—chitosan	Influenza A virus	9; 5 p.m.	[150]
Electrochemical	Graphene oxide—Pd nanoparticles	Dopamine	0.3–196.3 μM	[151]
Electrochemical	Reduced Graphene oxide	PSA	1–36 ng/mL	[152]

wall, which does not come into direct (i.e., electrical) contact with the graphene surface. The sensitivity of this sensor is quoted as being higher than that for a one-dimensional nano-tube-based device [143] and was able to detect the metabolic activities of the bacteria when exposed to glucose in real time.

A brief summary of the different electrochemical sensor materials that have been demonstrated based on graphene-like materials is given in Table 9.6. From the data in the table, it can be seen that graphene oxides and reduced graphene oxide are commonly used for the creation of biosensors, with a wide range of target analytes. In both cases, the sp^2 bonded carbon is chemically bonded to oxygen, and these materials can be considered as limiting cases of the functionalization of a graphene surface with oxygen. Hence, the data summarized next is an extension of the technology summarized in the early part of the chapter that does not take advantage of whole wafer processing in a semiconductor environment.

5. Conclusions

The superlative material properties of graphene offer a paradigm shift in the field of biological sensing, for a range of compounds and cell lines of interest. To maximize these advantages and realize the potential of the material to support the healthcare of the wider population, the repeatable manufacture of sensors using conventional semiconductor processing is imperative. The control of the graphene surface, through functionalization, is a further key step in the development of a viable route to manufacture and is a key enabler in the ability to chemically attach a range of different antibodies and metal nanoparticles that have demonstrated the ability to detect biological materials at the Femto level.

References

[1] K. Novoselov, A. Geim, S. Morozov, D. Jiang, Y. Zhang, S. Dubonos, I.V. Grigorieva, A. Firsov, Electric field effect in atomically thin carbon films, Science (2004) 2–6.
[2] J.S. Moon, D.K. Gaskill, Graphene: its fundamentals to future applications, IEEE Transactions on Microwave Theory and Techniques 59 (2011) 2702–2708.
[3] Y.-M. Lin, K.A. Jenkins, A. Valdes-Garcia, J.P. Small, D.B. Farmer, P. Avouris, Operation of graphene transistors at gigahertz frequencies, Nano Letters 9 (1) (2009) 422–426.
[4] M. Grande, G.V. Bianco, M.A. Vincenti, D. De Ceglia, P. Capezzuto, V. Petruzzelli, M. Scalora, G. Bruno, A. D'Orazio, Graphene-based devices: a platform for high

frequency applications?, in: International Conference on Transparent Optical Networks, Vol. 2016-Augus, 2016, pp. 5–8.
[5] Z. Cheng, Q. Zhou, C. Wang, Q. Li, C. Wang, Y. Fang, Toward intrinsic graphene surfaces: a systematic study on thermal annealing and wet chemical treatment of SiO_2 supported graphene devices, Nano Letters 11 (2) (2011) 2–6.
[6] J. Moon, D. Curtis, M. Hu, D. Wong, C. McGuire, P. Campbell, et al., Epitaxial graphene RF field-effect transistors on Si-face 6H-SiC substrates, IEEE Electron Device Letters 30 (2009) 650–652.
[7] J. Kedzierski, H. Pei-Lan, P. Healey, P.W. Wyatt, C.L. Keast, M. Sprinkle, et al., Epitaxial graphene transistors on SiC substrates, IEEE Transactions Electron Devices 55 (2008) 20782085.
[8] Y.J. Shin, Y. Wang, H. Huang, G. Kalon, A.T.S. Wee, Z. Shen, et al., Surface energy engineering of graphene, Langmuir 26 (2010) 3798–3802.
[9] R. Pearce, T. Iakimov, M. Andersson, L. Hultman, A.L. Spetz, R. Yakimova, Epitaxially grown graphene based gas sensors for ultra sensitive NO_2 detection, Sensors and Actuators B: Chemical 155 (2011) 451–455.
[10] F. Schedin, A. Geim, S. Morozov, E. Hill, P. Blake, M. Katsnelson, et al., Detection of individual gas molecules adsorbed on graphene, Nature Mater 6 (2007) 652–655.
[11] A.K. Geim, K.S. Novoselov, The rise of graphene, Nature Materials 6 (3) (2007) 183–191.
[12] V. Panchal, D. Cox, R. Yakimova, O. Kazakova, Epitaxial graphene sensors for detection of small magnetic moments, IEEE Transactions on Magnetics 49 (1) (2013) 97–100.
[13] A. Peters, "Graphene Hall Sensors for Harsh Environment Current Sensing" PhD Thesis, University of Durham, 2021.
[14] Y. Dong, Y. Xie, C. Xu, Y. Fu, X. Fan, X. Li, L. Wang, F. Xiong, W. Guo, G. Pan, Q. Wang, F. Qian, J. Sun, Transfer-free, lithography-free and fast growth of patterned CVD graphene directly on insulators by using sacrificial metal catalyst, Nanotechnology 29 (36) (2018).
[15] M. Batzill, The surface science of graphene: metal interfaces, CVD synthesis, nanoribbons, chemical modifications and defects, Surface Science Reports 67 (3–4) (2012) 83–115.
[16] K. Biswas, S. Kal, Etch characteristics of KOH, TMAH and dual doped TMAH for bulk micromachining of silicon, Microelectronics Journal 37 (6) (2006) 519–525.
[17] G. Giovannetti, P.A. Khomyakov, G. Brocks, V.M. Karpan, J. Van Den Brink, P.J. Kelly, Doping graphene with metal contacts, Physical Review Letters 101 (2) (2008) 4–7.
[18] J.M. Wofford, "Graphene Growth on Low Carbon Solubility Metals," PhD Thesis, University of California, 2012.
[19] Y. Dong, S. Guo, H. Mao, C. Xu, Y. Xie, C. Cheng, X. Mao, J. Deng, G. Pan, J. Sun, The growth of graphene on NiCu alloy thin films at a low temperature and its carbon diffusion mechanism, Nanomaterials 9 (11) (2019) 1–11.
[20] V. Miseikis, S. Xiang, S. Roddaro, S. Heun, C. Coletti, Perfecting the growth and transfer of large single-crystal CVD graphene: a platform material for optoelectronic applications, Carbon Nanostructures 0 (2017) 113–124, no. 9783319581323.
[21] H.Y. Jeong, J.Y. Kim, J.W. Kim, J.O. Hwang, J.-E. Kim, J.Y. Lee, et al., Graphene oxide thin films for flexible nonvolatile memory applications, Nano Lett 10 (2010) 4381–4386.
[22] L.M. Malard, M.A. Pimenta, G. Dresselhaus, M.S. Dresselhaus, Raman spectroscopy in graphene, Physics Reports 473 (5–6) (2009) 51–87.

[23] H. Park, C. Lim, C.-J. Lee, J. Kang, J. Kim, M. Choi, H. Park, Optimized Poly-MethylMethacrylate -mediated graphene transfer process for fabrication of high-quality graphene layer, Nanotechnology (2018) 11−14.

[24] Y. Jia, X. Gong, P. Peng, Z. Wang, Z. Tian, L. Ren, Y. Fu, H. Zhang, Toward high carrier mobility and low contact resistance: laser cleaning of PMMA residues on graphene surfaces, Nano-Micro Letters 8 (4) (2016) 336−346.

[25] Z. Ni, Y. Wang, T. Yu, Z. Shen, Spectroscopy and imaging of graphene, Nano Research 1 (4) (2008) 273−291.

[26] B. Tang, H. Guoxin, H. Gao, Raman spectroscopic characterization of graphene, Applied Spectroscopy Reviews 45 (5) (2010) 369−407.

[27] S. Revo, S. Hamamda, K. Ivanenko, O. Boshko, A. Djarri, A. Boubertakh, Analysis of Al + 0.1% CNT ribbon, Nanoscale Research Letters 10 (1) (2015) 1−7.

[28] V.T. Nguyen, H.D. Le, V.C. Nguyen, T.T.T. Ngo, D.Q. Le, X.N. Nguyen, N.M. Phan, Of multi-layer graphene films on copper tape by atmospheric pressure chemical vapor deposition method, Advances in Natural Sciences: Nanoscience and Nanotechnology 4 (3) (2013) 2−7.

[29] A. Das, S. Pisana, B. Chakraborty, S. Piscanec, S. Saha, U. Waghmare, K.S. Novoselov, H.R. Krishnamurthy, A.K. Geim, A.C. Ferrari, A.K. Sood, Monitoring dopants by Raman scattering in an electrochemically top-gated graphene transistor, Nature Nanotech 3 (2008) 210−215.

[30] A.C. Ferrari, Raman spectroscopy of graphene and graphite: disorder, electron-phonon coupling, doping and nonadiabatic effects, Solid State Communications 143 (1−2) (2007) 47−57.

[31] B. Li, L. Zhou, D. Wu, H. Peng, K. Yan, Y. Zhou, et al., Photochemical chlorination of graphene, ACS Nano 5 (2011) 5957−5961.

[32] R. Fates, J.P. Raskin, Linear and non-linear electrical behaviors in graphene ribbon based devices, Journal of Science: Advanced Materials and Devices 3 (3) (2018) 366−370.

[33] L. Wang, X. Chen, Y. Hu, A. Yu, W. Lu, Nonlinear current voltage characteristics and enhanced negative differential conductance in graphene field effect transistors, Nanoscale 6 (21) (2014) 12769−12779.

[34] C.A. Chavarin, A.A. Sagade, D. Neumaier, G. Bacher, W. Mertin, On the origin of contact resistances in graphene devices fabricated by optical lithography, Applied Physics A: Materials Science and Processing 122 (2) (2016) 1−5.

[35] S.M. Sze, Physics of Semiconductor Devices, 1981.

[36] T. Cusati, G. Fiori, A. Gahoi, V. Passi, M.C. Lemme, A. Fortunelli, G. Iannaccone, Electrical properties of graphene-metal contacts, Scientific Reports 7 (1) (2017) 5109.

[37] Y. Sharon, B. Khachatryan, D. Cheskis, Towards a low current Hall effect sensor, Sensors and Actuators, A: Physical 279 (2018) 278−283, no. January 2019.

[38] B. Chen, L. Huang, X. Ma, L. Dong, Z. Zhang, L.-M. Peng, Exploration of sensitivity limit for graphene magnetic sensors, Science Direct 94 (2015) 585−589, no. November.

[39] L. Huang, Z. Zhang, B. Chen, X. Ma, H. Zhong, L.M. Peng, UltraSensitive graphene Hall elements, Applied Physics Letters 104 (18) (2014) 2012−2016.

[40] J. Dauber, A.A. Sagade, M. Oellers, K. Watanabe, T. Taniguchi, D. Neumaier, C. Stampfer, Ultra-sensitive Hall sensors based on graphene encapsulated in hexagonal boron nitride, Applied Physics Letters 106 (19) (2015).

[41] M.A. Khan, J. Sun, B. Li, A. Przybysz, J. Kosel, Magnetic sensors-A review and recent technologies, Engineering Research Express 3 (2021) 022005.

[42] S. Sanfilippo, Hall probes: physics and application to magnetometry, in: CAS 2009 - CERN Accelerator School: Magnets, Proceedings, 2010, pp. 423−462.

[43] R.G. Mani, K.V. Klitzing, F. Jost, K. Marx, S. Lindenkreuz, H.P. Trah, Method for simultaneously reducing the misalignment offset and separating the Hall voltage from the off-diagonal piezoresistive voltage in Hall effect and piezoresistive devices based on silicon, Applied Physics Letters 67 (1995) 2223, no. October.
[44] J.E. Johns, M.C. Hersam, Atomic covalent functionalization of graphene, Accounts of Chemical Research 46 (2012) 77–86.
[45] V. Georgakilas, M. Otyepka, A.B. Bourlinos, V. Chandra, N. Kim, K.C. Kemp, et al., Functionalization of graphene: covalent and non-covalent approaches, derivatives and applications, Chemical Review 112 (2012) 6156–6214.
[46] J.M. Englert, C. Dotzer, G. Yang, M. Schmid, C. Papp, J.M. Gottfried, et al., Covalent bulk functionalization of graphene, Nature Chem 3 (2011) 279–286.
[47] D. Boukhvalov, M. Katsnelson, Chemical functionalization of graphene, Journal of Physics: Condensed Matter 21 (2009) 344205.
[48] H. Bai, Y. Xu, L. Zhao, C. Li, G. Shi, Non-covalent functionalization of graphene sheets by sulfonated polyaniline, Chemical Communications (2009) 1667–1669.
[49] T. Kuila, S. Bose, A.K. Mishra, P. Khanra, N.H. Kim, J.H. Lee, Chemical functionalization of graphene and its applications, Progress in Materials Science 57 (2012) 1061–1105.
[50] M. Song, D. Cai, Graphene functionalization: a review, in: V. Mittal (Ed.), Polymer Graphene Composites, vol. 26, RSC Nanoscience and Nanotechnology, 2012.
[51] H. Liu, Y. Liu, D. Zhu, Chemical doping of graphene, Journal of Materials Chemistry 21 (2011) 3335–3345.
[52] J. Liu, J. Tang, J.J. Gooding, Strategies for chemical modification of graphene and applications of chemically modified graphene, Journal of Materials Chemistry 22 (2012) 12435–12452.
[53] F.e. Karlický, K. Kumara Ramanatha Datta, M. Otyepka, R. Zbořil, Halogenated graphenes: rapidly growing family of graphene derivatives, ACS Nano 7 (2013) 64346464.
[54] L. Yan, Y.B. Zheng, F. Zhao, S. Li, X. Gao, B. Xu, et al., Chemistry and physics of a single atomic layer: strategies and challenges for functionalization of graphene and graphene-based materials, Chemical Society Reviews 41 (2012) 97–114.
[55] T. Sreeprasad, V. Berry, How do the electrical properties of graphene change with its functionalization? Small 9 (2013) 341–350.
[56] R. Balog, B. Jørgensen, L. Nilsson, M. Andersen, E. Rienks, M. Bianchi, et al., Bandgap opening in graphene induced by patterned hydrogen adsorption, Nature Materials 9 (2010) 315–319.
[57] K.-J. Jeon, Z. Lee, E. Pollak, L. Moreschini, A. Bostwick, C.-M. Park, et al., Fluorographene: a wide bandgap semiconductor with ultraviolet luminescence, ACS Nano 5 (2011) 1042–1046.
[58] T. Gokus, R. Nair, A. Bonetti, M. Bohmler, A. Lombardo, K. Novoselov, et al., Making graphene luminescent by oxygen plasma treatment, ACS Nano 3 (2009) 3963–3968.
[59] A. Nourbakhsh, M. Cantoro, A.V. Klekachev, G. Pourtois, T. Vosch, J. Hofkens, et al., Single layer vs bilayer graphene: a comparative study of the effects of oxygen plasma treatment on their electronic and optical properties, The Journal of Physical Chemistry C 115 (2011) 16619–16624.
[60] A. Nourbakhsh, M. Cantoro, T. Vosch, G. Pourtois, F. Clemente, M.H. van der Veen, et al., Bandgap opening in oxygen plasma-treated graphene, Nanotechnology 21 (2010) 435203.
[61] P.E. Hopkins, M. Baraket, E.V. Barnat, T.E. Beechem, S.P. Kearney, J.C. Duda, et al., Manipulating thermal conductance at metal–graphene contacts via chemical functionalization, Nano Letters 12 (2012) 590–595.

[62] D.R. Dreyer, S. Park, C.W. Bielawski, R.S. Ruoff, The chemistry of graphene oxide, Chemical Society Reviews 39 (2010) 228–240.

[63] S. Park, R.S. Ruoff, Chemical methods for the production of graphenes, Nature Nanotechnology 4 (2009) 217–224.

[64] N. Xiao, X. Dong, L. Song, D. Liu, Y. Tay, S. Wu, et al., Enhanced thermopower of graphene films with oxygen plasma treatment, ACS Nano 5 (2011) 2749–2755.

[65] A. Ganguly, S. Sharma, P. Papakonstantinou, J. Hamilton, Probing the thermal deoxygenation of graphene oxide using high-resolution in situ X-ray-based spectroscopies, The Journal of Physical Chemistry C 115 (2011) 17009–17019.

[66] A. Bagri, C. Mattevi, M. Acik, Y.J. Chabal, M. Chhowalla, V.B. Shenoy, Structural evolution during the reduction of chemically derived graphene oxide, Nature Chem 2 (2010) 581–587.

[67] A. Felten, A. Eckmann, J. Pireaux, R. Krupke, C. Casiraghi, Controlled modification of mono-and bilayer graphene in O_2, H_2 and CF_4 plasmas, Nanotechnology 24 (2013) 355705.

[68] A. Felten, B.S. Flavel, L. Britnell, A. Eckmann, P. Louette, J.J. Pireaux, et al., Single and double[U+2010]Sided chemical functionalization of bilayer graphene, Small 9 (2013) 631–639.

[69] M.Z. Hossain, J.E. Johns, K.H. Bevan, H.J. Karmel, Y.T. Liang, S. Yoshimoto, et al., Chemically homogeneous and thermally reversible oxidation of epitaxial graphene, Nature Chemistry 4 (2012) 305–309.

[70] D.C. Kim, D.-Y. Jeon, H.-J. Chung, Y. Woo, J.K. Shin, S. Seo, The structural and electrical evolution of graphene by oxygen plasma-induced disorder, Nanotechnology 20 (2009) 375703.

[71] J.T. Robinson, J.S. Burgess, C.E. Junkermeier, S.C. Badescu, T.L. Reinecke, F.K. Perkins, et al., Properties of fluorinated graphene films, Nano Letters 10 (2010) 30013005.

[72] D. Elias, R. Nair, T. Mohiuddin, S. Morozov, P. Blake, M. Halsall, et al., Control of graphene's properties by reversible hydrogenation: evidence for graphane, Science 323 (2009) 610–613.

[73] O.J. Guy, A. Castaing, Z. Tehrani, S.H. Doak, Fabrication of ultrasensitive graphene nanobiosensors, in: Sensors, 2010 IEEE, 2010, pp. 907–912.

[74] J.T. Robinson, F.K. Perkins, E.S. Snow, Z. Wei, P.E. Sheehan, Reduced graphene oxide molecular sensors, Nano Letters 8 (2008) 3137–3140.

[75] H. Jeong, W.T. Hwang, Y. Song, J.K. Kim, Y. Kim, J. Hihath, S. Chung, T. Lee, Highly uniform monolayer graphene synthesis: via a facile pretreatment of copper catalyst substrates using an Ammonium persulfate solution, RSC Advances 9 (36) (2019) 20871–20877.

[76] V.K. Nagareddy, Fabrication, Functionalisation and Characterisation of Epitaxial Graphene Devices, PhD Thesis, University of Newcastle upon Tyne, UK, 2014.

[77] A. Lerf, H. He, M. Forster, J. Klinowski, Structure of graphite oxide revisited, Journal of Physical Chemistry B 102 (1998) 4477–4482.

[78] W. Cai, R.D. Piner, F.J. Stadermann, S. Park, M.A. Shaibat, Y. Ishii, et al., Synthesis and solid-state NMR structural characterization of 13C-labeled graphite oxide, Science 321 (2008) 1815–1817.

[79] B.L. VanMil, R.L. Myers-Ward, J.L. Tedesco, C.R. Eddy Jr., G.G. Jernigan, J.C. Culbertson, P.M. Campbell, J.M. McCrate, S.A. Kitt, D.K. Gaskill, Graphene formation on SiC substrates, Materials Science Forum 615–617 (2009) 211.

[80] L.G. Cancado, A. Jorio, E.M. Ferreira, F. Stavale, C. Achete, R. Capaz, et al., Quantifying defects in graphene via Raman spectroscopy at different excitation energies, Nano Letters 11 (2011) 3190–3196.

[81] A. Das, S.P.T. Mohiuddin, A. Lombardo, R. Nair, A. Bonetti, G. Savini, R. Jalil, et al., Uniaxial strain in graphene by Raman spectroscopy: G peak splitting, Grüneisen parameters, and sample orientation, Physical Review B 79 (2009) 205433.

[82] R. Murali, K. Brenner, Y. Yang, T. Beck, J.D. Meindl, Resistivity of graphene nanoribbon interconnects, IEEE Electron Device Lett 30 (2009) 611–613.

[83] X. Chen, D. Akinwande, K.-J. Lee, G.F. Close, S. Yasuda, B.C. Paul, et al., Fully integrated graphene and carbon nanotube interconnects for gigahertz high-speed CMOS electronics, IEEE Transactions on Electron Devices 57 (2010) 3137–3143.

[84] A.A. Balandin, S. Ghosh, W. Bao, I. Calizo, D. Teweldebrhan, F. Miao, et al., Superior thermal conductivity of single-layer graphene, Nano Letters 8 (2008) 902–907.

[85] S. Ghosh, I. Calizo, D. Teweldebrhan, E. Pokatilov, D. Nika, A. Balandin, et al., Extremely high thermal conductivity of graphene: prospects for thermal management applications in nanoelectronic circuits, Applied Physics Letters 92 (2008) 151911–151913.

[86] P. Blake, P.D. Brimicombe, R.R. Nair, T.J. Booth, D. Jiang, F. Schedin, et al., Graphene based liquid crystal device, Nano Letters 8 (2008) 1704–1708.

[87] F. Xia, T. Mueller, Y.-m. Lin, A. Valdes-Garcia, P. Avouris, Ultrafast graphene photodetector, Nature Nanotechnology 4 (2009) 839–843.

[88] T. Mueller, F. Xia, P. Avouris, Graphene photodetectors for high-speed optical communications, Nature Photonics 4 (2010) 297–301.

[89] X. Wang, L. Zhi, K. Mullen, Transparent, conductive graphene electrodes for dye sensitized solar cells, Nano Letters 8 (2008) 323–327.

[90] G. Jo, M. Choe, S. Lee, W. Park, Y.H. Kahng, T. Lee, The application of graphene as electrodes in electrical and optical devices, Nanotechnology 23 (2012) 112001.

[91] Y. Ji, S. Lee, B. Cho, S. Song, T. Lee, Flexible organic memory devices with multilayer graphene electrodes, ACS Nano 5 (2011) 5995–6000.

[92] V. Nagareddy, H. Chan, S. Hernandez, V. Wheeler, R. Myers-Ward, L. Nyakiti, et al., Detection of polar chemical vapors using epitaxial graphene grown on SiC (0001), Applied Physics Letters 102 (2013) 173103.

[93] X. Wang, S.M. Tabakman, H. Dai, Atomic layer deposition of metal oxides on pristine and functionalized graphene, Journal of the American Chemical Society 130 (2008) 8152–8153.

[94] S.M. Song, B.J. Cho, Investigation of interaction between graphene and dielectrics, Nanotechnology 21 (2010) 335706.

[95] N. Lu, Z. Li, J. Yang, Electronic structure engineering via on-plane chemical functionalization: a comparison study on two-dimensional polysilane and graphane, The Journal of Physical Chemistry C 113 (2009) 16741–16746.

[96] S. Ryu, M.Y. Han, J. Maultzsch, T.F. Heinz, P. Kim, M.L. Steigerwald, et al., Reversible basal plane hydrogenation of graphene, Nano Letters 8 (2008) 4597–4602.

[97] H. Yang, M. Chen, H. Zhou, C. Qiu, L. Hu, F. Yu, et al., Preferential and reversible fluorination of monolayer graphene, The Journal of Physical Chemistry C 115 (2011) 16844–16848.

[98] X. Zhang, A. Hsu, H. Wang, Y. Song, J. Kong, M.S. Dresselhaus, et al., Impact of chlorine functionalization on high-mobility chemical vapor deposition grown graphene, ACS Nano 7 (2013) 7262–7270.

[99] J. Choi, K.-j. Kim, B. Kim, H. Lee, S. Kim, Covalent functionalization of epitaxial graphene by azidotrimethylsilane, The Journal of Physical Chemistry C 113 (2009) 9433–9435.

[100] E. Bekyarova, M.E. Itkis, P. Ramesh, C. Berger, M. Sprinkle, W.A. de Heer, et al., Chemical modification of epitaxial graphene: spontaneous grafting of aryl groups, Journal of the American Chemical Society 131 (2009) 1336–1337.
[101] S.-H. Cheng, K. Zou, F. Okino, H.R. Gutierrez, A. Gupta, N. Shen, et al., Reversible fluorination of graphene: evidence of a two-dimensional wide bandgap semiconductor, Physical Review 81 (2010) 205435.
[102] B.R. Matis, J.S. Burgess, F.A. Bulat, A.L. Friedman, B.H. Houston, J.W. Baldwin, Surface doping and band gap tunability in hydrogenated graphene, ACS Nano 6 (2012) 17–22.
[103] Y. Wei, Y. Zhang, Z. Liu, Y. Wang, F. Ke, J. Meng, Y. Guo, P. Ma, Q. Feng, Z. Gan, High quality and large-scale manually operated monolayer graphene pasters, Nanotechnology 25 (27) (2014).
[104] Y. Liu, D. Yu, C. Zeng, Z. Miao, L. Dai, Biocompatible graphene oxide-based glucose biosensors, Langmuir 26 (2010) 6158–6160.
[105] J.H. Jung, D.S. Cheon, F. Liu, K.B. Lee, T.S. Seo, A graphene oxide based immuno biosensor for pathogen detection, Angewandte Chemie International Edition 49 (2010) 5708–5711.
[106] V. Nagareddy, H. Chan, S. Hernandez, V.D. Wheeler, L. Nyakiti, R. Myers-Ward, et al., Improved chemical detection and ultra-fast recovery using oxygen functionalized epitaxial graphene sensors, IIEEE Sensors Journal 13 (2013) 2810–2817.
[107] J.D. Fowler, M.J. Allen, V.C. Tung, Y. Yang, R.B. Kaner, B.H. Weiller, Practical chemical sensors from chemically derived graphene, ACS Nano 3 (2009) 301–306.
[108] S. Wang, Y. Zhang, N. Abidi, L. Cabrales, Wettability and surface free energy of graphene films, Langmuir 25 (2009) 11078–11081.
[109] J.A. Robinson, M. LaBella, M. Zhu, M. Hollander, R. Kasarda, Z. Hughes, et al., Contacting graphene, Applied Physics Letters 98 (2011) 053103–053103-3.
[110] S. Kumar, N. Peltekis, K. Lee, H.-Y. Kim, G.S. Duesberg, Reliable processing of graphene using metal etchmasks, Nanoscale Research Letters 6 (2011) 1–4.
[111] J. Yuan, L.-P. Ma, S. Pei, J. Du, Y. Su, W. Ren, et al., Tuning the electrical and optical properties of graphene by ozone treatment for patterning monolithic transparent electrodes, ACS Nano 7 (2013) 4233–4241.
[112] F. Alzina, H. Tao, J. Moser, Y. Garcia, A. Bachtold, C. Sotomayor-Torres, Probing the electron-phonon coupling in ozone-doped graphene by Raman spectroscopy, Physical Review B 82 (2010) 075422.
[113] N. McEvoy, H. Nolan, N. Ashok Kumar, T. Hallam, G.S. Duesberg, Functionalisation of graphene surfaces with downstream plasma treatments, Carbon 54 (2013) 283–290.
[114] S. Zhao, S.P. Surwade, Z. Li, H. Liu, Photochemical oxidation of CVD-grown single layer graphene, Nanotechnology 23 (2012) 355703.
[115] N. Mitoma, R. Nouchi, K. Tanigaki, Photo-oxidation of graphene in the presence of water, The Journal of Physical Chemistry C 117 (2013) 1453–1456.
[116] S. Pei, H.-M. Cheng, The reduction of graphene oxide, Carbon 50 (2012) 3210–3228.
[117] G. Eda, G. Fanchini, M. Chhowalla, Large-area ultrathin films of reduced graphene oxide as a transparent and flexible electronic material, Nature Nanotech 3 (2008) 270274.
[118] W. Gao, L.B. Alemany, L. Ci, P.M. Ajayan, New insights into the structure and reduction of graphite oxide, Nature Chem 1 (2009) 403–408.
[119] C. Gómez-Navarro, J.C. Meyer, R.S. Sundaram, A. Chuvilin, S. Kurasch, M. Burghard, et al., Atomic structure of reduced graphene oxide, Nano Letters 10 (2010) 1144–1148.

[120] K. Ostrikov, E. Neyts, M. Meyyappan, Plasma nanoscience: from nano-solids in plasmas to nano-plasmas in solids, Advances in Physics 62 (2013) 113–224.
[121] M. Eliáš, Z. Kučerová, O. Jašek, L. Zajíčková, V. Buršíková, H. Maršíková, et al., Functionalization of Carbon Nanotubes in low pressure capacitive coupled FR Discharge, in: CESPC II Book of Extended Abstracts, first ed., Masarykova Univerzita, Brno, 2008, pp. 156–157.
[122] A. Felten, C. Bittencourt, J.J. Pireaux, G. Van Lier, J.C. Charlier, Radiofrequency plasma functionalization of carbon nanotubes surface O_2, NH_3, and CF_4 treatments, Journal of Applied Physics 98 (2005).
[123] A. Kumar, A. Voevodin, R. Paul, I. Altfeder, D. Zemlyanov, D.N. Zakharov, et al., Nitrogen-doped graphene by microwave plasma chemical vapor deposition, Thin Solid Films 528 (2013) 269–273.
[124] C. Shen, G. Huang, Y. Cheng, R. Cao, F. Ding, U. Schwingenschlögl, et al., Thinning and functionalization of few-layer graphene sheets by CF4 plasma treatment, Nanoscale Research Letters 7 (2012) 1–8.
[125] M. Baraket, S. Walton, E. Lock, J. Robinson, F. Perkins, The functionalization of graphene using electron-beam generated plasmas, Applied Physics Letters 96 (2010) 1501.
[126] S.C. Hernandez, C.J. Bennett, C.E. Junkermeier, S.D. Tsoi, F.J. Bezares, R. Stine, et al., Chemical gradients on graphene to drive droplet motion, ACS Nano 7 (2013) 4746–4755.
[127] D.R. Boris, G.M. Petrov, E.H. Lock, T.B. Petrova, R.F. Fernsler, S.G. Walton, Controlling the electron energy distribution function of electron beam generated plasmas with molecular gas concentration: I. Experimental results, Plasma Sources Science Technology 22 (2013) 065004.
[128] M. Baraket, R. Stine, W.K. Lee, J.T. Robinson, C.R. Tamanaha, P.E. Sheehan, et al., Aminated graphene for DNA attachment produced via plasma functionalization, Applied Physics Letters 100 (2012) 233123.
[129] Y.-C. Lin, C.-Y. Lin, P.-W. Chiu, Controllable graphene N-doping with ammonia plasma, Applied Physics Letters 96 (2010) 133110–133110-3.
[130] I. Childres, L.A. Jauregui, J. Tian, Y.P. Chen, Effect of oxygen plasma etching on graphene studied using Raman spectroscopy and electronic transport measurements, New Journal of Physics 13 (2011) 025008.
[131] A.L. Walter, K.-J. Jeon, A. Bostwick, F. Speck, M. Ostler, T. Seyller, et al., Highly p-doped epitaxial graphene obtained by fluorine intercalation, Applied Physics Letters 98 (2011) 184102.
[132] S.V. Morozov, K.S. Novoselov, M.I. Katsnelson, F. Schedin, D.C. Elias, J.A. Jaszczak, et al., Giant intrinsic carrier mobilities in graphene and its bilayer, Physics Review Letter 100 (2008) 016602.
[133] New Reference.
[134] J. Pena-Bahamonde, H.N. Nguyen, S.K. Fanourakis, D.F. Rodrigues, "title,", Journal of Nanobiotechnology 16 (2018) 75.
[135] M.J.E. Fischer, Amine coupling through EDC/NHS: a practical approach, in: N.J. Mol, M.J.E. Fischer (Eds.), Surf Plasmon Reson Methods Protoc, Humana Press, Totowa, 2010, pp. 55–73.
[136] C. Sign, G. Sumana, Antibody conjugated graphene nanocomposites for pathogen detection, Journal of Physics 704 (2016) 7.
[137] A. Valipour, M. Roushani, Using silver nanoparticle and thiol graphene quantum dots nanocomposite as a substratum to load antibody for detection of hepatitis C virus core antigen: electrochemical oxidation of riboflavin was used as redox probe, Biosensors and Bioelectronics 89 (2017) 946–951.

[138] J. Huang, Z. Xie, Z. Xie, S. Luo, L. Xie, L. Huang, et al., Silver nanoparticles coated graphene electrochemical sensor for the ultrasensitive analysis of avian influenza virus H7, Analytica Chimica Acta 913 (2016) 121–127.
[139] T. Demeritte, N.B.P. Viraka, R. Kanchanapally, S.S. Sinha, A. Pramanik, S.R. Chavva, et al., Hybrid graphene oxide based plasmonic-magnetic multifunctional nanoplatform for selective separation and label-free identification of Alzheimer's disease biomarkers, ACS Application Mater Interfaces 7 (2015) 13693–13700.
[140] M. Sharafeldin, G.W. Bishop, S. Bhakta, A. El-Sawy, S.L. Suib, J.F. Rusling, Fe_3O_4nanoparticles on graphene oxide sheets for isolation and ultrasensitive amperometric detection of cancer biomarker proteins, Biosensors and Bioelectronics 91 (2017) 359–366.
[141] Y. Liu, X., Dong, P. Chen, Biological and chemical sensors based on graphene materials, Chemical Society Reviews 41 (2012) 2283–2307.
[142] Y. Huang, X. Dong, Y. Liu, L.-J. Li, P. Chen, "title,", Journal of Materials Chemistry 21 (2011) 12358–12362.
[143] Y., Huang, H.G. Sudibya, P. Chen, "title,", Biosensors and Bioelectronics 26 (2011) 4257–4261.
[144] E.K.G. Trindade, B.V.M. Silva, R.F. Dutra, A probeless and label-free electrochemical immunosensor for cystatin C detection based on ferrocene functionalized-graphene platform, Biosensors and Bioelectronics 138 (2019) 111311.
[145] R. Batool, M.A. Akhtar, A. Hayat, D. Han, L. Niu, M.A. Ahmad, M.H. Nawaz, A nanocomposite prepared from magnetite nanoparticles, polyaniline and carboxy-modified graphene oxide for non-enzymatic sensing of glucose, Microchimica Acta 186 (2019) 267.
[146] I. Kallashiya, N. Singh, S.K. Singh, V. Agrawal, D. Dash, Graohene-Oxide based biosensor for detection of platelet tool for thrombus risk identification, Biosensors and Bioelectronics 65 (2015) 274.
[147] G. Martinez-Garcia, I. Agul, P. Yanez-Sedeno, J.M. Pingarron, Multiplexed electrochemical immunosensor for obesity related hormones using grafted graphene modifuied electrodes as platforms for antibodies immobilisation, Proecdia Technology 27 (2017) 187.
[148] E. Akbari, A. Nikoukar, Z. Buntat, A. Afroozeh, A. Zeinalinexhad, Escenchia Coli bacterium detection using graohene based biosensor, IET Nano-Biotechnology 9 (2015) 273.
[149] B. Thakur, G. Zhou, J. Chang, H. Pu, B. Jin, X. Sui, Biosensors and bioelectronics rapid detection of single E Coli bacteria using a graphene based field effect transistor device, Biosensors and Bioelectronics 110 (2018) 16.
[150] M. Veerapandian, R. Hunter, S. Neethirajan, Dual immunosensor based on methylene – blue electroadsorbed graphene oxide for rapid detection of the influenza A virus antigen, Talanta 155 (2016) 250.
[151] S. Palanisamy, V. Velusamy, S. Ramaraj, S.W. Chen, T.C.K. Yang, S. Balu, C.E. Banks, Facile synthesis of cellulose microfibers supported palladium nanospindles on graphene oxide for selective detection of dopamine in pharmaceutical and biological samples, Materials Science and Engineering: C 98 (2019) 256–265.
[152] P. Assari, A.A. Rafati, A. Feizollahi, R.A. Joghani, An electrochemical immunosensor for the prostate specific antigen based on the use of reduced graphene oxide decorated with gold nanoparticles, Microchimica Acta 186 (2019) 484.

CHAPTER 10

Antimicrobial properties of SiC nanostructures and coatings

William Chiappim[1], Rodrigo Sávio Pessoa[1] and Mariana Amorim Fraga[2]
[1]Departamento de Física, Laboratório de Plasmas e Processos, Instituto Tecnológico de Aeronáutica, São José dos Campos, Brazil; [2]Escola de Engenharia, Universidade Presbiteriana Mackenzie, São Paulo, Brazil

Contents

1. Introduction

Microbial infections are a serious concern to healthcare. Their control and prevention in hospitals and other healthcare settings continue to be a significant challenge. Also, the treatment of these infections can be difficult due to antibiotic or multidrug resistance. Another concern is that the use of biomedical devices, such as catheters, stents, and implants, among others, can result in an increased risk of infection [1]. Furthermore, pathogenic microorganisms are known to affect the optimal functioning of medical devices, surgical devices, and bone cements [2]. This has motivated the research on materials that fight against contamination by microorganisms on their surface and are divided into microbiostatic and microbiocidal

Silicon Carbide Technology for Advanced Human Healthcare Applications
ISBN 978-0-323-90609-8
https://doi.org/10.1016/B978-0-323-90609-8.00004-1

materials [3]. Microbiostatic materials inhibit the adhesion of microorganisms, while microbiocidal material is used to eliminate them in case of contamination.

In recent years, the development of antimicrobial surfaces has been greatly explored for implants and biomedical devices. Different types of nanomaterials have been synthesized and studied for such applications. Among them, silicon carbide (SiC) nanostructures and coatings, due to their well-known outstanding properties, have attracted attention as potential candidates for antimicrobial surfaces.

SiC is a carbon-based ceramic material used since the 19th century due to its excellent cutting properties [4]. However, the great leap in its use occurred in the 20th century, mainly in the area of semiconductors, due to its high thermal, chemical, and mechanical stability, in addition to other unique characteristics [5]. The consolidation of SiC took place in the 21st century, with applications in sensors, photovoltaic devices, photocatalysis, electrodes for supercapacitors, water splitting, energy storage devices, conversion of CO_2 into fuels, in addition to improving the performance of nanomaterials for use in biological applications [6–8]. The interest in biological applications gained prominence after the discovery of its biocompatibility in mammalian cells [9], and the finding that SiC on a micrometric scale does not cause destructive impacts to biological tissue [10]. This evidence helped make SiC-based materials one of the primary biomaterials of the future, mainly due to their properties at the frontier of knowledge, such as operating in aggressive environments and under physiological conditions for long time periods [11].

Based on the properties mentioned earlier, and on studies by various groups worldwide, it is evident that SiC-based materials can and should be applied as an antimicrobial agent [12] and in biomedical devices [13].

As shown in Fig. 10.1, SiC has characteristics that change according to its physical structure, making it a material of great appeal for biomedical applications [14]. And, as a basic example, we can mention the hexagonal polytype structures of the semiinsulating and porous SiC, which have distinct characteristics but are of paramount importance for the construction of biosensors. On the other hand, the amorphous form, generally used as a coating, also has properties that are of technological appeal in biodevices. Therefore, an overview of the different structures and their antimicrobial effect should bring together the main works in a more concise and guiding way.

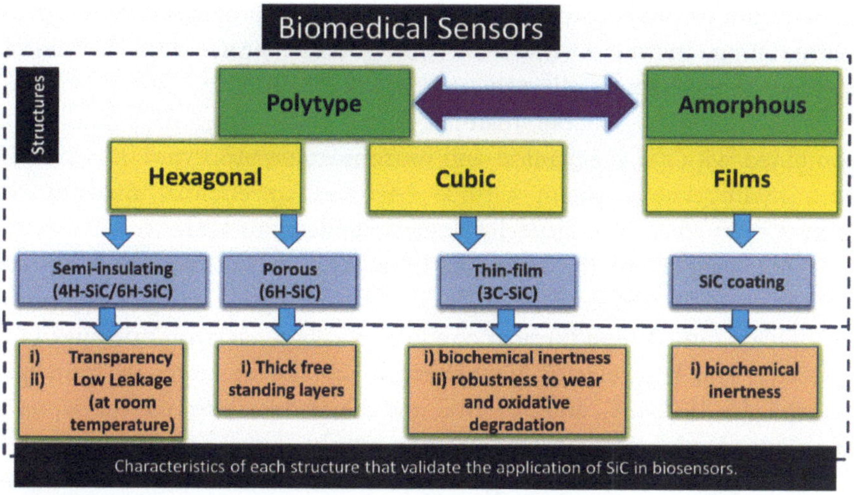

Figure 10.1 Amorphous and polytype SiC-based materials and their main characteristics for biosensor applications.

Therefore, this chapter will serve as a quick guide for health scientists, particularly nurses, doctors, and researchers in related fields who apply their knowledge in medical areas such as physicists, chemists, and engineers. To fulfill the purpose of a quick guide to antimicrobial applications, this chapter has been structured as follows: Section 2 focuses on the properties and synthesis of SiC nanostructures and coatings, Sections 3 and 4 discuss the antimicrobial effect and the main functionalities of SiC nanostructures and coatings and, respectfully, and Section 5 focuses on advanced devices and their applications in modern biomedicine.

2. Synthesis of SiC coatings and nanostructures for biomedical applications

2.1 Silicon carbide properties

Silicon carbide can be produced in amorphous and crystalline forms. SiC presents a wide bandgap in both forms that can be exploited for applications in several areas, mainly as sensors and biosensors [15]. As a substrate, SiC has excellent tribological, chemical, and electrical properties [16], making it possible to integrate it with technological devices in the field of micro and nanodevices. Due to its wide range of properties, SiC can be used as an active or passive material to construct biosensors [17].

Amorphous silicon carbide (*a*-SiC) can have its properties modified by incorporating hydrogen into its composition (*a*-SiC: H). Therefore, hydrogenation serves to adjust the optical and electronic properties of *a*-SiC films, making it a suitable material for a wide range of applications. Combined with the mechanical and biocompatible properties of *a*-SiC: H films, hydrogenated silicon carbide becomes an essential material for modern biomedical and biotechnological applications [18].

On the other hand, the crystalline form of SiC (*c*-SiC) is used for devices that require high temperature, high power, and high-frequency operation [19]. This is due to high thermal conductivity, high electron drift speed on its surface, and high electric field strength [20]. In this case, the principle polytypes are 4H-, 6H-, and 3C—SiC, and the reader is referred to Chapter 1 for an introduction to these important materials.

At this point, it is interesting to highlight the main crystalline compositions of silicon carbide. Fig. 10.2A shows the tetrahedral coordination of the bonds between Si and C. Fig. 10.2B shows the tetrahedral structure of Si—C clusters in a hexagonal structure arranged in the form of bilayers,

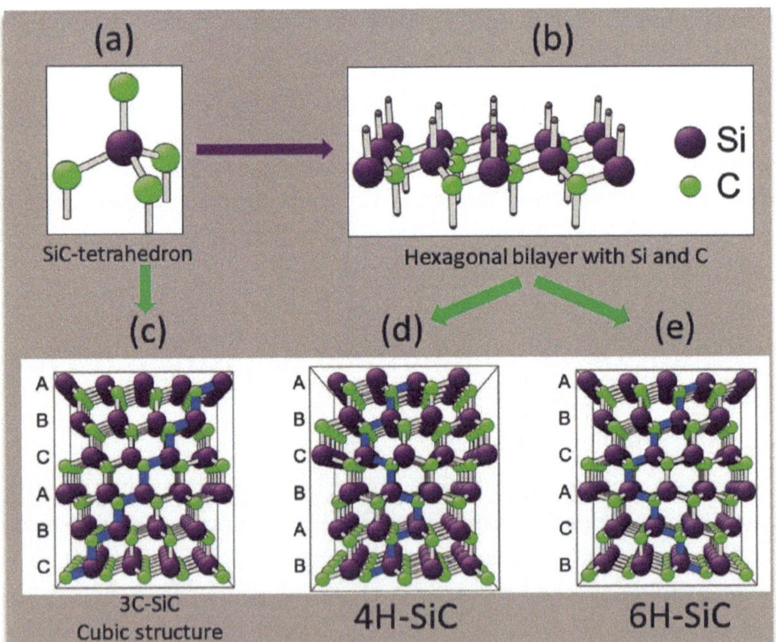

Figure 10.2 Physical structure of different SiC polytypes: (A) tetrahedrally bonding of Si and C, (B) hexagonal bilayer, (C) 3C—SiC (zinc blende structure), (D) 4H—SiC (hexagonal structure), and (E) 6H—SiC (hexagonal structure) [21].

similar to the diamond crystal structure, albeit with Si and C occupying sublayers of the bilayer [21]. Fig. 10.2C–E show the SiC crystal polytypes. These polytypes arise due to the near degeneracy of the total energies that generate mutual orientations in adjacent bilayers [22]. Fig. 10.2C shows the crystal structure of a cubic zinc blende (3C–SiC) structure, characterized by identical orientations of all bilayers in the crystal. Due to the repetition of the atomic geometry every three bilayers around the axis called c, this 3C polytype represents three layers in the cubic form [21]. Another possible crystal structure is Wurtzite, which in the case of SiC is not stable. Fig. 10.2D and E show polytypes with hexagonal lattice symmetry (4H- and 6H–SiC, respectively). 4H–SiC features identically and periodically oriented bilayer plates with four layers along the c axis. On the other hand, 6H–SiC consists of three bilayer plates oriented along the c axis with a periodicity of six layers [23].

2.2 Synthesis methods of silicon carbide coatings

The manufacture of SiC in the form of crystalline substrates (wafers with 150 and 200 mm diameter) of the n-, p-type, and in the form of "semi-insulating" with high purity composition, takes place at temperatures above 2000°C [24]. The growth method for crystalline SiC wafers is high-temperature chemical vapor deposition (see Fig. 10.3). SiC wafers can

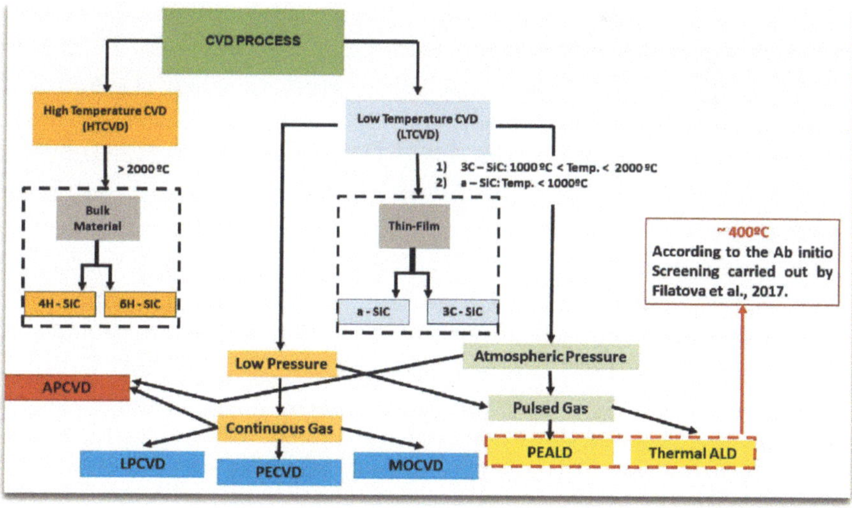

Figure 10.3 Main types of chemical vapor deposition (CVD) reactors and processes used to grow amorphous and crystalline silicon carbide thin films. *(Adapted from Ref. [33]; Creative Commons Attribution License.)*

have a 4H–SiC and 6H–SiC structure, depending on the seed crystal, that is, when the growth is seeded with 4H–SiC, the polytype obtained is 4H–SiC the same behavior occurs for 6H–SiC [25].

SiC in the form of thin films can be grown by magnetron sputtering [26,27], liquid phase epitaxy [28], molecular beam epitaxy [29], and chemical vapor deposition (CVD) processes [30,31]. However, the process that stands out for this application is CVD, which consists of the insertion of molecular gases in the reaction chamber, where they are dissociated and react on the substrate surface, forming a film. The CVD technique stands out for producing high-quality films, having an associated low cost, and having excellent growth uniformity with high-purity films with excellent adhesion [7]. As seen in Fig. 10.3, a wide variety of systems can be used in this technique for thin-film growth. The CVD technique can produce crystalline films of the 3C -SiC type and the amorphous type (*a*-SiC). Below is a summary of the main existing CVD systems.

LPCVD: Low-pressure chemical vapor deposition (LPCVD) is the most widely used CVD system for the growth of 3C–SiC films, mainly due to a larger surface coverage area. This is due to good uniformity in temperature distribution across the substrate. The good conformality and uniformity of the deposited films can also be highlighted [32], which are a consequence of the pressure used in the process being some orders of magnitude below atmospheric pressure, which increases the diffusivity of the vapor phase, leading to a rate-limited deposition with low gas-phase nucleation rate which generates resulting low particulates [32,33]. It is noteworthy that for the growth of SiC films, both LPCVD reactors are used: (1) cold wall (mandrel and substrate are heated), and (2) hot wall (the entire reactor is externally heated). Notably, the LPCVD reactor has the versatility to operate with a wide range of precursors, making it an essential tool in the growth of SiC films and enabling its doping [33]. Precursors can be divided into two types, namely single source and dual source. The most used single source Si and C precursors are 1,3-disilabutane (DSB) [34,35], disilacylane [36,37], dimethyldichlorosilane (DMDCS, $(CH_3)_2$ SiClutane [36], silacyclobutane (C_3H_6Si) [38], ditertiarybutylsilane ($C_8H_{18}Si$) [39], hexamethyldisilane (HMDS, $Si_2C_6H_{18}$) [40,41], tetramethylsilane (TMS, $C_4H_{12}Si$) [41], diethylmethylsilane (DEMS, $C_5H_{13}Si$) [42], diethylsilane ($(C_2H_5)_2SiH_4)$) [43], methylsilane (CH_6Si) [44,45], and methyl trichlorosilane (MTS) [46]. Regarding the doping process, ammonia (NH_3), nitrogen (N_2), and disilabutane [47] can be used, all these gases as nitrogen doping sources. On the other hand, for dual-source precursors, SiH_4 is the most used Si source and C_3H_8 or acetylene (C_2H_2) is used as a carbon source [31,48–51].

PECVD: Plasma-enhanced chemical vapor deposition (PECVD) is a modification of the conventional CVD system, where plasma is used as a source of reactive gas decomposition. This process occurs at lower temperatures (between 200 and 600°C) compared to conventional CVD, mainly due to the mechanism of chemical reactions generated in the plasma by ionization and dissociation by the impact of electrons that diffuse toward the substrate, causing surface chemical reactions that lead to the growth of the film. Three plasma sources are used, namely microwave discharge, pulsed discharge, and radio frequency (RF) discharge [7]. SiC films grown through PECVD at low temperatures are generally amorphous (*a*-SiC). Depending on the application, postdeposition annealing is required for crystallization. The most used precursors of single sources of Si and C are, respectively, silane (SiH_4) and methane (CH_4) [52], and of dual sources they are DSB, methylsilane, MTS, or tetramethylsilane (HMDS) [7,53].

MOCVD: Metal-organic chemical vapor deposition (MOCVD) was developed as a variant of the CVD method by Manasevit and Simpson [54]. MOCVD is based on organometallic chemistry with the use of one or more precursors. This CVD variant is widely applied for the synthesis of SiC thick films [55]. A "cold wall" reactor is generally used with the precursors being carried to a heated substrate with a carrier gas. The reactions occur at temperatures between 700 and 1100°C and pressures between 10 and 760 torrs [56]. In 3C–SiC crystalline film growth, the single-source precursor DEMS can be used [55]. On the other hand, in the development of homoepitaxial SiC of the 6H–SiC type, bis-trimethylsilylmethane can be used [57].

APCVD: Atmospheric pressure chemical vapor deposition (APCVD) was the dominant CVD variant in the 1980s and early 1990s to grow SiC films [7,33]. The literature reports 3C–SiC polycrystalline films deposited by this variant of CVD at temperatures above 1300°C and at atmospheric pressure [33]. Currently, APCVD has been replaced by LPCVD reactors, basically because it has better growth control and better nucleation [7,19]. APCVD is still a technique widely used in research laboratories, as it is a relatively simple system, consisting of a gas or steam flow injection system, a reaction chamber and gas mixture (which can be heated), and a system from the exhaustion of byproducts and precursors [58]. As a single precursor source, MTS is the most used precursor, as it produces high-quality films [59–61]. We can also mention HDMS [62]. Dual-source precursors have commonly used silane (SiH_4) and propane (C_3H_8) as sources of Si and C, respectively [63]. Other widely used precursors are dichlorosilane and trichlorosilane (HCl_3Si) [64].

ALD: Atomic layer deposition (ALD) and plasma-enhanced atomic layer deposition are specific modifications of CVD [65], with its main difference being the mode of exposure to gases. In CVD, we have the precursor, and the reaction gas dissociated simultaneously in the reactor/substrate. In ALD, precursors are alternately exposed, and the reactor is purged with an inert gas between reaction gas and precursor [66]. Therefore, ALD has a cyclic process that consists of a sequence of precursor exposure, inert gas purging, reaction gas exposure, and new purging [67]. This layer-by-layer film growth process is the fundamental characteristic of ALD. This specific modification of CVD is applied in a wide range of fields of science, from applications in the area of food packaging protection [66], to microelectronics [67–69], biomedicine [3], and solar cells [70], among others.

ALD as a SiC film growth tool was recently studied through the density functional theory by Filatova et al. [71,72]. Recent articles have discussed the possibilities of SiC growth by the ALD technique [33,73]. And all authors agree that the process of growing SiC by ALD is challenging. The few strategies related to the development of SiC by thermal ALD are found in a specific period between 1989 and 1995 [74–80]. LPCVD reactors operating as ALD systems and using the precursors SiH_2Cl_2, Si_2H_6, C_2H_2, and C_2H_4 as Si and C sources, respectively, were used. Except for Sadayuki et al. [80], who used temperatures on the order of 600°C, all the other works mentioned earlier used temperatures between 750 and 1200°C for the growth of SiC films. Fraga and Pessoa [33] suggest that due to the growth per cycle change with the increase of the temperature, occurs parasitic CVD in all works mentioned earlier, which shows that the processes do not fit as a real ALD process. According to Filatova et al. [71,72], H desorption occurs from Si surfaces above 350°C and desorption of methyl groups occurs above 423°C, which are temperatures higher than the thermal decomposition of the precursors Si_2H_6, C_2H_2, and C_2H_4. Therefore, this supports the idea that there is a parasitic CVD process in the works mentioned earlier [75–80].

Despite the great challenge to deposit SiC films by ALD, it is necessary to overcome it to improve all application areas, especially concerning bionanotechnology and its applications. In this sense, Fitalova et al. [71,72] used the ab initio theory to calculate the Gibbs free energy of reactions for a wide range of Si and C precursors using thermal ALD at 400°C. They showed that silicon precursors, namely SiH_3Cl, SiH_4, and Si_2H_6 combined with carbon precursors, namely $CHCl_3$, CCl_4, and C_2H_2 proved to be the most promising precursors for the growth of uniform and conformal SiC films at 400°C. However, novel chemical routes for new silicon and carbon precursors are needed to enhance and establish the development of SiC by ALD.

2.3 Synthesis methods of silicon carbide nanostructures

2.3.1 Nanoparticles

It is expected that, by reducing the characteristic size of SiC nanomaterials, some new properties, such as quantum confinement, arise because of this characteristic size. Consequently, SiC nanomaterials can be applied in different fields of engineering and science. For example, these materials can exhibit potential applications in electronic devices, sensors, catalysts, and biological technologies [81]. These nanometric SiC materials can also be very useful for building bulk materials, such as SiC nanoparticles, which can provide great advantages for preparing dense SiC bulk materials, significantly in lowering the sintering temperature [81,82].

Currently, many techniques have been developed or applied for the synthesis of SiC nanoparticles. The most common methods are CVD of CH_4 and SiH_4 containing compounds [83], laser pyrolysis and ablation [84], carbonization of the reaction mixture of silicon- and carbon-containing powders [85], and carbothermal reduction of fine sources of carbon and silicon, which are either natural or artificial sources [86].

2.3.2 Nanofibers, nanowires, and nanorods

An increasing amount of interest has been devoted to 1D nanostructures because of their significance in fundamentally scientific research works as well as their prospective technological utilization, especially for sensing applications [87]. The combination of the inherent characteristics of the SiC material with various 1D nanostructured morphologies has demonstrated the generation of numerous promising applications [81]. Usually, 1D SiC nanostructures with designed shape and aspect ratio are one of the most important aspects to investigate the unique behaviors at the nanoscale as well as size- and dimensionality-dependent physical/chemical characteristics. In addition, they can be used as interconnects and crucial units for the exploration of electronic, electrochemical, optoelectronic, and electromechanical micro/nanodevices [88]. The synthesis of fruitful 1D SiC nanostructures has been accomplished over the past decades, for example, nanowires, nanorods, nanoneedles, nanotubes, nanobelts, hierarchical nanoarchitectures, beaded nano chains, bamboo-like, twinned, and bi-crystalline structures, nanosprings, core—shell structures, and nanoarrays [81].

As reported in previous research works, several techniques, such as pyrolysis of polymeric precursors, carbothermal reduction, CVD, and thermal evaporation, have been used for the fabrication of SiC nanowires [89,90], nanorods [89], and nanoneedles [88]. On other hand, SiC nanotubes are grown by two main strategies. One is template-assisted growth, and the other is described as direct synthesis without a template. For other 1D SiC nanostructures with complex morphologies, the reader is recommended to visit the review article of Chen et al. [81].

Among the applications for 1D SiC nanostructures, photocatalysis is one of the most interesting with respect to the antimicrobial properties of SiC. Generally, the typical process of a photocatalytic reaction can be described as follows: (1) the generation and separation of charges induced by the absorbed light, (2) the transfer of charges, and (3) the reaction between the solution and photo-generated charge carriers [7]. The charge separation and shift across interfaces are regarded as crucial factors for the exploration of novel and efficient photocatalysts. The charge separation is governed by the band structure of photolytic materials. Accordingly, careful design of the structures, which results in efficient charge separation and transport, is a popular strategy to obtain the desired photocatalytic properties. To achieve this target, several methods have been developed, such as selective doping, surface decoration, structure, or morphology modifications. SiC materials are indirect semiconductors, which have wide band gaps of ~2.3—3.3 eV as well as robust chemical stability against hydrolysis. Hence, 1D nanostructures of SiC are attractive candidates for photocatalysts, where they would be subjected to aggressive conditions. It is an established fact that the bandgap of SiC semiconductors is readily regulated by doping and surface decoration, rendering them promising photocatalysts under visible light irradiation [81].

Another possible antimicrobial application of 1D SiC nanostructures may be due to superhydrophobic surfaces and intrinsic chemical robustness in hostile environments [91]. To manipulate the superhydrophobic behavior of 1D SiC nanostructure surfaces, their surface roughness and chemistry are considered the two crucial points. Increasing the surface roughness enhances the number of air-trapping pores. On the other hand, the chemical layer lowers the free energy. Fascinating superhydrophobic properties might be achieved through a combination of enhanced surface roughness and reduced surface energy via chemical coatings [81]. In addition to the intrinsic properties of 1D SiC nanostructures, some external treatments such as UV irradiation and electrowetting are also effective strategies to tune superhydrophobic properties [81].

3. Interaction mechanisms between microorganisms and SiC nanostructured surfaces

At this point, the types of SiC structures in bulk and film form, and the main growth tools based on the chemical vapor deposition method, have been reviewed. Now, it is necessary to understand the mechanism of interaction between microorganisms and SiC nanostructured surfaces. As reported in the literature, SiC is utterly inert to biological systems in its amorphous form (*a*-SiC) [92,93]. However, in nanostructured form, interaction with living cells occurs as in other nanostructured materials. Fig. 10.4 summarizes the primary main effects of the interaction between SiC nanostructured surfaces and bacteria. Two main mechanisms of bactericidal effects can be defined; namely, mechanical damage to the bacterial membrane and oxidative stress caused by the release of ions [94].

As seen in Fig. 10.4, mechanical damage can cause pit formation, lipid peroxidation, mechanical adhesion, alteration of bacterial metabolism, and

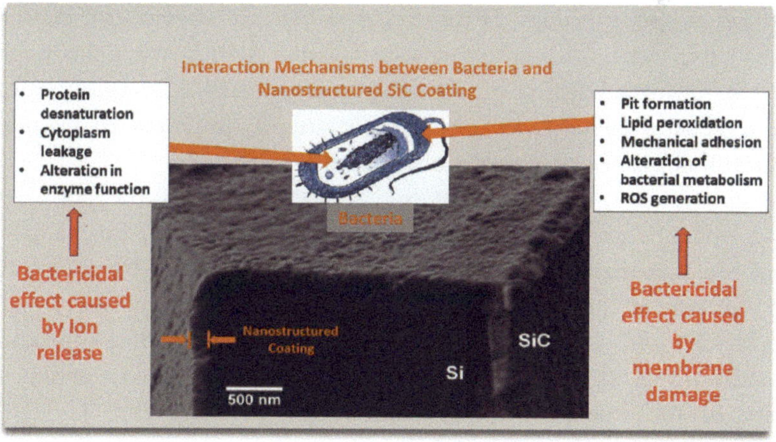

Figure 10.4 Schematic representation of a bacteria on the surface of a nanostructured SiC coating with the fundamental mechanisms of interaction between the coating and the bacteria summarized. *(Adapted from Ref. [35].)*

reactive oxygen species (ROS) generation. It is important to note that ROS can be present on the surface of SiC nanostructures by spontaneous SiC oxidation or by the addition of oxide thin films [95]. The effects of ROS tend to be enhanced due to the high catalytic activity of nanostructured materials and their large surface areas [96]. On the other hand, oxidative stress can cause protein denaturation, cytoplasm leakage, and alteration in enzyme function. According to Cadet et al., ROS is responsible for forming highly reactive radicals that cause DNA damage [97]. Therefore, the next topic will explore the different types of SiC nanostructures, namely, nanoparticles, nanofibers, nanowires, nanorods, and their antimicrobial applications.

4. Antimicrobial properties of SiC nanostructures and coatings

The antibacterial activity of SiC and palladium-loaded SiC nanoparticles was reported in 2018 [11]. This study evaluated their antibacterial action against gram-negative (*E. coli*) and gram-positive (*S. aureus*) bacteria by determining the minimal inhibitory concentration and minimal bactericidal concentration using standard agar dilution methods. In addition, scanning electron microscopy analyses were employed to evaluate the morphological change caused by these nanoparticles against *E. coli* and *S. aureus*. The antibacterial performance of pure SiC and Pd-loaded SiC materials was compared. The results indicated that the pure SiC nanoparticles had no effects on the morphology of the *S. aureus* cells. However, the Pd-loaded SiC had excellent antibacterial activity against pathogenic gram-negative and gram-positive bacteria preventing the attachment and colonization of these infectious bacteria, which demonstrates its potential to be used as antimicrobial agents for coating of medical devices.

More recently, the effect of SiC nanoparticles on the antibacterial activity of Ti—Cu alloy was investigated and discussed [98]. To evaluate the role of SiC nanoparticles on the antibacterial activity, two types of samples were synthesized: Ti—Cu alloy and Ti—Cu/SiC nanocomposite (using SiC nanoparticles with a particle size of less than 40 nm). The disc diffusion was the antibacterial detection method used for measuring the antibacterial activity of the studied materials. Both Ti—Cu alloy and Ti—Cu/SiC nanocomposite samples exhibited a strong antibacterial behavior for *E. coli*. On the other hand, Ti—Cu/SiC nanocomposite exhibited higher antibacterial activity rather than the Ti—Cu alloy, which confirms a higher antibacterial activity due to the presence of SiC nanoparticles. In a later study, the same authors observed an enhanced antibacterial effect of TiCu/SiC nanocomposite against *S. aureus* and *E. coli* of TiCu/SiC as a function of SiC content increase, that is, with increasing SiC content the antibacterial behavior was improved [98]. This behavior was attributed to high Cu^{2+} ion release as a result of particle size refinement with increasing SiC nanoparticles.

Along the same lines of adding SiC nanoparticles to increase the antibacterial activity in nanocomposites, Ahmed et al. addressed the structural, electrical, and electronic properties of PVA−MgO−SiC for antibacterial applications [99]. PVA−MgO−SiC nanocomposites were prepared with different SiC nanoparticles content. It was observed that the inhibition zone for *S. aureus* and *E. coli* is increased with an increase in the SiC nanoparticle concentration.

The incorporation of iron nanoparticles into SiC nanoparticles as novel antimicrobial bimetallic nanoparticles was proposed by Lemraski et al. [100]. For this system, they modified SiC nanoparticles by using zero-valent iron nanoparticles (ZVI). The ZVI/SiC bimetallic nanoparticles, due to their proper pore sizes, high specific areas, and high mechanical and chemical stabilities, exhibit high antibacterial activity against human pathogenic bacteria, such as *E. coli*, *Bacillus subtilis*, and *Pseudomonas putida*, demonstrating to be a potential antimicrobial agent.

Regarding the antibacterial properties of SiC nanofibers and nanorods, they were reported in an interesting study developed by Szala et al. [101]. The SiC nanofiber and nanorods used were produced by combustion synthesis. These nanostructures exhibited strong antibacterial activity. It was also observed that the presence of SiC nanostructures in bacterial cultures might not be the only factor leading to the decrease in microbial activity because a strong toxic effect was achieved when the examined suspensions of bacteria with SiC nanostructures were subjected to stirring. In their conclusions, the authors highlighted that, based on the issues addressed in the study, the chemical and thermal stability of SiC nanofibers and nanorods makes them more advantageous than carbon nanotubes indicating many potential applications of SiC nanostructures.

In another article, Borkowski et al. [92] observed that SiC nanofibers and nanorods can induce oxidative stress in *Pseudomonas putida* (Fig. 10.5). They concluded that nanostructured SiC may affect the activity of microorganisms by increasing the formation of highly reactive radicals and disrupting cell membrane integrity.

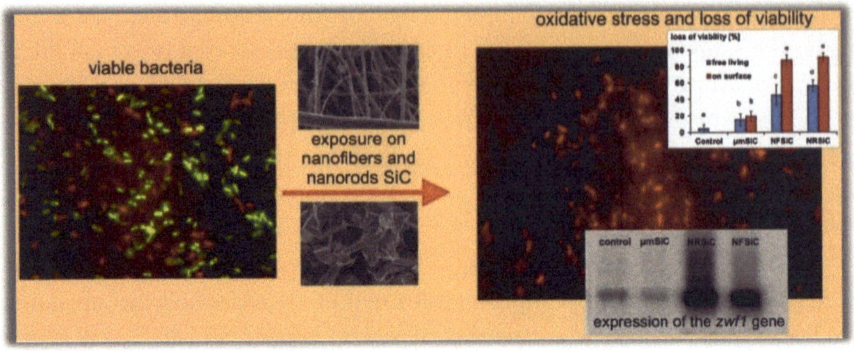

Figure 10.5 Overview of oxidative stress mechanisms in bacteria *Pseudomonas putida* exposed to SiC nanostructures. *(Reproduced with permission from Ref. [92] published by Elsevier, 2015.)*

The inhibitory effects of SiC nanowires against *E. coli* and *L. monocytogenes* were explored recently [102]. In this research, hexagonal SiC nanowires were produced using a versatile method of combining the waste from silicon wafers and graphite powder by robust high-energy ball milling and heat treatment approaches. Excellent antibacterial activity results were obtained: 90% against pathogenic *E. coli* and 75% against *L. monocytogenes* bacteria (Fig. 10.6A and B. A corresponding schematic representation of bacterial inhibition mechanisms by the synthesized SiC nanowires was elaborated (Fig. 10.6C). The results confirm the potential of SiC nanowires for medical applications to avoid add-on and colonization of transferrable bacteria.

The antibacterial properties of SiC coatings deposited on dental ceramics by PECVD were also investigated [103]. The objective was to evaluate that SiC coatings promote the decreased adhesion of mono-microbial and polymicrobial biofilms on the surface of the ceramic and exhibit biocompatibility without signs of cytotoxicity. The obtained results show that the SiC coating exhibited bactericidal activity against *S. mutans* and *S. sanguinis* after 24 h of culture. The coating also did not induce cytotoxic effects on periodontal ligament fibroblasts. Thus, SiC coatings can be used to improve the clinical performance of ceramic restorations.

A comparative study evaluated titanium nitride (TiN) and SiC adhesion properties to biofilms and the proliferation of human osteoblasts [104]. It was shown that TiN and SiC coatings significantly reduce the bacterial adhesion and prevent dental biofilm formation. Furthermore, they promote osteoblast adhesion and proliferation, that is, both exhibited osseointegration and antimicrobial properties.

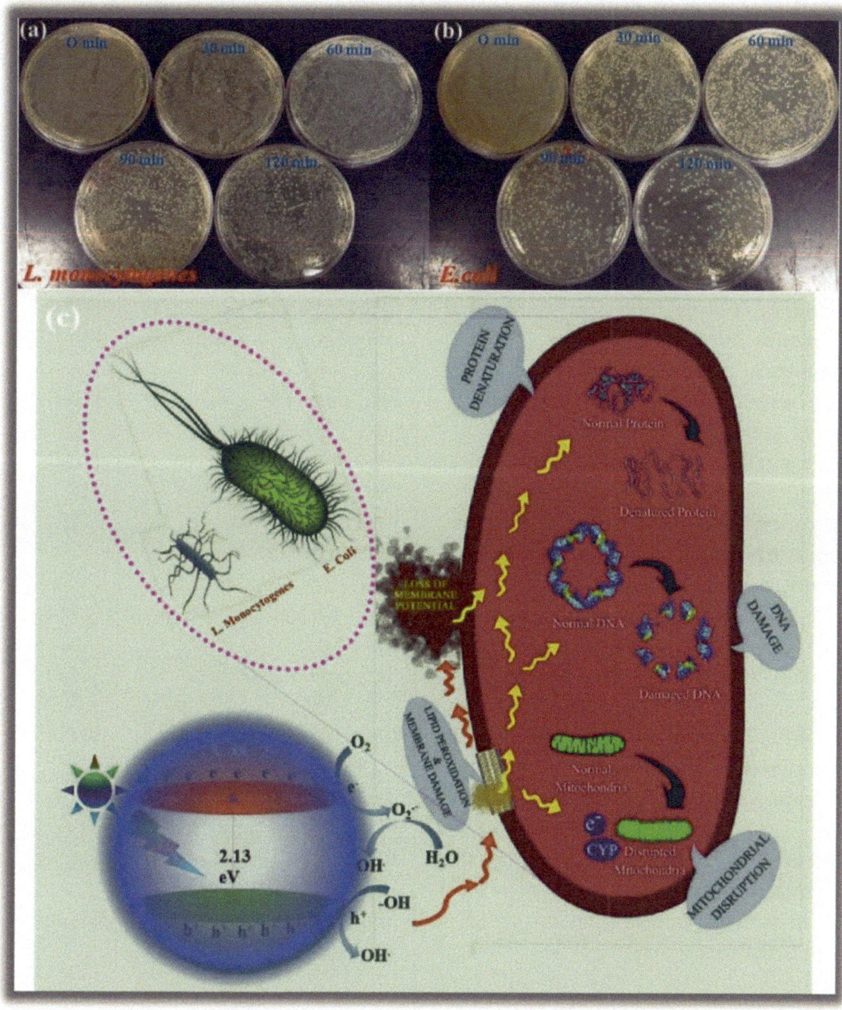

Figure 10.6 (A) and (B) Bacterial inhibition kinetics of SiC nanowires for *E. coli* and *L. monocytogenes* under visible-light irradiation and (C) Schematic of the antibacterial mechanism of SiC nanowires. *(Adapted from [102].)*

5. Applications of SiC in modern biomedicine

In addition to antimicrobial applications, SiC has a wide range of applications in biomedicine and biomedical engineering. This topic presents a list of main applications of the various forms of existing SiC nanomaterials (see Table 10.1). From this table, it can be noted that SiC applications range

Table 10.1 Summary of the main applications of silicon carbide in its various forms in modern biomedicine.

Applications	Type of SiC	Authors/ year
As bactericide	SiC nanofibers and nanorods	[92]
Neural stem cells plated on 3C–SiC substrate as clinical tool for lesioned neural areas	3C–SiC substrate	[105]
Protective coating for implanted retinal	a-SiC: H	[106]
SiC planar microelectrode for intracortical neural interface (INI)	4H–SiC and a-SiC	[107]
Electrocatalyst for nonenzymatic glucose sensing	SiC particles	[108]
Electrochemical enzymatic glucose sensor	SiC nanoparticles	[109]
Photothermal antitumor treatment has been performed to treat oral squamous carcinoma by photothermal therapy	Metallic carbon-defective silicon carbide (SiC_{1-x})	[110]
SiC RF antenna for in vivo biosensors	Poly-crystalline 3C–SiC	[111]
SiC nanowire devices for electrical DNA detection	3C–SiC nanowires	[112]
SiC/SiO_x nanowires for X-ray-excited photodynamic therapy	Core-shell SiC/SiO_x	[113]
SiC applied for coating coronary heart stent	a-SiC: H	[114]
SiC-based microprobe for myocardial ischemia monitoring	6H- and 4H–SiC substrates	[115]
SiC for healthy bone regeneration in femoral fracture	SiC nanoparticles	[116]
SiC for coating for dental ceramic prostheses	SiO_2/SiC	[117]
SiC for brain-machine interface applications	3C–SiC	[118]
SiC-based electrode devices for central nervous system biomedical implants	3C–SiC	[119]
Porous SiC for microdialysis technology	Porous SiC	[120]
SiC for anaerobic ceramic membrane bioreactor to co-manage domestic wastewater and food waste recycling wastewater	SiC ceramic membrane	[121]

Table 10.1 Summary of the main applications of silicon carbide in its various forms in modern biomedicine.—cont'd

Applications	Type of SiC	Authors/ year
Polymer-derived SiC foams for adsorption of non-steroidal antiinflammatory drugs	SiC foams	[122]
SiC quantum dots for cellular imaging and transport	SiC quantum dots	[123]
3C–SiC NEMS for biosensors	3C–SiC	[124]
SiC for magnetic resonance imaging	Epitaxial SiC films	[125]

from brain implants to biomedical devices used as stents or quantum dots for cellular imaging. Note that most works date from the last decade, showing the potential of this semiconductor as a biomaterial.

6. Summary

This chapter aimed to describe the antimicrobial properties of silicon carbide nanostructures and coatings, as well as to discuss their importance for the development of biomedical devices based on this material. The idea was to contribute to broadening the understanding of the characteristics that make SiC-based technologies promising for applications in areas such as biomedicine and health. A brief overview of why inhibiting infections in biomedical devices is critical, and how SiC material has the potential to be used as antimicrobial surfaces was presented. For this, recent publications dedicated to the antimicrobial properties of SiC nanostructures and coatings were discussed. The different methods of synthesis of 0D and 1D SiC coatings and nanostructures were described in detail. In addition, fundamental properties, application examples, and the potential of the SiC material in its different forms, nanoparticles, nanofibers, nanowires, nanorods, and coatings, for advances in the biomedical field were summarized. Finally, a listing of the applications of SiC-based devices in modern biomedicine was presented.

In summary, this chapter focused on an interesting and current application of the SiC material, which is its use as an antimicrobial surface in biomedical devices and implants.

Acknowledgments

The financial support of the Brazilian agency program FAPESP (grant no. 2018/01265-1), CNPq (grant nos. 446545/2014-7 and 437921/2018-2), and the Brazilian Space Agency (AEB/Uniespaço) is also gratefully acknowledged. W. Chiappim thanks the individual grant financed by FAPESP grant no. 20/10450-7.

References

[1] M. Zare, M. Zare, J.A. Butler, S. Ramakrishna, Nanoscience-led antimicrobial surface engineering to prevent infections, ACS Applied Nano Materials 4 (5) (May 19, 2021) 4269–4283, https://doi.org/10.1021/acsanm.1c00466.

[2] S. Mahira, A. Jain, W. Khan, J. Abraham, Domb, Chapter 1. Antimicrobial Materials—An Overview, Antimicrobial Materials for Biomedical Applications, 2019, pp. 1–37, https://doi.org/10.1039/9781788012638-00001.

[3] R.S. Pessoa, V.P. dos Santos, S.B. Cardoso, A.C.O.C. Doria, F.R. Figueira, B.V.M. Rodrigues, G.E. Testoni, M.A. Fraga, F.R. Marciano, A.O. Lobo, H.S. Maciel, TiO_2 coatings via atomic layer deposition on polyurethane and polydimethylsiloxane substrates: properties and effects on C. albicans growth and inactivation process, Applied Surface Science 422 (November, 2017) 73–84, https://doi.org/10.1016/j.apsusc.2017.05.254.

[4] F. Eblagon, B. Ehrle, T. Graule, J. Kuebler, Development of silicon nitride/silicon carbide composites for wood-cutting tolls, Journal of the European Ceramics Society 27 (2007) 419–428, https://doi.org/10.1016/j.jeurceramsoc.2006.02.040.

[5] P.G. Neudeck, Progress in silicon carbide semiconductor electronics technology, Journal of Electronic Materials (April, 1995), https://doi.org/10.1007/BF02659688.

[6] M.A. Gondal, M.A. Ali, M.A. Dastageer, X. Chang, CO_2 conversion into metanol using granular silicon carbide (a6H-SiC): a comparative evaluation of 355 nm laser and xenon mercury broad band radiation sources, Catalysis Letters 143 (2013) 108–117, https://doi.org/10.1007/s10562-012-0916-z.

[7] R.S. Pessoa, M.A. Fraga, L.V. Santos, M. Massi, H.S. Maciel, Nanostructured thin films based on TiO_2 and/or SiC for use in photoelectrochemical cells: a review of the material characteristics, synthesis and recent applications, Materials Science in Semiconductor Processing 29 (January, 2015) 56–68, https://doi.org/10.1016/j.mssp.2014.05.053.

[8] M.A. Gondal, A.M. Ilyas, U. Baig, Facile synthesis of silicon carbide-titanium dioxide semiconducting nanocomposite using pulsed laser ablation technique and its performance in photovoltaic dye sensitized solar cell and photocatalytic water purification, Applied Surface Science 378 (August, 2016) 8–14, https://doi.org/10.1016/j.apsusc.2016.03.135.

[9] S. Barillet, A. Simon-Deckers, N. Herlin-Boime, M. Mayne-L'Hermite, C. Reynaud, B. Gouget, M. Carrière, Toxicological consequences of TiO_2, SiC nanoparticles and multi-walled carbon nanotubes exposure in several mammalian cell types: an in vitro study, Journal of Nanoparticle Research 12 (2010) 61–73, https://doi.org/10.1007/s11051-009-9694-y.

[10] J. Bruch, B. Renh, H. Song, E. Gono, W. Malkusch, Toxicological investigations on silicon carbide. 1. Inhalation studies, British Journal of Industrial Medicine 50 (1993) 797–806, https://doi.org/10.1136/oem.50.9.797.

[11] U. Baig, M.A. Gondal, M.A. Ansari, A. Sultan, Facile synthesis, characterization and antibacterial activity of nanostructured palladium loaded silicon carbide, Ceramics International 44 (14) (October, 2018) 16908–16914, https://doi.org/10.1016/j.ceramint.2018.06.129.

[12] A.A. Askar, M.S. Selim, S.A. El-Safty, A.I. Hashem, M.M. Selim, M.A. Shenashen, Antimicrobial and immunomodulatory potential of nanscale hierarchical one-dimensional zinc oxide and silicon carbide materials, Materials Chemistry and Physics 263 (April, 2021) 124376, https://doi.org/10.1016/j.matchemphys.2021.124376.
[13] A. Oliveros, A. Guiseppi-Elie, S.E. Saddow, Silicon carbide: a versatile material for biosensor applicatrions, Biomedical Microdevices 15 (January, 2013) 353–368, https://doi.org/10.1007/s10544-013-9742-3.
[14] P. Godignon, SiC materials and technologies for sensors development, Materials Science Forum 483–485 (May, 2005) 1009–1014, https://doi.org/10.4028/www.scientific.net/msf.483-485.1009.
[15] N. Yang, H. Zhuang, R. Hoffmann, W. Smirnov, J. Hees, X. Jiang, C.E. Nebel, Nanocrystalline 3C-SiC electrode for biosensing applications, Analytical Chemistry 83 (15) (June, 2011) 5827–5830, https://doi.org/10.1021/ac201315q.
[16] W. Zhang, S. Yamashita, H. Kita, Progress in tribological research of SiC ceramics in unlubricated slidind – a review, Material and Design 190 (May, 2020) 108528, https://doi.org/10.1016/j.matdes.2020.108528. https://doi.org/10.1039/C9AN02390A.
[17] Y. Wang, H. Feng, H. Zhang, Y. Chen, W. Huang, J. Zhang, X. Jiang, M. Wang, H. Jiang, X. Wang, Nanoelectrochemical biosensors for monitoring ROS in cancer cells, Analyst 145 (December, 2020) 1294–1301, https://doi.org/10.1016/S0921-5107(02)00204-0.
[18] S. Kaci, A. Keffous, S. Hakoum, A. Mansri, Hydrogen sensitivity of the sensors based on nanostructured lead sulfide thin films deposited on a-SiC: H and p-Si(100) substrates, Vacuum 116 (June, 2015) 27–30, https://doi.org/10.1016/j.vacuum.2015.02.024.
[19] G. Foti, Silicon carbide: from amorphous to crystalline, Applied Surface Science 184 (December, 2001) 20–26, https://doi.org/10.1016/S0169-4332(01)00751-6.
[20] T. Kimoto, Material science and device physics in SiC technology for high-voltage power devices, Japanese Journal of Applied Physics 54 (March, 2015) 040103, https://doi.org/10.7567/jjap.54.040103.
[21] U. Starke, J. Bernhardt, J. Schart, K. Heinz, SiC surface reconstruction: relevancy of atomic structure for growth technology, Surface Review and Letters 6 (1999) 1129–1141, https://doi.org/10.1142/S0218625X99001256.
[22] V. Heine, C. Cheng, R.J. Needs, A computacional study into the origin of SiC polytipes, Material Science and Engineering: B 11 (January, 1992) 55–60, https://doi.org/10.1016/0921-5107(92)90190-K.
[23] R.S. Mitchell, Studies on a group of silicon carbide structures, The Journal of Chemical Physics 22 (12) (1954) 1977, https://doi.org/10.1063/1.1739978.
[24] A. Ellison, J. Zhang, J. Peterson, A. Henry, Q. Wahab, J.P. Bergman, Y.N. Makarov, A. Vorobev, A. Vehanen, E. Janzén, High temperature CVD growth of SiC, Materials Science and Engineering: B 61–62 (July, 1999) 113–120, https://doi.org/10.1016/S0921-5107(98)00482-6.
[25] A. Wada, T. Kimoto, K. Nishikawa, H. Matsunami, Epitaxial growth of 4H-SiC on 4° off-axis (0001) and (0001-) substrates by hot-wall chemical vapor deposition, Journal of Crystal Growth 291 (2006) 370–374.
[26] H.S. Medeiros, R.S. Pessoa, J.C. Sagás, M.A. Fraga, L.V. Santos, H.S. Maciel, M. Massi, A.S. da Silva Sobrinho, SixCy thin films deposited at low temperature by DC dual magnetron sputtering: effect of power supplied to Si and C cathode targets on film physicochemical properties, Materials Science Forum 717 (2012) 197–201, https://doi.org/10.4028/www.scientific.net/MSF.717-720.197.
[27] N. Galvão, M. Guerino, T. Campos, K. Grigorov, M. Fraga, B. Rodrigues, R. Pessoa, J. Camus, M. Djouadi, H. Maciel, The influence of AlN intermediate layer on the structural and chemical properties of SiC thin films produced by high-power impulse magnetron sputtering, Micromachines 10 (March, 2019) 202, https://doi.org/10.3390/mi10030202.

[28] M. Syväjärvi, R. Yakimova, H.H. Radamson, N.T. Son, Q. Wahab, E. Janzén, Liquid phase epitaxial growth of SiC, Journal of Crystal Growth 197 (February, 1999) 147–154, https://doi.org/10.1016/S0022-0248(98)00878-1.
[29] J. Chen, A.J. Steckl, Molecular beam epitaxy growth of SiC on Si(111) from silacyclobutane, Journal of Vacuum Science and Technology B: Microelectronics and Nanometer Structures Processing, Measurement, and Phenomena 16 (June, 1998) 1305, https://doi.org/10.1116/1.590006.
[30] M. Zielinski, M. Portail, T. Chassagne, S. Juillguet, H. Peyre, Nitrogen doping of 3C − SiC thin films grown by CVD in a resistively heated horizontal hot-wall reactor, Journal of Crystal Growth 310 (June, 2008) 3174–3182, https://doi.org/10.1016/j.jcrysgro.2008.03.022.
[31] C.-F. Wang, D.-S. Tsai, Low pressure chemical vapor deposition of silicon carbide from dichlorosilane and acetylene, Materials Chemistry and Physics 63 (3) (March, 2000) 196–201.
[32] M. Mehregany, C.A. Zorman, S. Roy, A.J. Fleischman, C.-H. Wu, N. Rajan, Silicon carbide for microelectromechanical systems, International Materials Reviews 45 (July, 2013) 85–108, https://doi.org/10.1179/095066000101528322.
[33] M. Fraga, R. Pessoa, Progress in synthesis and applications of SiC films: from CVD to ALD and from MEMS to NEMS, Micromachines 11 (August, 2020) 799, https://doi.org/10.3390/mi11090799.
[34] J.-H. Boo, K.-S. Yu, Y. Kim, S.H. Yeon, I.N. Jung, Growth of cubic SiC films using 1,3-disilabutane, Chemistry of Materials 7 (4) (April, 1995) 694–698, https://doi.org/10.1021/cm00052a014.
[35] C.R. Stoldt, C. Carraro, W.R. Ashurst, D. Gao, R.T. Howe, R. Maboudian, A low-temperature CVD process for silicon carbide MEMS, Sensors and Actuators A: Physical 97–98 (April, 2002) 410–415, https://doi.org/10.1016/S0924-4247(01)00810-X.
[36] K.A. Jacobson, Growth, texture, and surface morphology of SiC layers, Journal of The Electrochemical Society 118 (1971) 1001, https://doi.org/10.1149/1.2408179.
[37] D.J. Larkin, L.V. Interrante, Chemical vapor deposition of silicon carbide from 1.3-disilacyclobutane, Chemistry of Materials 4 (1) (January, 1992) 22–24, https://doi.org/10.1021/cm00019a009.
[38] A.J. Steckl, C. Yuan, J.P. Li, Growth of crystalline 3C-SiC on Si at reduced temperatures by chemical vapor deposition from silacyclobutane, Applied Physics Letters 63 (September, 1993) 3347, https://doi.org/10.1063/1.110140.
[39] J.M. Grow, R.A. Levy, M. Bhaskaran, H.J. Boeglin, R. Shalvoy, Low pressure chemical vapor deposition of silicon carbide form ditertiarybutylsilane, Journal of The Electrochemical Society 140 (10) (1993) 3001, https://doi.org/10.1149/1.2220947.
[40] K. Takahashi, S. Nishino, J. Saraie, Low-temperature growth of 3C-SiC on Si substrate by chemical vapor deposition using hexamethyldisilane as a source material, Journal of The Electrochemical Society 139 (1992) 3565, https://doi.org/10.1149/1.2069122.
[41] B.T. Lee, D.K. Kim, C.K. Moon, J.K. Kim, Y.H. Seo, K.S. Nahm, H.J. Lee, K.W. Lee, K.S. Yu, Y. Kim, S.J. Jang, Microstructural investigation of low temperature chemical vapor deposited 3C-SiC/Si thin films using single-source precursors, Journal of Materials Research 14 (1999) 24–28, https://doi.org/10.1557/JMR.1999.0006.
[42] D.-C. Lim, H.-G. Jee, J.W. Kim, J.-S. Moon, S.-B. Lee, S.S. Choi, J.-H. Boo, Deposition of epitaxial silicon carbide films using high vacuum MOCVD method for MEMS, Thin Solid Films 459 (1–2) (July, 2004) 7–12, https://doi.org/10.1016/j.tsf.2003.12.140.

[43] Y. Avigal, M. Schieber, R. Levin, The growth of hetero-epitaxial SiC films by pyrolysis of various alkyl-silicon compounds, Journal of Crystal Growth 24–25 (October, 1974) 188–192, https://doi.org/10.1016/0022-0248(74)90302-9.
[44] C.W. Liu, J.C. Sturm, Low temperature chemical vapor deposition growth of b-SiC on (100) Si using methylsilane and device characteristics, Journal of Applied Physics 82 (July, 1997) 4558, https://doi.org/10.1063/1.366192.
[45] F. Liu, C. Carraro, J. Chu, R. Maboudian, Residual stress characterization of polycrystalline 3C – SiC films on Si(100) deposited from methylsilane, Journal of Applied Physics 106 (May, 2009) 013505, https://doi.org/10.1063/1.3157184.
[46] W.-C. Lien, N. Ferralis, C. Carraro, R. Maboundian, Growth of epitaxial 3C – SiC films on Si(100) via low temperature SiC buffer layer, Crystal Growth and Design 10 (1) (December, 2009) 36–39, https://doi.org/10.1021/cg901189k.
[47] M.T. Clavaguera-Mora, J. Rodriguez-Viejo, Z. El Felk, E. Hurtós, S. Berberich, J. Stoemenos, N. Clavaguera, Growth of SiC films obtained by LPCVD, Diamond and Related Materials 6 (10) (August, 1997) 1306–1310, https://doi.org/10.1016/S0925-9635(97)00084-8.
[48] S. Nishino, Y. Hazuki, H. Matsunami, T. Tanaka, Chemical vapor deposition of single crystalline b-SiC films on silicon substrate with sputtered SiC intermediate layer, Journal of The Electrochemical Society 127 (1980) 2674, https://doi.org/10.1149/1.2129570.
[49] P. Liaw, R.F. Davis, Epitaxial growth and characterization of b-SiC thin films, Journal of The Electrochemical Society 132 (1985) 642, https://doi.org/10.1149/1.2113921.
[50] K. Yagi, H. Nagasawa, 3C-SiC growth by alternate supply of SiH_2Cl_2 and C_2H_2, Journal of Crystal Growth 174 (1–2) (April, 1997) 653–657, https://doi.org/10.1016/S0022-0248(97)00055-9.
[51] X.-A. Fu, J.L. Dunning, M. Mehregany, C.A. Zorman, Low stress polycrystalline SiC thin films suitable for MEMS applications, Journal of The Electrochemical Society 158 (April, 2011) H675, https://doi.org/10.1149/1.3575160.
[52] M.V. Pelegrini, G.P. Rehder, I. Pereyra, a-SiC:H films deposited by PECVD for MEMS applications, Physica Status Solidi C 7 (3–4) (March, 2010) 786–789, https://doi.org/10.1002/pssc.200982888.
[53] A. Klumpp, U. Schaber, H.L. Offereins, K. Kühl, H. Sandmaier, Amorphous silicon carbide and its applications in silicon micromachining, Sensors and Actuators A: Physical 41 (1–3) (April, 1994) 310–316.
[54] H.M. Manasevit, W.I. Simpson, The use of metal-organics in the preparation of semiconductor materials: I. Epitaxial gallium-V compounds, Journal of The Electrochemical Society 116 (1969) 1725, https://doi.org/10.1149/1.2411685.
[55] R.E. Beisenov, R. Ebrahim, Z.A. Mansurov, S.T. Tokmoldin, B.Z. Mansurov, A. Ignatiev, Growth of 3C-SiC films on Si(111) and sapphire (0001) substrates by MOCVD, Eurasian Chemico-Technological Journal 15 (1) (January, 2013) 25–29, https://doi.org/10.18321/ectj136.
[56] R. Zuo, H. Zhang, X.-l. Liu, Transport phenomena in radial flow MOCVD reactor with three concentric vertical inlets, Journal of Crystal Growth 293 (2) (August, 2006) 498–508, https://doi.org/10.1016/j.jcrysgro.2006.05.063.
[57] J.K. Jeong, H.J. Na, J. Choi, C.S. Hwang, H.J. Kim, W. Bahng, Homoepitaxial growth of 6H-SiC thin films by metal-organic chemical vapor deposition using bis-trimethylsilylmethane precursor, Journal of Crystal Growth 210 (4) (March, 2000) 629–636, https://doi.org/10.1016/S0022-0248(99)00744-7.
[58] M.J. Powell, I.P. Parkin, Titania coated mica via chemical vapour deposition, post N-doped by liquid ammonia, Physics Procedia 46 (2013) 111–117, https://doi.org/10.1016/j.phpro.2013.07.052.

[59] G.D. Papasouliotis, S.V. Sotirchos, Experimental study of atmospheric pressure chemical vapor deposition of silicon carbide from methyltrichlorosialne, Journal of Materials Research 14 (August, 1999) 3397–3409, https://doi.org/10.1557%2FJMR.1999.0460.
[60] K. Schillinger, S. Janz, S. Reber, Atmospheric pressure chemical vapour deposition of 3C-SiC for silicon thin-film solar cells on various substrates, Journal of Nanoscience and Nanotechnology 11 (9) (September, 2011) 8108, https://doi.org/10.1166/jnn.2011.5062.
[61] Y. Funato, N. Sato, Y. Fukushima, H. Sugiura, T. Momose, Y. Shimogaki, Fundamental evaluation of gas-phase elementar reaction models for silicon carbide chemical vapor deposition, ECS Journal of Solid State Science and Technology 6 (May, 2017) P399, https://doi.org/10.1149/2.0141707jss.
[62] K.-S. Kim, G.-S. Chung, Mechanical properties of in-situ doped polycrystalline 3C-SiC thin films by APCVD, Journal of the Korean Institute of Electrical and Electronic Material Engineers 22 (3) (January, 2009) 235–238, https://doi.org/10.4313/JKEM.2009.22.3.235.
[63] C.A. Zorman, A.J. Fleischman, A.S. Dewa, M. Mehregany, Epitaxial growth of 3C-SiC films on 4 in. diam(100) silicon wafers by atmospheric pressure chemical vapor deposition, Journal of Applied Physics 78 (June, 1995) 5136, https://doi.org/10.1063/1.359745.
[64] M. Otani, T. Takahashi, H. Habuka, Y. Ishida, S.-I. Ikeda, S. Hara, Quartz Crystal microbalance for evaluating gas motion differences between dichlorosilane and trichlorosilane in ambient hydrogen in a slim vertical cold wall chemical vapor deposition reactor, Advances in Chemical Engineering and Science 10 (3) (July, 2020) 190–200, https://doi.org/10.4236/aces.2020.103014.
[65] W. Chiappim, M.A. Fraga, H.S. Maciel, R.S. Pessoa, An experimental and theoretical study of the impact of the precursor pulse time on the growth per cycle and crystallinity quality of TiO2 thinn films grown by ALD and PEALD technique, Frontiers in Mechanical Engineering 6 (October, 2020) 551085, https://doi.org/10.3389/fmech.2020.551085.
[66] V.M. Dias, W. Chiappim, M.A. Fraga, H.S. Maciel, F.R. Marciano, R.S. Pessoa, Atomic layer deposition of TiO_2 and Al_2O_3 thin films for electrochemical study of corrosion protection in aluminum alloy cans used in beverage, Material Research Express 7 (July, 2020) 076408, https://doi.org/10.1088/2053-1591/aba557/meta.
[67] W. Chiappim, G. Testoni, F. Miranda, M. Fraga, H. Furlan, D.A. Saraiva, A. da Silva Sobrinho, G. Petraconi, H. Maciel, R. Pessoa, Effect of plasma-enhanced atomic layer deposition on oxygen overabundance and its influence on the morphological, optical, structural, and mechanical properties of Al-doped TiO_2 coating, Micromachines 12 (6) (May, 2021) 588, https://doi.org/10.3390/mi12060588.
[68] R.S. Pessoa, M.A. Fraga, W. Chiappim, H.S. Maciel, Exploring the properties and fuel cell applications of ultrathin atomic layer deposited metal oxide films, in: K.Y. Cheong, G. Impellizzeri, M.A. Fraga (Eds.), Emerging Materials for Energy Conversion and Storage, first ed. vol. 1, Elsevier, Amsterdam, The Netherlands, 2018, pp. 83–114, https://doi.org/10.1016/B978-0-12-813794-9.00003-X.
[69] W. Chiappim, M. Watanabe, V. Dias, G. Testoni, R. Rangel, M. Fraga, H. Maciel, S. dos Santos Filho, R. Pessoa, MOS capacitance measurements for PEALD TiO_2 dielectric films grown under different conditions and the impact of Al_2O_3 partial-monolayer insertion, Nanomaterials 10 (2) (February, 2020) 338, https://doi.org/10.3390/nano10020338.

[70] M.A. Curado, J.P. Teixeira, M. Monteiro, E.F.M. Ribeiro, R.C. Vilão, H.V. Alberto, J.M.V. Cunha, T.S. Lopes, K. Oliveira, O. Donzel-Gargand, A. Hultqvist, S. Calderon, M.A. Barreiros, W. Chiappim, J.P. Leitão, A.G. Silva, T. Prokscha, C. Vinhais, P.A. Fernades, P.M.P. Salomé, Front passivation of Cu(In,Ga)Se_2 solar cells using Al_2O_3: culprits and benefits, Applied Materials Today 21 (December, 2020) 100867, https://doi.org/10.1016/j.apmt.2020.100867.

[71] E.A. Filatova, D. Hausmann, Investigating routes toward atomic layer deposition of silicon carbide: ab initio screening of potential silicon and carbon precursors, Journal of Vacuum Science and Technology A 35 (October, 2016) 01B103, https://doi.org/10.1116/1.4964890.

[72] E.A. Filatova, D. Hausmann, S.D. Elliott, Understanding the mechanism of SiC plasma-enhanced chemical vapor deposition (PECVD) and developing routes toward SiC atomic layer deposition (ALD) with density functional theory, ACS Applied Materials and Interfaces 10 (17) (2018) 15216–15225, https://doi.org/10.1021/acsami.8b00794.

[73] R.A. Ovanesyan, E.A. Filatova, S.D. Elliott, D.M. Hausmann, D.C. Smith, S. Agarwal, Atomic layer deposition of silicon-based dielectrics for semiconductor manufacturing: current status and future outlook, Journal of Vacuum Science and Technology A 37 (August, 2009) 060904, https://doi.org/10.1116/1.5113631.

[74] H. Nagasawa, Y. Yamaguchi, Atomic level epitaxy of 3C-SiC low pressure vapour deposition with alternating gas supply, Thin Solid Films 222 (1–2) (March, 1993) 230–234, https://doi.org/10.1016/0040-6090(93)90160-Q.

[75] H. Nagasawa, Y.-i. Yamaguchi, Mechanisms of SiC growth by alternate supply of SiH_2Cl_2 and C_2H_2, Applied Surface Science 82–83 (December, 1994) 405–409, https://doi.org/10.1016/0169-4332(94)90249-6.

[76] T. Fuyuki, M. Nakayama, T. Yoshinobu, H. Shiomi, H. Matsunami, Atomic layer epitaxy of cubic SiC by gas source MBE using surface superstructure, Journal of Crystal Growth 95 (1–4) (February, 1989) 461–463, https://doi.org/10.1016/0022-0248(89)90442-9.

[77] T. Fuyuki, T. Yoshinobu, H. Matsunami, Atomic layer epitaxy controlled by surface superstructures in SiC, Thin Solid Films 225 (1–2) (March, 1993) 225–229, https://doi.org/10.1016/0040-6090(93)90159-M.

[78] S. Hara, Y. Aoyagi, M. Kawai, S. Misawa, E. Sakuma, S. Yoshida, Self-limiting growth on the b-SiC(001) surface, Surface Science 273 (3) (July, 1992) 437–441, https://doi.org/10.1016/0039-6028(92)90080-P.

[79] J.J. Sumakeris, L.B. Rowland, R.S. Kern, S. Tanaka, R.F. Davis, Layer-by-layer growth of SiC at low temperatures, Thin Solid Films 225 (1–2) (March, 1993) 219–224, https://doi.org/10.1016/0040-6090(93)90158-L5.

[80] E. Sadayuki, S. Imai, M. Matsumura, Sub-atomic layer growth of SiC at low temperatures, Japanese Journal of Applied Physics 34 (1995) 6166, https://doi.org/10.1143/JJAP.34.6166.

[81] S. Chen, W. Li, X. Li, W. Yang, One-dimensional SiC nanostructures: designed growth, properties, and applications, Progress in Materials Science 104 (April 13, 2019) 138–214, https://doi.org/10.1016/j.pmatsci.2019.04.004.

[82] I. Khan, K. Saeed, I. Khan, Nanoparticles: properties, applications and toxicities, Arabian Journal of Chemistry 12 (7) (November, 2019) 908–931, https://doi.org/10.1016/j.arabjc.2017.05.011.

[83] D. Kim, D.-Y. Kim, J.-H. Kwon, N.-M. Hwang, Effects of the size of charged nanoparticles on the crystallinity of SiC films prepared by hot wire chemical vapor deposition, Coatings 10 (2020) 726, https://doi.org/10.3390/coatings10080726.
[84] X. Yu, S. Terakawa, S. Hayashi, T. Asaka, F. Itoigawa, S. Ono, J. Takayanagi, Carbonization of silicon nanoparticles via ablation induced by femtosecond laser pulses in hexane, Arabian Journal for Science and Engineering 42 (May 25, 2017) 4221–4226, https://doi.org/10.1007/s13369-017-2619-7.
[85] Y. Yang, Z.-M. Lin, J.-T. Li, Synthesis of SiC by silicon and carbon combustion in air, Journal of the European Ceramic Society 29 (1) (January, 2009) 175–180, https://doi.org/10.1016/j.jeurceramsoc.2008.06.013.
[86] Y.L. Chiew, K.Y. Cheong, A review on the synthesis of SiC from plant-based biomasses, Materials Science and Engineering: B 176 (13) (August 15, 2011) 951–964, https://doi.org/10.1016/j.mseb.2011.05.037.
[87] M.A. Fraga, R.S. Pessoa, D.C. Barbosa, V.J. Trava Airoldi, One-Dimensional carbon nanostructures—from synthesis to nano-electromechanical systems sensing applications, Sensors and Materials 29 (1) (August, 2017) 39–56, https://doi.org/10.18494/SAM.2017.1366.
[88] J.Y. Fan, X.L. Wu, P.K. Chu, Low-dimensional SiC nanostructures: fabrication, luminescence, and electrical properties, Progress in Materials Science 51 (8) (November, 2006) 983–1031, https://doi.org/10.1016/j.pmatsci.2006.02.001.
[89] J. Fan, P.K. Chu, SiC nanowires, in: Silicon Carbide Nanostructures: Fabrication, Structure, and Properties, 2014, pp. 195–269, https://doi.org/10.1007/978-3-319-08726-9.
[90] B.-Y. Chen, C.-C. Chi, W.-K. Hsu, H. Ouyang, Synthesis of SiC/SiO2 core–shell nanowires with good optical properties on Ni/SiO2/Si substrate via ferrocene pyrolysis at low temperature, Scientific Reports 11 (January 8, 2021) 233, https://doi.org/10.1038/s41598-020-80580-y.
[91] B. Li, B. Mao, H. Huang, X. Yuan, X. Wang, T. He, A novel superhydrophobic coating consisting of SiC nanowires, Material and Research Express 6 (2019) 105094, https://doi.org/10.1088/2053-1591/ab3ec5.
[92] A. Borkowski, M. Szala, P. Kowalczyk, T. Cłapa, D. Narożna, M. Selwet, Oxidative stress in bacteria (Pseudomonas putida) exposed to nanostructures of silicon carbide, Chemosphere 135 (September, 2015) 233–239, https://doi.org/10.1016/j.chemosphere.2015.04.066.
[93] A. Borkowski, M. Szala, T. Clapa, Adsorption studies of the gram-negative bacteria onto nanostructured silicon carbide, Applied Biochemistry and Biotechnology 175 (November, 2014) 1448–1459, https://doi.org/10.1007/s12010-014-1374-4.
[94] G. Benetti, E. Cavaliere, F. Banfi, L. Gavioli, Antimicrobial nanostructured coatings: a gas phase deposition and magnetron sputtering perspective, Materials 13 (February, 2020) 784, https://doi.org/10.3390/ma13030784.
[95] A. Huczko, M. Bystrzejewski, H. Lange, A. Fabianowska, S. Cudzilo, A. Panas, M. Szala, Combustion synthesis as a novel method for production of 1-D SiC nanostructures, The Journal of Physical Chemistry B 109 (34) (August, 2005) 16244–16251, https://doi.org/10.1021/jp050837m.
[96] W. Jiang, H. Mashayekhi, B. Xing, Bacterial toxicity comparison between nano- and micro-scaled oxide particles, Environmental Pollution 157 (5) (May, 2009) 1619–1625, https://doi.org/10.1016/j.envpol.2008.12.025.
[97] J. Cadet, T. Delatour, T. Douki, D. Gasparutto, J.-P. Pouget, J.-L. Ravanat, S. Sauvaigo, Hydroxyl radicals and DNA base damage, Mutation Research/Fundamental and Molecular Mechanics of Mutagenesis 424 (1–2) (March, 1999) 9–21, https://doi.org/10.1016/S0027-5107(99)00004-4.

[98] S.M. Javadhesari, S. Alipour, M.R. Akbarpour, Effects of SiC nanoparticles on synthesis and antimicrobial activity of TiCu nanocrystalline powder, Ceramics International 46 (1) (January, 2020) 114–120, https://doi.org/10.1016/j.ceramint.2019.08.240.
[99] H. Ahmed, H. Ahmed, H. Abduljalil, Analysis of structural, electrical and electronic properties of (polymer nanocomposites/silicon carbide) for antibacterial application, Egyptian Journal of Chemistry 0 (0) (January 14, 2019), https://doi.org/10.21608/ejchem.2019.6241.1522.
[100] Lemraski, E. Ghasemian, Z. Tahmasebi, T. Valadbeigi, M. Hajjami, Incorporation of iron nanoparticles into silicon carbide nanoparticles as novel antimicrobial bimetallic nanoparticles, Silicon 11 (2) (May 8, 2018) 857–867, https://doi.org/10.1007/s12633-018-9872-6.
[101] M. Szala, Andrzej Borkowski, Toxicity assessment of SiC nanofibers and nanorods against bacteria, Ecotoxicology and Environmental Safety 100 (February, 2014) 287–293, https://doi.org/10.1016/j.ecoenv.2013.10.030.
[102] I.N. Reddy, Adem Sreedhar, M. Reddy Pallavolu, L. Veeranjaneya Reddy, M. Cho, D. Kim, N. Jayashree, J. Shim, Photoelectrochemical water oxidation kinetics and antibacterial studies of one-dimensional SiC nanowires synthesized from industrial waste, Journal of Solid State Electrochemistry (June 16, 2021), https://doi.org/10.1007/s10008-021-04991-1.
[103] S.E. Camargo, A.S. Mohiuddeen, C. Fares, J.L. Partain, P.H. Carey, R. Fan, S.-M. Hsu, A.E. Clark, J.F. Esquivel-Upshaw, Anti-bacterial properties and biocompatibility of novel SiC coating for dental ceramic, Journal of Functional Biomaterials 11 (2) (May 20, 2020) 33, https://doi.org/10.3390/jfb11020033.
[104] S.E.A. Camargo, T. Roy, P.H. Carey IV, C. Fares, R. Fan, A.E. Clark, J.F. Esquivel-Upshaw, Novel coatings to minimize bacterial adhesion and promote osteoblast activity for titanium implants, Journal of Functional Biomaterials 11 (2) (June 16, 2020) 42, https://doi.org/10.3390/jfb11020042.
[105] G. Bonaventura, R. Iemmolo, V. La Cognata, M. Zimbone, F. La Via, M.E. Fragalà, M.L. Barcellona, R. Pellitteri, S. Cavallaro, Biocompatibility beteween silicon or silicon carbide and neural stem cells, Scientific Reports 9 (August, 2019) 11540, https://doi.org/10.1038/s41598-019-48041-3.
[106] X. Lei, S. Kane, S. Cogan, H. Lorach, L. Galambos, P. Huie, K. Mathieson, T. Kamins, J. Harris, D. Palanker, SiC protective coating for photovoltaic retinal prosthesis, Journal of Neural Engineering 13 (June, 2016) 046016, https://doi.org/10.1088/1741-2560/13/4/046016.
[107] E. Bernadin, C.L. Frewin, A. Dey, R. Everly, J. Ul Hassan, E. Janzén, J. Pancrazio, S.E. Saddow, Development of an all-SiC neuronal interface device, MRS Advances 1 (May, 2016) 3679–3684, https://doi.org/10.1557/adv.2016.360.
[108] P. Yang, X. Tong, G. Wang, Z. Gao, X. Guo, Y. Qin, NiO/SiC nanocomposite prepared by atomic layer deposition used as a novel electrocatalyst for nonenzymatic glucose sensing, ACS Applied Materials and Interfaces 7 (8) (February, 2015) 4772–4777, https://doi.org/10.1021/am508508m.
[109] K. Puttananjegowda, A. Takshi, S. Thomas, Silicon carbide nanoparticles electrospun nanofibrous enzymatic glucose sensor, Biosensors and Bioelectronics 186 (August, 2021) 113285, https://doi.org/10.1016/j.bios.2021.113285.
[110] H. Mu, H. Pang, C. Zheng, K. Wang, N. Hu, B. Zhang, Photothermal treatment of oropharyngeal cancer with carbon-defective silicon carbide, Journal of Materials Chemistry B 9 (26) (2021) 5284–5292, https://doi.org/10.1039/d1tb00876e.

[111] S. Afroz, S.W. Thomas, G. Mumcu, C.W. Locke, S.E. Saddow, A biocompatible SiC RF antenna for In-vivo sensing applications, MRS Online Proceedings Library 1433 (March, 2012) 119–124, https://doi.org/10.1557%2Fopl.2012.1150.
[112] L. Fradetal, E. Bano, L. Montes, G. Atolini, V. Stambouli, Silicon carbide nanowire devices for label-free electrical DNA detection, Materials Science Forum 821–823 (June, 2015) 855–858, https://doi.org/10.4028/www.scientific.net/MSF.821-823.855.
[113] F. Rossi, E. Bedogni, F. Bigi, T. Rimoldi, L. Cristofolini, S. Pinelli, R. Alinovi, M. Negri, S.C. Dhanabalan, G. Attolini, F. Fabbri, M. Goldoni, A. Mutti, G. Benecchi, C. Ghetti, S. Ianotta, Salviati, Porphyrin conjugated SiC/SiOx nanowires for X-ray-excited photodynamic therapy, Scientific Reports 5 (January, 2015) 7606, https://doi.org/10.1038/srep07606.
[114] C. Hehrlein, Stent passivation with silicon carbide as a possible alternative to drug-eluting stents – a comprehensive review of pre-clinical and clinical results, International Cardiology Review 4 (1) (August, 2009) 60–63, https://doi.org/10.15420/icr.2009.4.1.60.
[115] J. Pascual, F. Valvo, P. Godignon, J. Aguiló, J. Millan, J. Camassel, N. Mestres, SiC base micro-probe for myocardial ischemia monitoring, Materials Science Forum 457–460 (June, 2004) 1483–1486, https://doi.org/10.4028/www.scientific.net/MSF.457-460.1483.
[116] T. Li, X.-L. Li, S.-X. Hu, J. Wu, Enhanced osteoporotic effect of silicon carbide nanoparticles combine with nano-hydroxyapatite coated anodized titanium implant on healthy bone regeneration in femoral fracture, Journal of Photochemistry and Photobiology B: Biology 197 (August, 2019) 111515, https://doi.org/10.1016/j.jphotobiol.2019.111515.
[117] Z. Chen, C. Fares, R. Elhassani, F. Ren, M. Kim, S.-M. Hsu, A.E. Clark, J.F. Esquivel-Upshaw, Demonstration of SiO2/SiC-based protective coating for dental ceramic prostheses, Journal of the American Ceramic Society 102 (11) (April, 2019) 6591–6599, https://doi.org/10.1111/jace.16525.
[118] S.E. Saddow, C.L. Frewin, F.A. Cespedes, M. Gazziro, E. Bernadin, S. Thomas, SiC for biomedical applications, Materials Science Forum 858 (May, 2016) 1010–1014, https://doi.org/10.4028/www.scientific.net/MSF.858.1010.
[119] C. Frewin, A. Oliveros, C. Locke, I. Filinova, J. Rogers, E. Weeber, S.E. Saddow, The development of silicon carbide based electrode devices for central nervous system biomedical implants, MRS Online Proceedings Library (January, 2011), https://doi.org/10.1557/PROC-1236-SS01-02. 1236-SS01-02.
[120] A.J. Rosenbloom, D.M. Sipe, Y. Shishkin, Y. Ke, R.P. Devaty, W.J. Choyke, Nanoporous SiC: a candidate semi-permeable materials for biomedical applications, Biomedical Microdevices 6 (December, 2004) 261–267, https://doi.org/10.1023/B:BMMD.0000048558.91401.1d.
[121] K. Cho, K.W. Seo, S.G. Shin, S. Lee, C. Park, Process stability and comparative rDNA/rRNA community abalyses in an anaerobic membrane bioreactor with silicon carbide ceramic membrane applications, Science of The Total Environmental 666 (May, 2019) 155–164, https://doi.org/10.1016/j.scitotenv.2019.02.166.
[122] P. Jana, M.C. Bruzzoniti, M. Appendini, L. Rivoira, M. Del Bubba, D. Rossini, L. Ciofi, G.D. Sorarù, Processing of Polymer-derived silicon carbide foams and their adsorption capacity for non-steroidal anti-inflammatory drugs, Ceramics International 42 (16) (December, 2016) 18937–18943, https://doi.org/10.1016/j.ceramint.2016.09.045.

[123] Y. Cao, H. Dong, S. Pu, X. Zhang, Photoluminescent two-dimensional SiC quantum dots for cellular imaging and transport, Nano Research 11 (January, 2018) 4074–4081, https://doi.org/10.1007/s12274-018-1990-3.
[124] V. Cimalla, J. Pezoldt, O. Ambacher, Group III nitride and SiC based MEMS and NEMS: materials properties, technology and applications, Journal of Physics D: Applied Physics 40 (October, 2007) 6386, https://doi.org/10.1088/0022-3727/40/20/s19.
[125] M. Beygi, W. Dominguez-Viqueira, C. Feng, G. Mumcu, C.L. Frewin, F. La Via, S.E. Saddow, Silicon carbide and MRI: towards developing a MRI safe neural interface, Micromachines 12 (2) (January, 2021) 126, https://doi.org/10.3390/mi12020126.

Index

Note: 'Page numbers followed by "f" indicate figures and those followed by "t" indicate tables.'

H

I

L

M

N

O

P

R

T

X

FSC
www.fsc.org
MIX
Papier | Fördert
gute Waldnutzung
FSC® C083411

Kolibri 360 GmbH
Ferdinand-Jühlke-Straße 7
99095 Erfurt, Deutschland
produktsicherheit@kolibri360.de